SM
DERMATOLOGY

General Editor
P Harvey Locke
BVSc MRCVS

Scientific Editors
Richard G Harvey
BVSc CertSAD CBiol MIBiol MRCVS

Ian S Mason
BVetMed PhD MRCVS

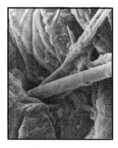

Cover Picture
*Scanning electron micrograph of
canine skin surface showing hairs
and hair follicle infundibulum.
Approximate magnification X8900.
Photo: Ian Mason*

Published by the
British Small Animal
Veterinary Association,
Kingsley House, Church Lane,
Shurdington, Cheltenham,
Gloucestershire GL51 5TQ.

Printed by J. Looker Printers Ltd,
Upton, Poole, Dorset.

The publishers cannot take any responsibility
for information provided on dosages and methods
of application of drugs mentioned in this publication.
Details of this kind must be verified by individual users
in the appropriate literature.

First published 1993

ISBN 0 905214 20 X

CONTENTS

SECTION I: BASICS

SECTION II: APPROACH TO COMMON CLINICAL PRESENTATIONS

CONTENTS

CONTRIBUTORS

Ross Bond, B.V.M.S., Cert.S.A.D., M.R.C.V.S.
Dermatology Unit, Department of Small Animal Medicine and Surgery,
Royal Veterinary College, Hawkshead Lane,
North Mymms, Hatfield, Herts, AL9 7TA

Ray L. Butcher, M.A., Vet.M.B., M.R.C.V.S.
Wylie and Partners,
196, Hall Lane, Upminster, Essex, RM14 1TD

Didier N. Carlotti, Docteur-Vétérinaire,
Cert. d'Etudes Supérieures de Dermatologie Vétérinaire
Les Places, Ste. Eulalie, F-33560, Carbon Blanc, France

John E. Cooper, B.V.Sc., D.T.V.M., C.Biol.,
F.I.Biol., Cert.L.A.S., M.R.C.Path., F.R.C.V.S
Faculty of Veterinary Medicine, P.O. Box 1387,
Morogoro, Tanzania, East Africa or
Durrell Institute of Conservation and Ecology,
The University, Canterbury, Kent

Ewan A. Ferguson, B.V.M.&S., Cert.S.A.D., M.R.C.V.S.
Veterinary Dermatology Consultancy,
37, Herongate Road, Wanstead, London, E12 5EJ

David I. Grant, B.Vet.Med., Cert.S.A.D., F.R.C.V.S.
R.S.P.C.A., Sir Harold Harmsworth Memorial Hospital,
Sonderburg Road, Holloway, London, N7 7QD

Craig E. Griffin, D.V.M., Diplomate A.C.V.D.
Animal Dermatology Clinic,
13240 Evening Creek Drive, Ste. 302, San Diego,
California 92128, U.S.A.

Richard G. Harvey, B.V.Sc., Cert.S.A.D., C.Biol., M.I.Biol., M.R.C.V.S.
The Veterinary Centre,
207, Daventry Road, Cheylesmore, Coventry, CV3 5HH

Julie I. Henfrey, B.V.M.&S., Cert.S.A.D., M.R.C.V.S.
Veterinary Dermatology Referral Services,
11, Woodlands Close, High Spen, Tyne and Wear, NE39 2AE

Kenneth W. Kwochka, D.V.M., Diplomate A.C.V.D.
Department of Veterinary Clinical Sciences,
College of Veterinary Medicine, The Ohio State University,
601, Vernon L Tharp Street, Columbus,
Ohio 43210, U.S.A.

CONTRIBUTORS

Martin P.C. Lawton, B.Vet.Med., Cert.V.Ophthal.,
Cert.L.A.S., G.I.Biol., F.R.C.V.S.
12, Fitzilian Avenue, Harold Wood, Romford, Essex, RM3 0QS

Janet D. Littlewood, B.V.Sc., M.A., Ph.D., D.V.R., Cert.S.A.D., M.R.C.V.S.
Animal Health Trust,
P.O. Box 5, Newmarket, Suffolk, CB8 7DW

David H. Lloyd, B.Vet.Med., Ph.D., F.R.C.V.S.
Dermatology Unit, Department of Small Animal Medicine and Surgery,
Royal Veterinary College, Hawkeshead Lane,
North Mymms, Hatfield, Herts, AL9 7TA

Patrick J. McKeever, D.V.M., M.S., Diplomate A.C.V.D.
Veterinary Comparative Dermatology,
Department of Small Animal Clinical Sciences,
College of Veterinary Medicine, University of Minnesota,
C339 Veterinary Hospitals, 1352 Boyd Avenue,
St Paul, Minnesota 55108, U.S.A.

Ian S. Mason, B.Vet.Med., Ph.D., M.R.C.V.S.
Veterinary Dermatology Referral Service,
6, Station Road, Hampton, Middlesex, TW12 2BX

David H. Scarff, B.Vet.Med., Cert.S.A.D., M.R.C.V.S
2, Highlands, Old Costessey, Norwich, NR8 5EA

David H. Shearer, B.Vet.Med., Cert.S.A.D., M.R.C.V.S.
University of Bristol,
Department of Pathology & Microbiology,
Comparative Pathology Laboratory,
School of Veterinary Science,
Langford, Bristol, Avon, BS18 7DU

Wayne S. Rosenkrantz, D.V.M., Diplomate A.C.V.D.
Animal Dermatology Clinic
13132 Garden Grove Boulevard, Unit B, Garden Grove,
California 92643, U.S.A.

Stephen D. White, D.V.M., Diplomate A.C.V.D.
Department of Clinical Science,
College of Veterinary Medicine, Colorado State University,
Fort Collins, Colorado 80523, U.S.A.

ACKNOWLEDGEMENTS

It is a pleasure to have the opportunity to thank everyone involved in the production of this latest addition to the successful BSAVA manual series.

I wish to express my grateful appreciation to all the contributors in meeting rigid deadlines. Without their full co-operation the book never would have met its planned publication date.

Matthew Poulson and the staff of J. Looker Printers have again been magnificent in helping advise on layout and production. The many demands made on their time have always been met with professionalism and good humour.

I am also indebted to my predecessor as the Chairman of BSAVA Publications Committee, Simon Orr, who has always been available to offer advice and encouragement whenever it was needed.

Last, but by no means least, I offer the greatest thanks to my co-editors, Richard Harvey and Ian Mason. Their combined depth of knowledge of their subject has been invaluable in helping cope with any potential problems posed by a multi author book such as this. There has been as excellent team spirit between us motivated by the desire to produce as high a quality publication as we were able in the time available.

None of this would have been possible without the support of our wives and families who have endured hours of losing their partner to the office upstairs with amazing understanding.

I hope you enjoy reading the book as much as we have enjoyed producing it.

Harvey Locke

FOREWORD

The diagnosis and management of skin disease has always represented a major component of small animal practice. Over the past two decades the discipline of veterinary dermatology has expanded quite markedly with the recognition of new diseases which has been paralleled by a greater understanding of the underlying disease processes involved along with the treatments that should be used. The picture is, however, still incomplete. The significant volume of new information produced each year is a testament to this and it is recognised that veterinary dermatology will be an ever expanding and changing field. It is essential therefore, for both the small animal practitioner and the veterinary student, to have access to texts that not only reflect the state of knowledge but also are easy to use as a reference.

The purpose of this manual is not to review material past and present that can be obtained in other reference books. It is much more to provide an informative and practical guide to the major dermatological conditions that are seen in small animal practice. The success of treatment, as with all systems, depends upon a logical approach to the presenting problems and arriving at the correct diagnosis. This manual has been designed specifically to allow a problem-based approach to the common dermatological problems in the species that are seen in companion animal practice and incorporating the salient scientific information on the subject material. The editors have ensured that this common theme is extended throughout the book.

The BSAVA would like to thank the editors, Richard Harvey, Harvey Locke and Ian Mason, and all the contributing authors who are to be congratulated on this very clear and informative text which is an invaluable addition to the manual series published by the Association.

Neil T. Gorman BVSc., PhD., DACVIM, FRCVS
President BSAVA 1992-93

INTRODUCTION

Small animal dermatology arguably forms the commonest, most frustrating and challenging area of clinical veterinary practice. This BSAVA manual has been produced with the aim of helping the overstretched practitioner deal with this burden although it is hoped that it will also provide useful guidance to veterinary students preparing for finals and for veterinary surgeons taking the RCVS Certificate in Veterinary Dermatology.

The book is divided into three sections. The first covers structure and function of the skin, the logical approach to the skin case and gives information on the laboratory tests applicable to this organ. Section Two deals with dermatological disorders from the point of view of the presenting sign rather than the aetological system favoured by most other textbooks. This approach has, inevitably, led to some repetition. However, it is our opinion that the alternative (extensive cross-referencing) would have rendered the manual less readable and less useful. The final section is on therapeutics.

It is intended that the manual can be used in two ways. Some readers will prefer to read it from cover to cover. Others may simply use an appropriate chapter to aid in the management of a specific case although it is preferable to have read Section One before adopting such an approach.

Richard G. Harvey
P. Harvey Locke
Ian S. Mason

CHAPTER ONE

STRUCTURE, FUNCTION AND MICROFLORA OF THE SKIN

David H Lloyd

INTRODUCTION

The skin is the largest of the organs and performs a wide variety of functions vital to maintenance of the homoeostatic status of the body (Table 1). In addition, different regions of the skin such as the ear, eyelids, lips, prepuce, footpads and nails have specialised functions and differ structurally from the skin covering the general body surface. A consideration of all of these topics is beyond the scope of this chapter. Attention will be concentrated therefore on those aspects of the skin and its inhabitants which are most relevant to the pathogenesis of skin disease and its diagnosis and treatment.

THE EPIDERMIS

The epidermis forms the superficial layer of the skin and is thus subjected to a wide variety of different chemical, physical and biological stresses. It is not, in itself, physically strong but preserves its integrity by continually secreting protective components. These include the hair coat, the keratinised cells of the stratum corneum and the secretions of the skin glands. The epidermis is firmly attached to the dermis, which forms the major part of the skin and is strong, flexible and elastic. It provides physical, vascular and nervous support to the epidermis.

Table 1
Skin activities associated with homoeostatis

Function	Range of Activities
Barrier	Controls loss of water, electrolytes etc. Excludes chemical, physical, biological agents.
Sensation	Heat, cold, pain, itch, pressure.
Temperature regulation	Insulation, variable blood flow, sweating.
Haemodynamic control	Peripheral vascular changes.
Secretion, excretion	Glandular function, hair and epidermal growth. Percutaneous loss of gasses, liquids and solutes.
Synthesis	Vitamin D.
Immune function	Surveillance, response.

Epidermal structure and proliferation of keratinocytes

The epidermis is a stratified squamous epithelium which is composed principally (c. 85%) of keratinocytes. A variety of dendritic cells is also present. Langerhans cells form 5 to 8% of the population and about 5% are melanocytes. The Langerhans cells are derived from the bone marrow and form a network in the epidermis. They are the chief epidermal antigen-presenting cells and are able to phagocytose antigen and migrate via the lymphatics to lymph node paracortical areas where they present processed antigenic material to antigen specific T-cells. Epidermotropic dendritic lymphocytes bearing the Thy-1 marker are also found in the canine epidermis. They act as presenters of antigen and may also have cytotoxic activity. They are believed to be capable of inducing tolerance, thus modulating the effects of Langerhans cells. Merkel cells, which act as slowly adapting type I mechanoreceptors, are found in or just below the basal layer of the epidermis but only in the tylotrich pads (epidermal papillae).

The keratinocytes are important both as structural components and as members of the skin immune system. They are phagocytic and are thought to process antigen more efficiently than the Langerhans cells; their role in epidermal immunity may be greater than has been recognised to date. Under the influence of gamma-interferon the keratinocytes are capable of both stimulating and dampening the immune response by their interaction with T-cells. They produce interleukin-1 constitutively and, following antigenic stimulation, can produce a wide range of cytokines which stimulate or inhibit the immune response. Diffusion of interleukin-1 from the epidermis into the dermis can also influence the dermal inflammatory response.

Keratinocytes are formed by the division of the tightly adherent columnar cells of the stratum basale which are attached to the epidermal basement membrane (Figure 1). Following cell division, daughter cells move out into the stratum spinosum where they are at first polyhedral but become flattened as they proceed into the overlying stratum granulosum.

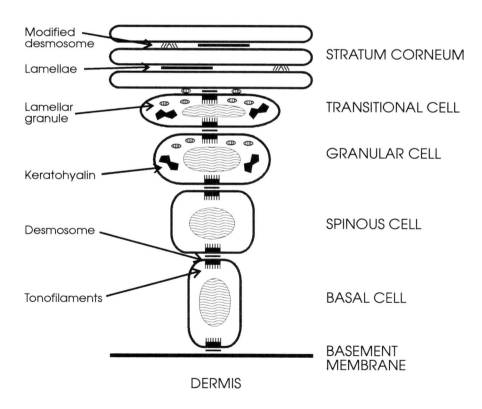

Figure 1
Diagram of the epidermis, illustrating the organisation of the cells and their maturation into fully cornified cells. Only the proximal three layers of the stratum corneum are shown.

The spinous cells are so called because of the abundant desmosomes which appear as spines in tissue processed for histology, following retraction of the cell borders. In this layer, keratin formation accelerates and the keratin filaments become organised into bundles (tonofibrils). More mature spinous cells contain granular membrane bound organelles known as lamellar granules (keratinosomes, Odland bodies, membrane coating granules) which are located at the cell margins. These granules discharge their contents into the intercellular spaces in both the spinous and granular layers.

The cells of the stratum granulosum are characterised by the presence of keratohyalin granules composed of profilaggrin, a precursor of the filaggrin which links and binds the keratin filaments prior to their crosslinking and incorporation into the cell envelope of the stratum corneum. The lamellar granule contents are extruded into the intercellular spaces where they are converted into lipid-rich hydrophobic lamellae which form an important part of the epidermal permeability barrier. Within the cells, the cytoplasmic organelles degenerate and the nucleus becomes flattened and inactive as the granular cells are converted into the dead stratum corneum.

The corneum in dogs has a thickness of 12-15 μm and is composed of 45-52 layers compared with the living epidermis which has 3 or 4 layers and is 8-12 μm thick over the general body surface (Plate 1 and Figure 2). The flattened, polyhedral cornified cells are principally composed of filaggrin and keratin and are embedded in the insoluble, lipid-rich cell envelope.

In the outer layers of the stratum corneum, loosening of the cells occurs and they acquire increased water-holding capacity. The intercellular spaces become permeated by sweat and sebum (Plate 1) and desquamation occurs at a rate which matches cell production, thus maintaining epidermal thickness.

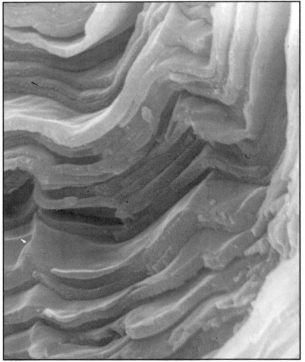

Photo: Ian Mason

Figure 2
Scanning electron micrograph of frozen hydrated canine stratum corneum showing the compact layered arrangement of the squames (Magnification x 6.7k).

Keratinocyte growth and differentiation

Migration of cells from the basal to the cornified layer takes about 22 days in normal beagles. This process can be shortened by damage or injury to the skin. Even minor procedures can affect this transit time; clipping reduces it to 15 days in the beagle.

Growth and differentiation in the epidermis are controlled by a complex variety of substances including growth factors, interleukins, adenosine triphosphate, interferon-α, vitamin D_3, retinoids and calcium availability. Some of these factors are produced within the dermis and it is clear that the dermal activity can have profound effects on epidermal development. During wound healing in the skin, the repair process is controlled by interaction between epidermal and dermal cells, including keratinocytes, fibroblasts, mast cells, neutrophils and macrophages, and is mediated by the production of cytokines, cell-to-cell contact and actions involving the extracellular matrix.

THE HAIR FOLLICLE AND ADNASCENT STRUCTURES

Simple hair follicles, as found in horses, cattle and in man, are each associated with an arrector pili muscle, a sweat gland and a sebaceous gland; these structures constitute the hair follicle unit. In dogs and cats, compound follicles are found, which incorporate both primary and secondary hairs (Figure 3). Here, a single large, central primary hair is surrounded by up to five lateral primary hairs, each with its arrector pili, sweat and sebaceous gland. The primary hairs are in turn surrounded by smaller secondary hairs, which may also have sebaceous glands. In each compound follicle, the hairs emerge together from the same pore. Contraction of the arrector pili muscles causes raising of the hairs, an action principally associated with signalling in the skin of the neck and back, in response to fright or anger ("raising of the hackles"). Erection of the hairs also influences ventilation of and heat loss from the skin surface.

The ratio of primary to secondary hairs and the hair density are important factors in determining the coat type. In dogs with normal coats, as seen in wild Canidae and the German shepherd dog,

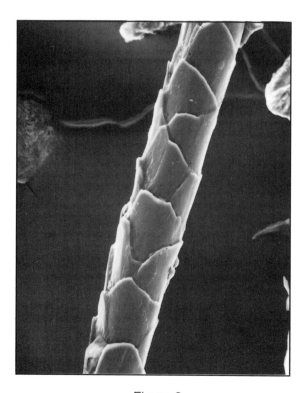

Figure 3
Scanning electron micrograph of a normal canine hair. The surface is tiled with cells of the cuticle which point away from the base of the hair.

13

the coarse primary (guard) hairs are accompanied by many finer secondary hairs. In comparison, breeds with short, coarse coats, typified by the terriers, have a higher ratio of primary hairs, and in short, fine coats e.g. boxers, the density of the secondary hairs is greater and the primary hairs are reduced in size. Mean hair density can vary between 100-600 per cm^2 and 800-1600 per cm^2 in dogs and cats respectively.

Hair follicle structure and the hair growth cycle

The hair follicle is described in three parts: the inferior segment extends from the attachment of the arrector pili to the hair papilla; the isthmus forms the mid-portion between the sebaceous duct opening and the arrector pili; the infundibulum, is the distal part and opens onto the skin surface. The structure of the hair follicle is presented in Table 2, Plate 2 and Figure 3. Hair growth commences in the inferior segment at the hair bulb matrix where the proliferative epithelial cell layer covering the hair papilla gives rise to cells forming the hair cortex, inner root sheath and the outer root sheath. Melanocytes present in the matrix may transfer pigment to the cells forming the cortices of the hairs at this stage.

Hairs grow in cycles with a period of active hair growth termed *anagen*, a transitional period, *catagen*, and a resting period, *telogen*, when the hair remains in the follicle until shed (Figure 5). The cycle is controlled and modified by a variety of factors including hormones, photoperiod, temperature,

Table 2
Structure and composition of the hair follicle

Structure	Characteristics
Dermal papilla	Dermal tissue including blood vessels; covered by basement membrane.
Hair matrix (hair bulb)	Proliferative epithelial cells covering the hair papilla; gives rise to inner and outer root sheaths and hair.
Hair – 3 regions:	Medulla: longitudinal rows of cuboidal cells; solid at hair root, vacuolated distally (air and glycogen).
	Cortex: cornified, spindle-shaped cells; contain pigment in coloured hairs.
	Cuticle: flat, cornified cells, like tiles, covering the hair surface.
Inner root sheath – 3 layers	Cuticle: flat, overlapping cells; interlock with hair cuticle.
	Huxley's layer: 1 to 3 layers of nucleate cells; contain trichohyalin granules.
	Henle's layer: 1 layer of anucleate cells; contain trichohyalin granules.
Outer root sheath	Below the isthmus: covered by inner root sheath; no keratinisation; clear vacuolated cells.
	At the isthmus: shows tricholemmal keratinisation.
	Above the isthmus: normal keratinisation with formation of keratohyaline granules and orthokeratotic keratin.
Basement membrane zone	Surrounds outer root sheath; includes the glassy membrane and fibrous root sheath.

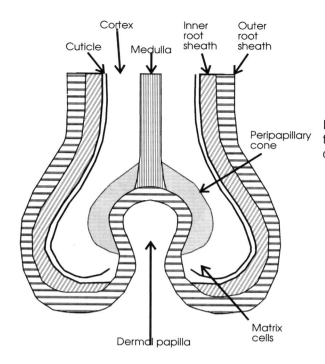

Figure 4
Diagrammatic representation of the inferior segment of the hair follicle showing the relationships of the different cellular layers. Only the epidermal tissue is illustrated.

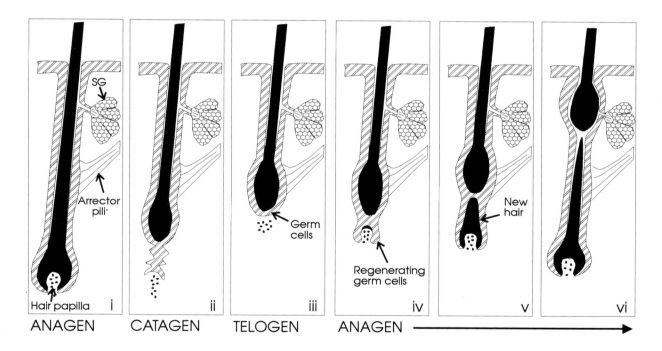

Figure 5
The hair growth cycle.

i) Maturing anagen hair with well-developed dermal papilla. SG, sebaceous gland.

ii) In catagen, hair growth ceases, the hair is moved out towards the skin surface, the base of the follicle below the hair shrinks and the papilla becomes detached.

iii) This process is completed in the telogen stage.

iv-vi) Growth of the new hair begins as germ cells at the base of the hair follicle again surround the papilla and form the hair bulb. (After Baden, 1991, figure 15-8).

Table 3
Exocrine skin glands and their properties

Skin type	Glands	Properties
Haired	Sweat	Tubular, epitrichial [1] Tubular, atrichial (dog, uncommon)
	Sebaceous	Alveolar, pilosebaceous
Glabrous e.g. footpads	Sweat	Tubular, atrichial [2]
Ear canal	Sweat	Tubular, epitrichial
	Sebaceous (ceruminous)	Alveolar, free
Eyelids	Moll's	Tubular, sweat glands
	Meibomian, tarsal	Alveolar, sebaceous,
Prepuce	Preputial glands	Specialised sweat gland, (sebaceous origin ?)
Tail	Tail gland	Alveolar, pilosebaceous Cells identical to those of perianal glands
Perianum	Circumanal ("hepatoid", perianal)	Alveolar, sebaceous. Cells identical to those of the tail gland.

[1] Formerly known as apocrine glands.   [2] Formerly known as eccrine glands.

nutrition, stress and genetic influences. In dogs and cats, hair replacement is mosaic in pattern; it is influenced particularly by photoperiod, but also by ambient temperature and nutrition. Hair shedding is prominent in the spring and autumn. Follicular activity is normally greatest in spring and early summer and least in winter when all primary and 50% of secondary follicles may be in telogen.

In addition to the normal body hair, there are two types of specialised hairs associated with sensation. The tylotrich hairs are large, single hairs surrounded by a complex of neurovascular tissue at the level of the sebaceous gland; they are thought to act as mechanoreceptors and are found scattered over the body surface in association with the tylotrich pads. The vibrissae are thick, stiff hairs which are associated with a blood sinus, lined with endothelium and containing nerve fibres, located between the follicle and the outer connective tissue capsule, in cats. They are thought to act as slow-adapting mechanoreceptors and are found on the head, throat, and in the feline carpal organ.

THE SKIN GLANDS

The skin incorporates a variety of tubular and alveolar exocrine glands (Table 3). These glands may emerge at the hair follicle (pilosebaceous or epitrichial glands) or independently in glabrous regions (free or atrichial glands).

The functions of the sweat glands include provision of moisture to the skin surface to aid in protection against friction in areas such as the footpads and eyelids, maintenance of skin surface pliability, excretion of waste products, and chemical defence through the production of substances including immunoglobulin A, transferrin and sodium chloride. The salts and proteins present in sweat also provide nutrients for the skin microflora and contribute towards the pH buffering capacity of the skin. Sweat is not a significant factor in thermoregulatory function in cats and dogs, as in other species eg. equidae, bovidae and some primates.

Sebaceous glands are larger in areas with low hair follicle density and have a higher density per unit area near mucocutaneous junctions, in interdigital spaces, on the dorsal neck and rump, on the chin (submental organ of cats) and on the dorsal part of the tail gland. Sebum helps to form the barrier at the skin surface, protecting against proliferation and invasion by pathogenic micro-organisms via the stratum corneum and into the hair follicles. Together with the sweat it aids in maintenance and control of the normal skin flora. It also helps to control water loss and maintain skin surface pliability. Sebum is probably responsible, in part, for maintenance of coat condition and sheen. It appears to form an emulsion with sweat and this may aid its penetration into the intercellular spaces of the superficial stratum corneum. In some species, specialised sweat and sebaceous glands produce pheremones.

Secretory activity in sweat and sebaceous glands

The mechanisms of sweat and sebum production appear to be basically the same. They have two main components - cell death and secretion. The process appears to be similar in principal to that involved in the production of the other epidermal tissues ie. the hair by the hair follicle and the interfollicular stratum corneum by the epidermis. This emphasises the unity of the epidermal components of the skin and helps to explain how the actions of one component are often paralleled by changes in the others.

Sebum is stored in the sebaceous gland duct and is excreted slowly. Radioactive tracer studies show that it takes days for freshly synthesised lipid to reach the skin surface. Control of glandular output is influenced by hormones and non-endocrine factors are also likely to be involved. Androgens tend to cause hypertrophy and hyperplasia whilst oestrogens and glucocorticoids cause involution.

The secretory actions of the sweat gland have been more fully explained and may involve the following processes: exocytosis, transcellular ion and water transport, microapocrine blebbing, paracellular transport, and cell death. Prolonged stimulation of the sweat gland leads to exhaustion and cessation of sweat production, particularly in sheep and goats. Chronic stimulation may lead to glandular degenerative changes as in equine anhidrosis.

A unified theory of sweat gland control has been advanced by Jenkinson and colleagues (Jenkinson, 1990). It is proposed that in the cat, dog, cow, sheep and goat, where blood vessels are in close proximity to the glands, the action of sympathetic adrenergic and cholinergic nerves on skin blood vessels elicits local transfer to the gland of a transmitter such as adrenaline or noradrenaline from the circulation or dopamine stores in mast cells close to the capillaries. In humans, horses and in the footpads of cats and dogs, where nerves are found very close to the glands and may be located within the glandular fibrocyte sheaths, there may also be a direct action on the gland by catecholamines and acetylcholine released from the sympathetic nerve endings.

THE DERMO-EPIDERMAL JUNCTION

This junction acts as a region of interaction and exchange of both cellular and humoral elements between the epidermis and dermis. The principal structural component is the dermo-epidermal basement membrane which functions as a foundation for the epidermis, a barrier zone between the epidermis and dermis, and a system anchoring the epidermis to the dermis. It extends around all of the epidermal components of the hair follicle units and has three zones. The first includes the tonofilament-hemidesmosome complex of the epidermal basal cells and the underlying lamina rara (lamina lucida) which contains heparan sulphate proteoglycan, laminin and bullous pemphigoid antigen. The second, the lamina densa, is principally composed of the type IV collagen. The third (sub-basal lamina) extends from the lamina densa to the superficial part of the dermis itself and is made up of anchoring fibrils and oxytalan filaments.

THE DERMIS

The dermis is the major structural component of the skin. It provides a matrix of supporting structures and secretions which maintain and interact with the epidermis and its adnexae. These include the connective tissue, blood and lymphatic vessels, nerves and receptors, and cellular components. It is an important thermoregulatory and sensory structure and also contributes significantly to body water storage.

DERMAL CONNECTIVE TISSUE

The dermal connective tissue matrix consists mainly of collagen and elastic fibres (Plates 3a and 3b) organised in a coherent pattern, composed principally of bundles of collagen bordered by the elastic fibres. The non-fibrous component consists of the proteoglycan ground substance and certain glycoproteins. The superficial dermis is composed of fine, irregularly distributed, loose, collagen fibres and a network of fine elastin fibres. Deeper in the dermis the collagen is thicker and denser and the fibres tend to run parallel to the skin surface; the elastin fibres are also thicker but less numerous.

Collagen is the major extracellular protein of the dermis and forms about 80% of the extracellular matrix. The fibres provide strength and elasticity. They are secreted by the skin fibroblasts in zymogen form (procollagen) which is converted into the active form in a variety of ways. The fibrillar form is very resistant to animal proteases but is broken down by collagenases. These are neutral metallo-endoproteases which require calcium as an activator and zinc as the intrinsic metal ion and are uniquely able to break down the native collagen triple helix. Collagen turnover in the dermis is slow. It is controlled by dermal cellular components which are able to respond to particular demands such as skin damage and wound healing. Hydroxyproline, an amino acid which is an abundant and vital component of collagen is released during collagen breakdown. Urinary hydroxyproline levels can be used as an indicator of this *in vivo*.

In mature individuals, the majority of dermal collagen is formed by types I (80-85%) and III (15-20%) which align into relatively large fibrils. Type IV is found forming a network in basement membranes. Type V collagen is found in nearly all connective tissues. Types VI and VII have also been described in skin and type VII may form anchoring fibrils below the basement membranes.

Elastic fibres form a network throughout the dermis and are also present in sheaths of hair follicles and in the walls of the blood and lymphatic vessels (Plate 3b). They are composed of two components, elastin and microfibrillar protein. The elastin is amorphous and, in fully mature elastic fibres forms the core, surrounded by an envelope of microfibrils. Microfibrillar material in the absence of elastin is called oxytalan. When small amounts of elastin are present it is called elaunin.

Elastin is a covalently crosslinked polypeptide with a very characteristic amino acid composition (rich in valine and alanine, low in cystine, absence of histidine and methionine). Like collagen it possesses much glycine and also contains hydroxyproline. It is synthesised by fibroblasts and smooth muscle cells. Metabolic turnover is slow but continuous. Degradation is by a variety of elastases including some calcium dependant metalloenzymes.

Much less is known of the microfibrillar material but the amino acid composition differs from that of elastin. Cystine, methionine and histidine are abundant whilst the amounts of alanine, glycine and valine are low; hydroxyproline is absent. The presence of hexose and hexosamines indicate that it is a glycoprotein.

Proteoglycans and Glycoproteins

Confusion exists over the nomenclature used for these substances. Originally called mucopolysaccharides (viscous polysaccharides), the term glycosaminoglycan was then introduced (glycan = polysaccharide; glycosamino = containing hexosamines). However, the polysaccharide is linked to protein and thus the term proteoglycan is now used.

The proteoglycans form the ground substance of the dermis and are composed chiefly of hyaluronic acid and dermatan sulphate with heparin-, chondroitin 4- and chondroitin 6- sulphates. Degradation and turnover of the dermal proteoglycans is not well understood but half-lives of 2-5 days and 7-14 days have been demonstrated for dermal hyaluronic acid and chondroitin sulphate. Hyaluronidase has been demonstrated in skin wounds and also in normal rat skin.

The proteoglycans appear to be involved in salt and water balance. They are very viscous in solution and may therefore provide support for other dermal components. They may also play a part in promoting growth, differentiation and cellular migration.

BLOOD AND NERVOUS SUPPLY, AND LYMPHATIC DRAINAGE

The skin has a well developed vascular supply in keeping with its role in thermoregulation and in haemodynamics; blood flow through the skin substantially exceeds that required merely to supply oxygen and metabolites. The cutaneous arteries ascend from the subcutaneous region and branch to form three networks (Plate 4). These are located 1) at the base of the dermis, supplying the hair papillae and sweat glands, 2) at the level of the follicular isthmus, supplying the sebaceous glands, arrector pili and mid-portion of the hair follicle, and 3) just below the epidermis (superficial plexus), giving rise to the superficial capillary network supplying the epidermis which is, itself, avascular. The veins draining the skin run parallel to the arteries. Arteriovenous anastomoses, which enable the capillary beds to be by-passed and are associated with thermoregulation, are concentrated in the deeper parts of the dermis and are particularly common in the extremities. They vary in form from the complex glomus to simple coiled structures. Control of blood flow in the capillaries is regulated by the contractile, fusiform pericytes which are aligned parallel to them.

The lymph vessels provide drainage for tissue fluid from the dermis. This fluid is collected in lymphatic capillary networks in the more superficial layers of the dermis and associated with components of the hair follicle units. The lymph vessels also provide a channel by which cellular traffic can flow to the lymph nodes. They differ from blood vessels in being flatter and wider, with thinner and flatter endothelial cells and no contractile components.

The general pattern of nerve distribution is similar to that of the blood vessels since they generally travel alongside one another. A plexus of nerves is present beneath the epidermis and free nerve endings also penetrate the epidermis itself. Nerve networks are also associated with the hair follicle, sweat and sebaceous glands, and the arrector pili muscle. Encapsulated nerve endings are found in mechanoreceptors such as the Pacinian corpuscles which are found deep in the dermis.

CELLULAR COMPONENTS OF THE DERMIS

A variety of cells is present in the dermis in addition to those of the glandular, muscular, nervous and vascular tissues. It is becoming clear that these cells are capable of performing a wide variety of different tasks and can interact with the dermal matrix and the other cellular components of the epidermis and dermis both by direct contact and by means of soluble mediators.

Fibroblasts are mesenchymal cells responsible for the synthesis and degradation of both fibrous and non-fibrous connective tissue matrix proteins. They are quite active and are capable of simultaneously secreting multiple matrix components. Attachment of fibroblasts to the fibrous matrix is mediated via fibronectin on the cell surface; collagen and fibronectin have complementary binding sites. Fibroblasts produce collagenase and gelatinase which degrade collagen. They migrate along the fibre bundles. Fibroblasts are also able to secrete a variety of cytokines and influence proliferative activity in the epidermis.

Mast cells are found throughout the dermis (rarely in the epidermis) particularly associated with the superficial vascular plexus and the epidermal adnexae. They contain abundant darkly staining secretory and lysosomal cytoplasmic granules. The secretory granules contain a predominance of histamine and heparin. The lysosomal granules contain acid hydrolases capable of degrading glycosaminoglycans, proteoglycans and glycolipids as well as some enzymes also found in the secretory granules. The cell surfaces possess microvilli and a coating of fibronectin may assist attachment to the connective tissue matrix. Skin mast cells belong to the connective tissue mast cell group and differ from mucosal mast cells both in morphology and staining reaction.

Mast cells are important mediators of immediate hypersensitivity reactions. In dog skin, two types, "typical" and "atypical", are found and are believed to be involved in the late and early phase responses, respectively. Recently the role of mast cells in delayed type hypersensitivity reactions has become apparent. Degranulation may occur four hours after antigenic exposure in contact hypersensitivity and thus precedes the T-cell reaction of the delayed response.

Basophils are not primarily found in the skin but are recruited during inflammatory and other pathological responses, including some IgE-dependant reactions. They are involved in cutaneous basophil hypersensitivity.

Macrophages are derived from monocytes which become terminally differentiated in the dermis. They can be difficult to differentiate from fibroblasts when they do not contain phagocytic vacuoles. They are capable of secreting a wide variety of substances including cytokines, complement components, hydrolytic enzymes and antimicrobial agents.

Dendritic cells, including melanocytes and Langerhans cells are found in both the epidermis and dermis. Antigen stimulated Langerhans cells migrate from the epidermis to the regional lymph nodes via the dermal lymphatics, in which they form cords, prior to their departure from the skin. Other dendritic antigen-presenting cells are found in the dermis, often in the perivascular spaces of the superficial dermal venules; their numbers are increased in inflammatory lesions. The term "veiled cells" has been used to describe these cells as well as the dermal Langerhans cells. Thy-1 positive dendritic cells are also found in the dermis.

MICROBIOLOGY OF NORMAL SKIN

The skin surface provides a habitat for a variety of flora and fauna which can survive and proliferate on the skin in the absence of clinical signs of disease as long there is an equilibrium with the host. Whilst this equilibrium exists, we speak of colonisation rather than infection, but it is well to remember that there are constant fluctuations in the relationship and that most 'healthy' animals have lesions of some sort on their skin. Thus even the definition of normality creates some difficulty. Furthermore, animal skin is frequently colonised by virulent pathogens but remains healthy; the mere presence of such pathogens does not constitute infection.

Residency status

The skin is exposed to constant contamination by a wide variety of micro-organisms. This contamination is derived from the environment, from contact with or grooming by other animals including the owners, and from the animal's own secretions and excretions (salivary, vaginal, preputial, anal, mammary). Thus it is difficult to determine which organisms are truly resident.

Residency implies prolonged establishment of colonies of micro-organisms on the skin and their continuing proliferation. Such organisms are likely to be present on the skin of most individuals in a group but may not be present on all parts of the skin and may be influenced by factors such as age, sex and environment. They are likely to be established in sectors of the skin where there are adequate supplies of nutrients and physical conditions are favourable.

Transient organisms are those which are deposited on the skin and are able to persist for short periods of time. If they are deposited on skin which is transiently favourable to their survival, some proliferation may occur. They are always superficially located but may be associated with skin infection if the skin becomes damaged or abnormal.

A third group of organisms, whose behaviour falls between that of the residents and transients, has been called the nomads. These are organisms which are readily able to take advantage of changes in the skin surface microenvironment and thus frequently become established and proliferate not only at the skin surface but also more deeply. Thus moderately large populations can occur sporadically at different very localised sites but do not persist. Coagulase-positive staphylococci seem well suited to nomadism on canine skin.

The microbial flora

Both aerobic and anaerobic bacteria are found on normal skin. Obligate anaerobes have been studied chiefly in relation to the occurrence of foot rot in the sheep and there is confusion as to which of these bacteria can exist as residents on skin; recent research by Harvey, Noble and Lloyd (1993) suggests that propionibacteria may be residents of the canine hair follicle. Amongst the Gram-positive genera, staphylococci, micrococci, streptococci and coryneform bacteria are commonly present and may be residents. Gram-negative species are probably not resident on normal skin.

Yeasts are commonly found on normal skin but their identity has not been studied in most species of animals. *Pityrosporum* (*Malassezia*) spp. can be isolated from the skin of dogs, particularly the ears in which it may be a true resident; it may also act as a nomad and is increasingly recognised as a cause of skin disease. Moulds are also often present, and dermatophytes can be isolated from clinically normal skin in some animals, but their status as residents is doubtful.

The skin as a microbial habitat

Skin presents a variety of different potential habitats for bacteria and fungi. The success or failure to colonise and persist in any of these sites depends the interaction of the microbes with one another and with the host. Marked differences in the surface microclimate, hair and glandular density, epidermal structure, levels of nutrient supply and skin contamination occur at different parts of the body. On densely haired and occluded regions, particularly where high rates of sweating occur, resident populations are likely to be higher. On skin areas open to contamination such as the groin and feet, the occurrence of nomads is more likely, whilst zones with sparse hair which remain relatively dry are likely to provide a poor microbial habitat. Areas which are frequently wet and remain moist (vulva, prepuce, lips, anus) may provide a habitat suitable for Gram-negative bacteria.

Changes in the composition of the flora will depend on alterations in the skin surface microenvironment. Such changes may make conditions more favourable for the proliferation of certain members of the existing flora, which can then overwhelm and exclude other inhabitants, or they may permit foreign microbes to become established. However, the normal flora, once established, is quite resistant to change. It will re-establish itself after short-term disturbance of the surface microenvironment and can play a significant role in protecting the skin against invasion by virulent micro-organisms. Indeed, it has been shown that staphylococcal skin infection in animals and man can be controlled by the establishment on normal skin of appropriate antagonistic bacteria.

Physical factors There is a limited amount of space which can be occupied by micro-organisms at the skin surface and the available niches rapidly become occupied by bacteria and yeasts which are adapted to survival and proliferation in them. In general, the moist, sheltered, nutrient-rich conditions prevailing in the hair follicle lumina and between the superficial cells of the stratum corneum provide a favourable environment whilst the relatively arid, nutrient-poor surfaces of the hairs are unfavourable. Little is known of the potential for colonisation of the skin glands.

Space available to microbes depends on the physical structure of the skin surface including the solid (keratinocytes, hairs) and fluid (sweat, sebum) components. Temperature and humidity are major factors in determining the success of colonisation. In general, when these are raised the populations will increase but the balance will also change and certain bacteria eg. streptococci in cattle, may change from being minor residents to being the dominant flora. In species in which sweating is significant in thermoregulation, temperature and humidity are linked by the response of the sweat gland.

Nutrients and Inhibitors The principal nutrients available to micro-organisms are derived from the sweat (water, proteins, inorganic substances) and the sebum (lipids, proteins). However, it is clear from studies in gnotobiotic animals that some microbes cannot survive at the skin surface in isolation; they depend on nutrients and growth factors made available by other organisms. Thus, use of nutrients derived from sebaceous lipid by non-lipophilic organisms may depend on the activities of the lipophiles, and so on. Chemical conditions including salt concentration and pH, the presence of substances such as transferrin (limiting the availability of iron) and lipids, particularly fatty acids, can act as inhibitors of microbial growth. It is likely that epidermal specific immune mechanisms also actively control some components of the skin surface flora but the mechanisms are not understood. Langerhans cells are continuously monitoring antigens at the superficial layers of the living epidermis and antibodies specific to soluble antigens present in the stratum corneum are found in many normal individuals. Immunoglobulins (IgG, IgA, IgM, IgE) derived from sweat and the epidermis are present at the skin surface and complement component C_3 has been demonstrated in the canine stratum corneum. The microbes also produce inhibitors which can be demonstrated *in vitro*. These include antibiotics eg. cyclic polypeptides, which usually have a relatively narrow spectrum, and oxidising agents such as hydrogen peroxide with a broad spectrum of activity.

Adhesion It has long been known that normal skin bacteria can adhere firmly to the cells of the stratum corneum but it is uncertain what advantage this confers. The skin makes use of this property to control the surface populations by the process of desquamation. This adherence presents considerable problems in counting surface bacterial populations since complete removal is practically impossible without bacterial disintegration. There is some evidence that ability to adhere is an important virulence factor in pathogenic microbes and recent evidence suggests that this may be a virulence factor in *Staphylococcus intermedius*. Much work still needs to be done to explain the role of this phenomenon in health and disease.

REFERENCES AND FURTHER READING

ALLAKER, R.P. (1993). Microbial interactions on the skin. In: *The Skin Microflora in Health and Disease*, (Ed. W.C. Noble), Cambridge University Press, Cambridge.

BADEN, H.P. (1991). Hair follicles and pathophysiology of certain hair disorders. In: *Pathophysiology of Dermatologic Diseases. 2nd Edn.*, (Eds. N.A. Soter and H.P. Baden), McGraw-Hill, New York.

GARTHWAITE, G., LLOYD, D.H. and THOMSETT, L.R. (1982) Location of immunoglobulins and complement (C_3) at the surface and within the skin of dogs. *Journal of Comparative Pathology* **93**, 185.

HARVEY, R.G., NOBLE, W.C. and LLOYD, D.H. (1993). The distribution of propionibacteria on dogs: a preliminary report. *Journal of Small Animal Practice.* **34**, 80.

JENKINSON, D. MCEWAN. (1990). Sweat and sebaceous glands and their function in domestic animals. In: *Advances in Veterinary Dermatology. Volume 1.*, (Eds. C. von Tscharner and R.E.W. Halliwell) Baillière Tindall, London.

JENKINSON, D. MCEWAN, MONTGOMERY, I. and ELDER, H.Y. (1978). Studies on the nature of the peripheral sudomotor control mechanism. *Journal of Anatomy* **125**, 625.

KWOCHKA, K.W. and RADEMAKERS, A.M. (1989). Cell proliferation of epidermis, hair follicles and sebaceous glands of Beagles and Cocker Spaniels with healthy skin. *American Journal of Veterinary Research* **50**, 587.

LLOYD, D.H. and GARTHWAITE, G. (1982). Epidermal structure and surface topography of canine skin. *Research in Veterinary Science* **33,** 99.

LLOYD, D.H. (1980). The inhabitants of the mammalian skin surface. *Proceedings of the Royal Society of Edinburgh* **79B,** 25.

MASON, I.S. and LLOYD, D.H. (1993). Scanning electron microscopical studies of the living epidermis and stratum corneum in dogs. In: *Advances in Veterinary Dermatology. Volume II*, (Eds. P.J. Ihrke, I.S. Mason and S.D. White) Pergamon Press, Oxford.

MULLER, G.H., KIRK, R.W. and SCOTT, D.W. (1989). *Small Animal Dermatology. 4th Edn.* W.B. Saunders, Philadelphia.

SCOTT, D.W. (1990). The biology of hair growth and its disturbances. In: *Advances in Veterinary Dermatology. Volume 1.*, (Eds. C. von Tscharner and R.E.W. Halliwell) Baillière Tindall, London.

SUTER, M., PANTANO, D. M., AUGUSTIN-VOSS, H. G., VARVAYANIS, M., CRAMERI, F.M. and WILKINSON, J.E. (1990). Keratinocyte differentiation in the dog. In: *Advances in Veterinary Dermatology. Volume 1.*, (Eds. C. von Tscharner and R.E.W. Halliwell) Baillière Tindall, London.

UITTO, J. and EISEN, A.Z. Biology of the dermis. In: *Dermatology in General Medicine. 3rd Edn.* (Eds. T.B. Fitzpatrick, A.Z. Eisen, K. Wolff, E.M. Freedberg and F.K. Austen) McGraw-Hill, New York.

APPROACH TO DERMATOLOGICAL DIAGNOSIS

David H Scarff

INTRODUCTION

One would think that making a dermatological diagnosis should be straightforward - the skin is the only organ that can be seen, touched and smelt! However, most referral centres suggest that at least forty minutes is needed for a full dermatological consultation and examination. This is neither practicable nor cost effective in first opinion practice.

In order to understand why a consultation of this duration is required, it is necessary to understand a fundamental of the pathogenesis of skin disease: despite the many insults it has to withstand, the skin has relatively few ways in which it may respond - thus many dermatoses appear identical. A working knowledge of the responses of the skin to various pathogens allows us to create a logical structure for dermatological examination and diagnosis which is applicable to general practice.

Structure of the Examination

In order to accomplish a thorough investigation in a realistic time, certain components must be included. The exact structure of the examination depends upon the individual case, but the following are essential:

1. History
2. Physical examination
3. Dermatological examination
4. Establishing the diagnosis
        Diagnostic tests
        Definitive diagnosis

HISTORY

One of the most important parts of making a dermatological diagnosis is taking a thorough history. Why should this be so? - again it is because of the limited number of reaction patterns available to the skin. Moreover, there is a high incidence of secondary changes which may mask the original disease.   In a referral consultation, the history may take from twenty to thirty minutes. It is reasonable to ask how this can be achieved in the first opinion setting - thirty minutes is a lot of time in a busy practice!

There are several ways of addressing this issue. Firstly, the general history may already be known if this is a longstanding client. It is important however not to assume any details that are not clear. Secondly, it may be possible to re-examine at a time in the day when more time is available, at the end of a surgery for instance. It is important however to realise that most cases will not be diagnosed on the first visit. It is more valuable to formulate a diagnostic plan at the first consultation to be achieved over several visits, rather than to conduct an inadequate examination leading to a presumptive or symptomatic approach to therapy.

History taking in dermatological cases, whether taken all at one time or continued as the case progresses has to be thorough and careful. The smallest omissions can be important - e.g. the diagnosis of sarcoptic mange rejected due to lack of response to gamma-BHC shampoo. In this case the owner may have omitted to say that the shampoo had not been used as the bottle said not to use the preparation on broken skin........

Whatever the structure of the consultation process, there are some parts of the history which are essential.

a)   Breed
b)   Age
c)   Sex
d)   General medical history
e)   Relevant dermatological history

Breed

The breed of dog can have major relevance to the diagnostic process. Whilst it is not possible to discuss all the breed susceptibilities to dermatological conditions, it may be useful to consider some examples (Table 1).

Age

The age of the patient when first affected by the skin disorder(s) in question may be of great help in limiting the differential diagnosis and determining the initial direction of the investigative process. Some examples of age related diagnoses are given in Table 2.

Sex

Sex related dermatoses should be easily apparent in most instances. Here are some examples:

Entire female   Ovarian imbalance 1, mammary neoplasia

Spayed female   Ovarian imbalance 2, mammary neoplasia, (flank alopecia)

Entire male   Sertoli cell tumour, perianal adenomata, tail gland hyperplasia, castration / growth hormone responsive dermatosis

Castrated male   Testosterone responsive dermatosis, (flank alopecia)

Clinicians should be careful not to overlook Sertoli cell tumour especially in monorchid or apparently castrated dogs. Changes to the coat may be seen following ovariohysterectomy; the coat may appear fine and wispy with extra curl - similar in appearance to the "puppy-coat" in other endocrinopathies. Such changes appear to have a breed predilection, with setters and spaniels commonly affected in the author's experience.

General medical history

The importance of taking a thorough general history cannot be over emphasised. There are two reasons for this - firstly, many systemic diseases may have dermatological signs and management of severe systemic disease may be more important to the patient than the dermatological diagnosis. Furthermore, some serious systemic diseases may show dermatological changes early in the course of disease. Two examples of the latter situation are leishmaniasis and hyperadrenocorticism.

Dermatological history

The importance of the dermatological history is obvious. What is more difficult to assess is the relevance of the past history in-toto - the author was once presented with a nine year bulldog with thirty five feet of computerised case history! On the other hand, the removal of an apparently innocuous mass in the skin may be of enormous importance when assessing possible mastocytosis.

Table 1
Some examples of diseases showing a strong breed predilection

DERMATOSIS	BREEDS AFFECTED
Acanthosis nigricans	Miniature dachshund
Acne	Doberman pinscher, boxer, longhair cats
Acral mutilation	Pointer
Atopic dermatitis	Retriever, boxer, English setter, Shar pei, terriers
Calcinosis circumscripta	German shepherd dog, boxer
Colour dilute alopecia	Doberman pinscher, setter, great Dane
Demodicosis	Boxer, bull terrier, Scottie, Westie, Shar pei, dachshund
Dermatophytosis	Jack Russell terrier, longhair cats
Discoid lupus erythematosus	German shepherd dog, rough collie
Facial intertrigo	Bulldog, longhair cats
Growth hormone / castration responsive dermatosis	Chow, Keeshond, Pomeranian, miniature poodle, Siberian husky, Malamute
Histiocytoma	Boxer, dachshund, great Dane
Hyperadrenocorticism	Boxer, retriever, dachshund, Yorkshire terrier, Cairn
Hypothyroidism	Boxer, setter, German shepherd dog, Doberman pinscher, Shar pei
Keratinisation defects	Spaniels, Doberman pinscher, Westie, schnauzer
Malassezia dermatitis	Westie, Basset hound, cavalier King Charles spaniel
Mast cell tumour	Boxer, bulldog, labrador retriever
Otitis externa	Spaniels, German shepherd dog
Perianal fistula	German shepherd dog, Irish setter
Pemphigus foliaceus	Cocker spaniel, vizsla
Psychogenic alopecia	Abyssinian, Siamese and Burmese cats
Sebaceous adenitis	Standard poodle, Samoyed, vizsla
Vitiligo	Rottweiler, Newfoundland, Doberman pinscher
Zinc responsive dermatitis	Siberian Husky, Malamute, Samoyed

Table 2
Examples of diseases with a strong age predilection include the following

AGE	DISEASE
Birth to six months	Acanthosis nigricans, demodicosis, dermatophytosis, juvenile impetigo/folliculitis, pituitary dwarfism, cutaneous asthenia
Before three years	Atopic dermatitis, castration/growth hormone responsive dermatosis, keratinisation defects, colour dilute alopecia, histiocytoma
Three to eight years	Flea bite allergy, hypothyroidism
Over six years	Neoplasia, hyperadrenocorticism

Whilst as complete a history as possible must be sought, there are several key questions, important both in their own right and in providing direction to further history taking:

1. To form an impression of the previous dermatological problem(s):

    a) Has the animal a history of chronic skin disease?
    b) Is the dermatosis now, or was it initially, seasonal?
    c) Have previous episodes been pruritic? - if so, have they always been so?
    d) What treatment has been administered in the past, and what was the response?

2. To gain an accurate history of the current problem:

    a) Is this the same problem as the animal has had previously?
    b) When was the problem first noticed, and what was the initial appearance?
    c) How have lesions progressed, and what is the rate of progression?
    d) Are the lesions pruritic, or the result of pruritus? (This one is difficult but, asked with care, can be very useful)
    e) Are any in-contact animals affected?
    f) Are any in-contact people affected? (This one is often denied and may have to be disguised, e.g. Has anyone in the household been affected by gnat-bites on their ankles?!)
    g) When (not if) was the last time you saw fleas on <u>any</u> of the animals in the household?
    h) Where does the animal live and exercise, now and before the problem started?
    i) What medication has been administered so far in this problem and what has been the response?

To gain accurate and helpful answers to these questions it is important to be attentive and not to interpret the answers according to preformed ideas about the case. From this point of view, it is often useful to have a list of preselected questions to be used in all cases. The presence of more than one member of the family in the consulting room can be helpful, especially if children are involved, as they are invariably more honest than their parents!

Following careful history taking, the clinician is able to proceed to firstly examine the patient as a whole, and then to carefully examine the skin. Whilst the history may have suggested differential diagnoses already, it is important to keep as open a mind as possible at this point.

Table 3
Some systemic diseases with dermatological features

Diabetes mellitus	Atrophy, pyoderma, *Malassezia* dermatitis
Drug eruption	Erythema multiforme, pemphigus-like eruption, papular eruptions
FeLV, FIV infection	Pyoderma, sarcoptic or demodectic mange
Hepato-cutaneous syndrome	Crusting, ulceration of skin, footpads and mucosae
Hyperadrenocorticism	Atrophy, alopecia, calcinosis cutis
Hypothyroidism	Alopecia, pyoderma, myxoedema
Leishmaniasis	Crusting, ulceration, erythema
Mast cell tumour	Erythema, nodules, poor healing
Mycosis fungoides	Exfoliative dermatitis, depigmentation
Pituitary dwarfism	Alopecia, scaling, hyperpigmentation
Sertoli cell tumour	Alopecia, feminisation, hyperpigmentation

PHYSICAL EXAMINATION

One of the most difficult parts of the examination of the dermatological case is the physical examination. The clinician, having had a myriad of possibilities suggested by the history, and itching (sorry!) to get at the skin glowing in front of him, must exercise restraint.

We all have our own routine for performing a full clinical examination, and in general practice, examinations will often be performed whilst conducting the history. This is ill-advised in the skin case however, as the history is often complex and should be recorded. The discipline of a routine is useful here, as again it encourages us to keep our hands off the skin at this time.

Signs of systemic disease must be noted, even if they do not appear to be relevant. Even if such disorders are not the cause of the skin disease, systemic illnesses may interfere with the diagnostic approach, either by preventing procedures such as anaesthesia for biopsy, or by producing conflicting results from laboratory tests.

DERMATOLOGICAL EXAMINATION

It may be thought that the skin is easily accessible for examination - try telling that to an irritated 45 kg German shepherd dog with ventral pyoderma! Obviously, for an adequate dermatological examination, the co-operation of the patient and owner must be achieved. If necessary, time must be found for sedation to allow the examination to be performed. Getting the co-operation of the owner can be difficult, as they are sometimes in a hurry, may be scared of their dog or cat, or are perhaps unable to afford chemical restraint. It is desperately important to explain both the procedure to be undertaken and its importance. If necessary, the financial advantages of procuring an early diagnosis may need to be explained.

I prefer to examine the dermatological patient (within reason) on an examination table. This achieves two objectives; it improves access and demonstrates to both dog and owner that the clinician is in charge.

The assessment of the skin is primarily visual (although manual and olfactory assessments are also of value) and so to conduct the examination in poor lighting is liable to give misleading results. Good lighting may be achieved in a number of ways; obviously the easiest is to have a well but evenly lit room. An illuminated magnifying glass may also be of value.

A logical approach to the examination of the skin is necessary; the author's approach is as follows:-

a)   Examine the coat, noting alopecia, oiliness, dryness and ease of epilation. Broken hairs may be of significance, indicating either pathology affecting the hair shaft or excessive grooming.

b)   The entire surface of the skin must be inspected - for example the only intact primary lesions of pemphigus foliaceus may be at the junction of the pad and skin on the ventral aspect of the foot! Clipping may form an important part of the examination, remembering to gain full consent from the owner - a show Yorkie or Afghan hound may take eighteen months to regain full coat!

c)   All primary lesions must be noted (Table 4), with some assessment of their distribution and number. However, some of the primary lesions such as pustules are very transient and may be few in number in comparison with precursors such as papules, or sequelae like epidermal collarettes. If in doubt do not hesitate to hospitalise the animal, and having clipped a window of affected skin, examine for new lesions at regular intervals - a "bulla watch". Secondary lesions, though less significant in their own right, may be helpful in the diagnostic process.

d)   The texture, thickness and elasticity of the skin must be assessed by palpation.

e) The presence or absence of ectoparasites, their eggs or faeces must be determined by examination and laboratory tests if necessary.

Table 4
Lesions found in the skin

PRIMARY LESIONS	SECONDARY LESIONS
Macule (patch if over 2 cm diameter)	Scale (epidermal collarette)
Papule (plaque if over 1 cm diameter)	Crust
Pustule	Scar
Vesicle (bulla if over 1 cm diameter)	Erosion (ulcer if full thickness)
Nodule (over 1 cm diameter)	Comedo
Tumour (cyst)	Fissure
Wheal	Excoriation
	Lichenification
	Hyper/hypo-pigmentation
	Hyperkeratosis (callus)

Primary Lesions

Macule: A circumscribed spot of normal skin thickness but with altered colour. Changes producing macules include not only pigmentary changes such as lentigo and vitiligo, but also changes due to erythema or haemorrhage.

Patch: A macule of greater than 2 cm diameter.

Papule: A small solid raised mass of less than 1 cm diameter. This is one of the most common lesions seen in the skin, and may result from any accumulation of inflammatory cells (Chapter 6). It is important to realise that superficial pyoderma may present as a solely papular rash.

Plaque: An elevated area of more than 1 cm diameter, often made up of a coalescence of papules.

Pustule: One of the most important lesions in small animal dermatology, which always justifies skin scraping and cytology (Chapter 3). Commonly found in superficial pyoderma, the pustule is also the primary lesion of the bullous auto-immune diseases in the dog and cat.

Vesicle: A small (<1 cm diameter) fluid filled blister. These lesions are very transient in the canine and feline epidermis, and may be difficult to demonstrate both clinically and histologically. Whilst they may suggest bullous autoimmune diseases, they can be formed by any acute inflammatory process in the skin.

Bulla: A larger vesicle, rarely found in small animal dermatology.

Nodule: A raised mass over 1 cm in diameter, often associated with an inflammatory process, such as nodular panniculitis or a granulomatous disease. Biopsy or fine needle aspirate cytology is often indicated when nodules are present.

Tumour: A neoplastic mass in the skin - may be difficult to differentiate from a nodule.

Cyst: A congenital or developmental lesion involving a fluid or keratinacious debris filled cavity.

Wheal: A sharply circumscribed, raised oedematous lesion which is often short lived. These lesions blanch when compressed by a glass slide (diascopy) demonstrating that they are neither pigmentary nor haemorrhagic.

Secondary lesions

Scale: An accumulation of partially shed stratum corneum cells on the surface of the skin or attached to hairs. May be indicative of a keratinisation defect.

Epidermal collarette: A circular peeling lesion often arising as a sequel to a pustule. An important lesion to look for in cases of suspected pustular disease.

Scar: An alopecic, often depigmented lesion arising from the fibrosis during the healing process following a full thickness lesion, such as an ulcer. Such lesions are prone to trauma and solar damage.

Erosion: A lesion involving less than full thickness epidermal loss. May be due to self trauma (see excoriation) or a severe pathological process. These lesions heal without scarring.

Ulcer: A full thickness break in the epidermis; indicative of severe inflammatory, vascular or neoplastic epidermal pathology. They heal with scarring, and are often investigated by cytology or biopsy of the rim.

Comedo: A comedo is a dilated, keratin plugged hair follicle which is usually devoid of hair. These lesions are secondary to any follicular pathology, whether inflammatory or due to a keratinisation defect. These lesions can be demonstrated in skin scrapings as follicular casts, even if not visible macroscopically.

Fissure: A fissure is a deep split through the epidermis, caused by trauma or swelling in the thickened epidermis found in footpads, nasal planum or pinnal tips.

Excoriation: When self trauma results in an erosion or ulceration, then this is termed excoriation. As long as the damage is less than full thickness, then healing will occur without scarring.

Lichenification: Thickening of the skin, sufficient to exaggerate the normal pavement-like markings. This lesion is extremely non-specific and may occur in any chronic dermatosis.

Hyperpigmentation: Increase in the pigmentation of the skin may occur as either a developmental disease such as lentigo (Chapter 9), or associated with inflammation.

Hypopigmentation: Decrease in the pigmentation of the skin is seen following full thickness damage to the epidermis or associated with inflammatory or neoplastic diseases. Acquired depigmentation may occur in vitiligo.

Hyperkeratosis: Any keratinisation defect leading to either decreased loss or increased production of stratum corneum will produce hyperkeratosis. This may present as either scaling or horny projections from footpads etc.

Having examined the skin carefully, it may be useful to record the findings on a skin chart (a lesion map). This allows an overall pattern of lesions to be assessed, facilitating comparison with previous or future examinations.

Examination for flea faeces

Flea are the commonest cause of skin disease in the dog and cat. For this reason the author takes coat brushings for evidence of fleas or their debris in virtually all small animal dermatology cases. The examination for evidence of flea contact has to be meticulous, and has to be performed on occasions in the presence of open hostility from the owners - in no other issue in veterinary dermatology are psycho-social factors so intrusive.

The author normally performs a hand brushing of the coat onto a large sheet of white paper, before gathering the material for examination on wet cotton wool. Careful examination of the cotton wool and of the paper left behind under good illumination is necessary, with demonstration of any flea faeces to the owners (Plate 5). The characteristic appearance of digested blood dissolving on the wet surface is helpful in differentiating flea faeces from other debris. Of course it must be remembered that the absence of fleas or their products never rules out their presence.

ESTABLISHING THE DIAGNOSIS

The next stage in the diagnostic process is the use of the information so far gathered to form a list of problems or differential diagnoses. In this way, the direction of further investigations is determined, allowing discussions with the owner about the priorities and financial constraints affecting the next step.

The initial list of differential diagnoses should start off being general, ruling in or out diseases such as parasitism, allergic skin disease or endocrine disease. In some cases, the list will begin with a description of the presenting lesions and will develop into a list of differentials. An heirarchical system can then be employed to sub-divide the headings; this can then be narrowed according to information already obtained along with that gathered from further diagnostic processes.

An example of the sort of list to be constructed would be as follows:

Patient: 5 year old spayed German shepherd bitch

Complaint: Pruritus for five months starting in May

Examination: Self trauma on dorsum and legs; ventral pyoderma

Skin examination: Papular and pustular rash on ventral abdomen. Areas of excoriation on the dorsum and proximal legs.

Problem / differential list

1.   Ventral pustular dermatitis   a)   pyoderma
                                                          b)   immune-mediated

1a: Secondary to:-

         i)   Ectoparasitism;   a)   fleas
                                                          b)   sarcoptic mange
                                                          c)   cheyletiellosis
                                                          d)   pediculosis
                                                          e)   demodectic mange

         ii)   Allergic;   a)   atopic dermatitis
                                                          b)   food intolerance
                                                          c)   drug eruption

         iii)   Metabolic   a)   hypothyroidism

1b: i)   bullous auto-immune   a)   pemphigus vulgaris
                                                          b)   pemphigus foliaceus

         ii)   sterile eosinophilic pustular dermatosis

         iii)   drug eruption

         iv)   sub-corneal pustular dermatosis

From this list, which is not exhaustive, it can be seen that further diagnostic effort is required if the problem is to be resolved. Symptomatic therapy with glucocorticoids for the pruritus and antibiotics for the spots is unlikely to be adequate!

Diagnostic Tests

Having constructed the differential list, the next step is to decide which diagnostic tests are likely to be the most useful in providing a definitive diagnosis. There is little value in applying tests randomly, hoping for a diagnosis, although there are some tests such as skin scrapings which are sufficiently valuable to be applied in most cases.

Factors to be taken into account when selecting which tests to select in each case include the following:

a)   Cost
b)   Specificity
c)   Sensitivity
d)   Applicability
e)   Speed of obtaining results

Cost: Although not the most important consideration clinically, this factor is often the first raised by the owner. In order to make judgements about cost considerations, it is important both to understand the value of each test to the diagnostic process and to be able to explain this. Owners often appear to wish all possible tests to be undertaken; until, that is, they get the account. It is better to explain the cost of a dermatological workup before the process is initiated.

Specificity: The ability of a test to provide a definitive diagnosis. For example, in a case of demodicosis, a bacterial culture may be of value but will not provide the diagnosis.

Sensitivity: A test may be very specific, i.e. a basal thyroxine estimation, but have a range in disease which overlaps with the normal values.

Applicability: Some tests, such as culture for dermatophytes, may be very specific and sensitive, but are only applicable to cases of dermatophytosis. On the other hand, tests such as skin scrapings, whilst often not providing a definitive diagnosis, are of value to most cases due to the diseases which they rule out as well as the ones that they diagnose.

Speed of results: In deciding the first tests to undertake, the speed of obtaining results is of importance, especially when the animal is distressed by its condition. In a case of sarcoptic mange, one would never wait for the results of a fungal culture before performing skin scrapings. Similarly, cytology may be of immense value due to the rapidity at which results may be obtained. Obviously this depends upon the in-house abilities - full biochemistry assays may not be considered worthwhile, but all practices should have the ability to examine skin scrapings.

Laboratory tests are discussed in more detail in Chapter 3.

Definitive Diagnosis

Having made a list of differentials and selected appropriate diagnostic tests, it should be possible to arrive at a definitive diagnosis. If this is the case, then the best possible advice can be given to the owner about the prognosis, and choices can be made about the management regimen to best suit the individual patient.

In some cases it is not possible to arrive at a definitive diagnosis. However, having followed a diagnostic process similar to the one described, the best approach to the management of the case is more likely to be determined. If rational, achievable goals are set and discussed fully with the owner at each stage, then there should rarely, if ever, be a need for a symptomatic approach.

APPLICATION OF THE DIAGNOSTIC APPROACH TO THE PRACTICE SITUATION

In the final section, we should return to where the chapter started - why should this approach be applied to the busy general practice?

There are three answers to this. The first is that this approach allows priorities for further investigation to be defined against the background of relevant history and thorough clinical examination. This may in some cases mean the judicious use of antibacterial therapy to remove secondary pyoderma prior to further examination. The time taken to remove the pyoderma may also be used to start to prepare for intradermal testing or to feed a test diet.

The second is that it facilitates the construction of a diagnostic plan to which any treatment given does not interfere. In this way the use of antibiotics would be acceptable, but the use of long acting glucocorticoids would not. In the same way, it is important that any treatment that is carried out is done adequately and the results of that therapy may be relied upon. Again, I cite the case of the gamma-BHC washes!

The third answer is one of belief - really believing that the diagnostic approach is necessary to the well being of the patient. In the dermatology case this is not the time for half-heartedness; anything less than meticulousness will allow the clinician to be misled. The carefully investigated dermatology case can be one of the most satisfying in small animal medicine - moreover a diagnostic approach can help to avoid the dread of seeing the same, familiar, scratching dog in the corner of the waiting room!

CHAPTER THREE

INVESTIGATIVE AND LABORATORY TECHNIQUES

Janet D Littlewood

INVESTIGATIVE TECHNIQUES

Whilst a complete history and thorough clinical examination are essential for dermatological cases, further diagnostic investigations are of paramount importance in reaching a definitive diagnosis. Many can be performed as part of, or at the conclusion of, the clinical examination.

Simple Magnification

Hand lens
Use of a hand held lens, in good natural light, or a combined light and magnifying lens allows closer examination of primary skin lesions. It is usually necessary to clip away surrounding hair to properly see the skin surface. This technique also enables identification of surface parasites such as fleas, lice, *Cheyletiella* mites (Plate 7), the larval stage of the harvest mite, *Neotrombicula autumnalis* and louse egg cases.

Otoscopy
Use of an otoscope is mandatory in any animal showing signs of aural irritation and inflammation and facial or head pruritus. Sedation, or even general anaesthesia, may be necessary to allow thorough examination in fractious patients. The examination permits identification of ear mites and rules out other causes of otitis externa, eg. foreign bodies or tumours.

Wood's lamp
These lamps emit violet and ultraviolet light and are used to identify those dermatophyte infections which fluoresce. Lamps currently available include a magnifying lens. The lamp must be allowed to become fully warm (at least 5 minutes) and the examination should be performed in a dark room. The haircoat is examined, looking for the typical apple green fluorescence of hairs infected with *Microsporum canis*. The technique allows selection of appropriate hairs for microscopy and culture to confirm the diagnosis. Unfortunately, not all strains of *M. canis* fluoresce, the number showing positive fluoresence varying between 30 and 50%, or even up to 90%, in published reports. Sometimes, the infected hairs need to warm up under the lamp before showing fluorescence and this may be a reason for false negative examinations. Other less common dermatophytes which may also show fluorescence include *M. distortum, M. audouinii* and *Trichophyton schoenlii*. False positive fluorescence may be observed due to certain topical medications, dead skin scales and certain bacteria.

Coat Brushings

Sample collection
The coat may be brushed to collect surface debris for closer examination using a flea comb or stiff plastic hair brush into a Petri dish for examination under a microscope or hand lens.

Wet paper test.
This is performed by brushing debris onto a piece of dampened white paper, for identification of

flea dirt. The black flea faeces stains the damp paper reddish brown, because of the presence of soluble blood pigments (Plate 5).

Mackenzie toothbrush technique
This is the method of choice for screening asymptomatic cats for the presence of dermatophyte infection. The whole coat is brushed with a new or sterilised toothbrush, which is then used to inoculate fungal culture medium. As an alternative a scalp massaging brush (Denman) may be used.

Samples for Direct Microscopy

Hair pluckings
Hair is plucked and placed on clear adhesive tape and affixed to a microscope slide, or mounted under a cover slip in liquid paraffin. The tips are examined for evidence of breaking and damage indicated by abrupt, blunt ends instead of the tapering tips of normal hairs, giving evidence of chewing and excessive grooming by the host or diseased hairs such as in dermatophytosis. The roots are examined to assess if hairs are in anagen (pronounced bulb present) or telogen (club root with barbs or frayed appearance). A count can be made of the number of hairs in anagen and telogen and an assessment made of the number of primary and secondary hairs present, ie. a **trichogram**. Abnormalities of hair structure may be detected in certain deficiency diseases, dysplasias and genetic abnormalities of the hair coat. The presence of comedones or follicular plugs can also be detected surrounding the shafts towards the root end of plucked hairs.

Examination of the roots of plucked hairs may reveal the presence of demodectic mange mites and is a better technique than skin scraping for the confirmation of demodicosis in pododermatitis. When fungal infection is suspected hair plucks can be taken for microscopical examination and for culture (see later).

Adhesive tape impressions
Strips of clear adhesive tape are applied to skin and then applied to slides for direct examination for surface parasites and eggs. Tape strips of the clipped skin surface may be stained (Diff Quick or Gram) to look for micro-organisms eg. *Malassezia*. This technique is particularly useful for small mammals where skin scraping can be difficult (Chapter 20).

Smears of expressed follicular contents
This is a useful method for extruding *Demodex* from hair follicles. The skin is squeezed and a clean microscope slide is drawn across the surface to smear extruded material for subsequent examination. Alternatively material may be collected on a scalpel blade and then transferred to a slide. No staining is necessary, although a little mineral oil (liquid paraffin) may be used for cover slip mounting.

Smears of aural wax/exudate
Debris from the external ear canal may be collected on a swab and placed on a slide for microscopical examination for identification of ear mites and their eggs. It may help material to adhere to the swab if it is dampened with liquid paraffin, which can also be used on the slide to disperse the sample and mount the coverslip.

Scrapings
The major secret to success, particularly in cases of suspected sarcoptic mange, is to scrape multiple sites, to choose the sites carefully and to scrape until capillary ooze is seen. Papules or crusts are the best sites for sampling. Overlying hair is clipped away and a blunted scalpel blade is used. The sites may be moistened with saline or mounting medium. Material can be collected directly onto microscope slides, or into a test tube if large amounts of material have been collected which require concentrating.

There is great debate amongst dermatologists with respect to which mounting medium is preferable for examination of skin scrapings. The choice is between liquid paraffin (mineral oil) and potassium hydroxide. Many prefer liquid paraffin since this allows immediate examination of slides and identification of live mites. It has the disadvantage of not clearing debris, in contrast to potassium hydroxide. Good separation of keratinocytes and clearing of material is obtained with 10% potassium hydroxide, but this is caustic to the skin itself and kills mites. Lower concentrations, eg. 6% potassium hydroxide, are not lethal to mites. Material on slides is cleared in about half an hour although this can be hastened by gentle heating. The use of a solution of 20% potassium hydroxide in 40% dimethyl sulphoxide (DMSO) will clear material on slides, without heating, in five to ten minutes. Large amounts of material may be concentrated and cleared by mixing with the same solution in a test tube and leaving to stand. The supernatant is discarded and the settled material transferred to a slide for microscopical examination. This method will also remove the bulk of liquid paraffin oil in samples, although some globules of oil tend to remain adherent to hairs. Use of other solvents first may aid·in removal of oil prior to clearing and concentration. Coverslips should always be used, no matter what the mounting medium.

If dermatophyte infection is suspected, samples should be taken from the advancing edge of a new lesion, to include hair and skin scale. Fungal elements are seen best in potassium hydroxide preparations, although the loss of glassy appearance of hairs which have become opaque indicative of dermatophytosis can be seen in liquid paraffin preparations. Hyphae may be seen inside hair shafts, which are often broken, or in squames. Spores may be inside (endothrix) or around hair shafts (ectothrix). Addition of a drop of Quink blue-black ink or lactophenol cotton blue to the slide may permit fungal structures to be more easily visualised.

Samples which are to be submitted to a diagnostic laboratory for fungal culture should be sent in paper envelopes or non-airtight containers such as Petri dishes since bacterial contaminants tend to overgrow the sample in a moist humid environment. Special envelopes are available for this purpose (Dermapak, Microbiological Supply Company, Toddington).

Stained smears from pustules / lesions
The microscopical examination of pustule and vesicle contents and the exfoliative cytology of the surface of lesions permits the identification of inflammatory cells, acantholytic cells, neoplastic cells and micro-organisms. Ideally an intact pustule should be ruptured with a sterile hypodermic needle, its contents aspirated and smeared onto a clean slide, fixed and stained. Impression smears of ulcerated lesions or of the cut surface of excised lesions can also be made. Rapid staining techniques using Diff Quick or Rapistain are ideal for practice laboratories. Other stains which may be helpful are Giemsa and methylene blue. Gram stain may be preferable for detecting micro-organisms.

Fine needle aspirates
Examination of stained smears of aspirated cells may be helpful, particularly in cases with multiple cutaneous masses and those with lymphadenopathy.

The hair over the lesion should be clipped and its surface aseptically prepared. Samples are obtained by inserting a 21 or 22 gauge needle attached to a 10 ml syringe into the mass, retracting the plunger briskly two or three times and withdrawing the needle from the mass. The syringe should then be detached, filled with a little air, and material in the needle and hub expressed onto a slide and smeared, prior to fixing and staining. Rapid air drying followed by fixing in absolute methanol is required for most of the Romanowsky (haematological) stains. However, certain pathologists have a preference for wet fixation of material, particularly with certain cytological staining methods. It as advisable to check with individual laboratories for their requirements.

This technique allows identification of the major cell type(s) involved in a lesion and may be diagnostic for mast cell tumours, but has the serious disadvantage of giving no information about structure and cellular organisation within the mass. It should not replace excision and routine histopathology, but can be a useful preoperative screening technique which, in the case of solitary mast cell tumours, might indicate the need to give a wide margin of excision.

Culture of Micro-organisms

Bacterial culture
Swabs should be taken from new lesions or recently ruptured pustules or vesicles, not old, crusted, excoriated lesions. An intact pustule is ruptured with a sterile needle and contents absorbed onto a sterile swab. Transport medium should be used for sending samples to a diagnostic

laboratory. Some authorities advise sterilisation of the skin surface with surgical spirit (alcohol) first, but this may lead to false negative cultures if spirit penetrates or ruptures the fragile stratum corneum overlying the pustule, or the pustule is opened before the spirit has evaporated. Biopsy tissue may also be submitted in a sterile container for bacterial culture. For deep pyodermas, a selective culture medium for Gram negative organisms should be inoculated in addition to routine blood agar plates, and anaerobic culture may also be indicated. For staphylococci coagulase production is an important indicator of pathogenicity. Ideally, further biochemical tests should be employed to further identify the species of *Staphylococcus* involved, although in dogs most are *S. intermedius*. In cases with granulomata both fungal and mycobacterial culture may be required. Some organisms are difficult to culture and tissue should be submitted to a mycobacterial reference laboratory.

Fungal culture

Sabouraud's dextrose agar in Petri dishes gives the best results allowing the development of good colony morphology and visible pigment changes. Addition of antibiotics such as gentamycin or chloramphenicol + actidione (cycloheximide) to the medium will prevent overgrowth of bacterial contaminants. In the UK incubation at room temperature, rather than in incubators, is usually adequate. Plates should be examined twice weekly and discarded after 3-4 weeks.

Dermatophyte test agar (bioMerieux UK Ltd, Basingstoke; Dermafyt, Kruuse) contains a pH colour indicator which turns red in the presence of pathogenic dermatophytes due to the production of alkaline metabolites. The medium remains yellow/orange with growth of contaminants until the cultures become aged. Therefore, these cultures should be examined daily for the first 10 days in order to pick up the early colour change of pathogenic fungi. This medium is useful as an early indicator of the presence of pathogens, but has the disadvantages of masking typical colony morphology and the reverse pigment changes. Thus subculture of positive colonies may be necessary for definitive identification of species from the reverse pigmentation and microscopical examination of macroaleurospores.

Skin Biopsy

Skin biopsy is all too often considered as a last line of investigation for chronic dermatoses. This is unfortunate since dermatohistopathology can be a valuable aid to diagnosis. In fact, it is better to consider biopsy sooner, rather than later in the course of investigating a case, since delay allows secondary changes to develop. Although the histological findings may not always be pathognomonic for a particular disease, the technique can be just as useful as a means of excluding some of the differential diagnoses.

Indications for skin biopsy include:

- masses or any possible neoplastic lesions
- persistent ulcerated lesions
- conditions failing to respond to appropriate therapy
- unusual or atypical dermatoses
- if a condition is suspected which requires therapy which may be expensive, of extended duration or hazardous

The procedure can be performed using gentle restraint and local analgesia. Local anaesthetic without adrenaline should be used to avoid the introduction of artefactual changes in the vasculature of the biopsied tissue. At times, sedation or general anaesthesia may be necessary, depending on the temperament of the patient, its state of health and the sites to be biopsied. Careful selection of lesions is important, choosing primary lesions such as pustules or vesicles and non-excoriated sites. Chronic secondary changes will often tend to obscure primary pathology. For suspected endocrine or atrophic conditions, fully developed, mature lesions give more typical histology. It is essential to take several samples and to include lesional and non-lesional skin. It is usually necessary to withdraw glucocorticoid medication and treat secondary bacterial infections for several weeks prior to taking biopsies to try and eliminate secondary or iatrogenic pathology. Two techniques for obtaining samples are described:

Punch biopsies

Disposable 4mm or 6mm diameter biopsy punches are available, which allow rapid sampling of multiple sites. The biopsy sample obtained with the smaller diameter punches may include only three or four hair follicle units and may be difficult to interpret histopathologically, but they are useful for sites such as the feet and the nose and for small, discreet lesions. However, the rotational force involved in obtaining the sample may disrupt vesicles or pustules. This method is inappropriate for masses or for the junctional area between lesional and normal skin. It is important, therefore, to take several biopsies of both affected and non-affected skin. Biopsy sites usually require only a single suture.

Excisional biopsies

An ellipse of tissue is excised using a surgical blade. Larger samples are thus obtained, requiring more lengthy surgical repair and therefore take more time. This technique enables removal of whole nodules or masses or bullae, or sampling of a wedge of tissue at junction of normal with abnormal skin. It is important that the orientation of the ellipse at such interfaces is correct, since samples are cut in half longitudinally during processing, and one half discarded. The lesion should be at one pole of the ellipse and normal tissue at the other so that examples of both are retained on the processed tissue.

The hair overlying biopsy sites should be carefully trimmed with scissors, with no surgical preparation, as clipping and scrubbing destroys vital surface structure. Full thickness of skin should be taken down to the subcutis. Excess blood should be removed and biopsies gently placed dermis side down onto stiff paper or cardboard before fixing to prevent curling and distortion. The usual fixative is 10% formal saline, unless immunofluorescence required, when Michel's medium should be used. Tissue can also be submitted for bacterial culture if infection is suspected.

It is vital that adequate information regarding the patient, the history (including medication), the clinical appearance of the condition, the sites biopsied and the possible differential diagnoses are supplied to the pathologist. Only with this information can the histopathological changes be interpreted appropriately and a meaningful conclusion drawn.

Allergy Testing

Restriction and provocative testing

This approach is appropriate for the diagnosis of contact allergies and food hypersensitivity.

Contact allergies - The patient is kept in a "safe" environment with no access to potential allergens for a period to determine whether pruritus resolves. This is difficult to achieve in the home environment. Admission to hospital kennels and bedding on newspaper, or white cotton sheeting, while allowing exercise only on paved surfaces is the best method, allowing frequent assessment of the patient. There is usually an improvement within seven to ten days in cases of contact allergy, although it should be noted that many cases of atopy will also improve with this regime. If improvement occurs the patient is returned home, to one room for the first week, then sequentially exposed to further rooms to identify the one which causes a return of symptoms. Attention can then be focused on individual items, carpets, fabrics and plants within that environment.

Food intolerance - The same principle applies, the patient being fed a novel diet consisting, if possible, of one protein and carbohydrate source, preferably to which the animal has never previously been exposed. All other foodstuffs should be excluded. Suitable proteins would be lamb, rabbit, chicken, egg or fish with boiled rice or potato as suitable choices of carbohydrate. The actual choice must depend on the previous dietary history of the individual case. An improvement whilst being fed this diet is suggestive of a food allergy. Ideally the food should be home prepared, although several commercial "hypoallergenic" diets are available. The duration of the restriction or elimination diet should be at least three months before the diagnosis is ruled out, although the majority of food allergic cases will improve within six to eight weeks. Once an improvement has been noted, foodstuffs may be reintroduced sequentially for a week at a time to identify the offending foodstuff. It may be desirable from a nutritional viewpoint to change to a commercially prepared diet during the provocative phase.

Intradermal skin tests

Intradermal skin testing is a valuable aid in the diagnosis of canine and feline atopy allowing identification of causal allergens and the formulation of appropriate vaccines for immunotherapy. Allergen solutions are available from a number of sources (Greer Laboratories Inc, North Carolina, USA; ARTU Biologicals NV, Leylstad, Holland; Veterinhal, Hal Allergen Laboratories BV, Haalem, Holland) and are supplied either as concentrated aqueous solutions which can be diluted to testing strength on a regular basis or ready diluted, although diluted allergens have a reduced shelf life. (Editor's note: these substances are not licenced for use in animals in the U.K.). Testing with allergen mixes is undesirable, since the concentration of individual allergens may not be sufficient to give a positive reaction. Selection of allergens which are relevant to the particular region is important. Table 1 shows a list of allergens selected on the basis of aeroallergens known to cause problems in man in the U.K.

Table 1
Allergens suitable for use in the UK

Environmental:
Ctenocephalides spp.
Tyrophagus putrescantiae
Acarus siro
Dermatophagoides farinae
Dermatophagoides pteronyssinus
Housedust
Human dander
Cat dander
Sheep epithelia
Kapok
Mixed feathers

Trees:
Birch mix
Alnus rugosa (Alder)
Corylus americana (Hazel)
Fagus americana (Beech)
Fraxinus americana (Ash)
Platanus occidentalis (Sycamore)
Pop. alba (Poplar)
Oak mix
Salix discolor (Willow)

Grasses:
Poa pratensis (Meadow grass)
Festuca elatior (Fescue)
Dactylis glomerata (Cocksfoot)
Agrostis alba (Bent-grass)
Lolium multiflorum (Italian rye grass)
Phleum pratensis (Timothy)

Weeds:
Artemisia vulgaris (Mugwort)
Brassica spp. (Rape)
Chenopodium botrys
Chenopodium album (Goosefoot)
Chrysanthemum spp. (Daisy)
Plantago lanceolata (Plantain)
Rumex acetosella (Sheep's sorrel)
Rumex crispus (Yellow dock)
Taxacara officionale (Dandelion)
Trifolium pratense (Red clover)
Urtica spp. (Nettle)

Moulds:
Alternaria alternata
Aspergillus fumigatus
Botrytis cinerae
Cladosporium herbarum
Epicoccum purpurascens
Fusarium moniliforme
Helminthosporum sativum
Penicilium notatum
Phoma betae

Pullularia pullulans
Rhodotorula rubra

Smuts:
Barley smut
Oat smut
Wheat smut

This comprises the panel of allergens used by most veterinary dermatologists in the UK. A multicentre study suggests that this is an appropriate panel for this country, although there are significant regional variations in reaction patterns, with more pollen and mould spore reactions reported in animals in the Southwest region (Ferguson, 1992). This study also demonstrated that environmental allergens such as *Dermatophagoides* spp. and housedust predominated in cases of canine atopy in the UK. Of the other groups of aeroallergens, weed pollens were found to be the most important overall.

Skin testing is performed with dogs in lateral recumbency, and the large number of test allergens usually necessitates the use of sedation. The choice of sedative is important, since many drugs will interfere with skin test reaction. Both xylazine and medetomidine are appropriate, and can be reversed with atipamezole. An area over the lateral trunk is clipped and injection sites can be identified by felt-tip marker pen. Most investigators inject a volume of 0.05 ml of each allergen into the dermis, using a 26 or 27 guage needle. Histamine diluted to 1/100,000 weight/volume is used as the positive control and phosphate buffered saline as the negative control. The injection sites are examined 10 to 20 minutes later for reactions. Although there is some individual variation in the definition of what constitutes a positive reaction, a wheal greater than the mean of those produced by the positive and negative controls is widely accepted as a positive skin test reaction. Test sites should be examined at 12, 24 and 48 hours for signs of late or delayed reactions.

The presence of a positive skin test reaction indicates that the patient has a skin sensitising antibody, but does not necessarily mean that the allergen is clinically significant for that patient. Positive reactions must be interpreted in conjunction with a full knowledge of the patient's history. Other factors which may lead to false positive reactions include irritant test solutions, contaminated allergen solutions, non-immunological histamine release, poor operator technique (traumatic needle placement, blunt needle, injection of too large a volume, injection of air) and dermatographism. Many factors may give rise to false negative reactions, the most common of which is the recent administration of drugs such as glucocorticoids and antihistamines. Although it is difficult to establish reliable withdrawal periods for such drugs one month off alternate day steroids and seven to ten days off antihistamines should be sufficient. Animals that have received depot steroids may need several months before reliable skin test results can be expected. It should be noted that a negative skin test does not necessarily mean that an animal is not atopic. Many workers have observed that a percentage of dogs (~10%) with classical signs of atopy may have negative skin tests and this may indicate a failure to challenge with the appropriate allergen(s) as well as the possible interference of factors known to produce false negative reactions.

The technique of intradermal skin testing and the interpretation of skin test reactions becomes much easier with increased experience of the operator, and is not a test which can be considered suitable for occasional use. It is preferable to refer cases to an experienced veterinary dermatologist, after other appropriate investigations have been completed.

Patch tests
Suspect materials in cases of contact allergy may be applied to the skin for 48 hours. The skin is then examined for erythema and induration which occurs with the causal allergen. It is necessary to distinguish irritant from allergic reactions and biopsy of the positive sites may be undertaken to document the typical histopathology of contact allergy. Specialised chambers (Finn chambers) containing potential allergens are used in human medicine and can also be used for veterinary patients. The haircoat must be clipped away the day before commencing the test and samples must be immobilised against the skin surface with bandages. This may not be tolerated by the patient and the owner may be unhappy about the removal of large areas of hair from their pet. Because contact allergy is relatively uncommon and due to the limitations of the procedure, patch testing is infrequently undertaken in veterinary dermatology.

Serological tests
Radio-allergosorbant tests (RAST) and enzyme-linked immunosorbant assays (ELISA) are available for the identification of allergen-specific antibodies circulating in the patients blood. The principle of the tests is similar: patient serum is added to wells containing antigens and species specific radiolabelled or enzyme-linked antisera (usually anti-IgE) is added. Bound antiserum remaining after washing indicates the presence of patient antibodies and is detected by measuring the radioactivity or colour change.

Work on the correlation between intradermal skin test results and a RAST test using anti-canine IgE showed great variability in test results, with a correlation of 82% for ragweed pollen, 64% for timothy grass, 42% for housedust mite and 12.5% to 39% correlation for other weeds (Halliwell and Kunkle, 1978). There was a good correlation (100%) between negative RAST tests and negative intradermal skin testing. Shirk (1986) reported an excellent correlation between RAST and skin test results in 50% of her patients, with a moderate correlation in 24% and only poor correlation in the remaining 26%. Immunotherapy based on RAST results in her series of cases resulted in an excellent response in 27%, moderate in 39%, fair in 24% and no response in 12% of patients, results broadly comparable with skin test-based vaccines.

The work of Willemse *et al* (1985) with an ELISA test using anti-IgGd antiserum showed similar variability, with positive correlations of 27% for housedust, 6 to 17% for various pollens and 1 to 16% for danders. With this ELISA test there was variable negative correlation, with some animals having positive ELISA results and negative skin test results. More recently an ELISA kit test marketed for use in a practice laboratory has been evaluated (Miller, *et al*, 1992). Whilst the results obtained with the kit showed good repeatability, comparison of results with a serological test available at a commercial laboratory showed high specificity (ie. good negative correlation) but poor sensitivity (positive correlation between test results). For most allergens the sensitivity was found to be considerably less than stated in the manufacturer's data sheets. The kit was felt to be of questionable value as a diagnostic aid.

The influence of drug therapy, and factors such as stress, oestrus, pregnancy, parasitism and intercurrent illness on serological tests in animals is unknown. The discrepancies between serological results and intradermal skin testing, the uncertainty regarding the relative importance of different immunoglobulins in canine atopy and the paucity of published studies documenting the accuracy of serological tests limits their usefulness as aids for the diagnosis and management of canine atopy at the present time. These tests cannot be considered to replace the intradermal skin test.

Little has been published about the usefulness of serological tests for food intolerance. The work of McDougal (1987) showed RAST to be unreliable for testing food hypersensitivity in dogs. Restriction to a hypoallergenic diet and provocative challenge remains the most specific test for food intolerance in animals.

Blood Samples

Routine haematological and biochemical investigations are not indicated in the majority of dermatological cases, but may give useful supportive information in certain situations; for example: eosinophilia in allergic conditions especially in cats; white cell responses in infections; haematological changes in certain endocrinopathies; changes in serum biochemistry in endocrinopathies and hepatic disorders; tests for malabsorption; FeLV and FIV titres of cats with recurrent infections. Such investigations may be of value in monitoring animals treated with immunosuppressive or chemotherapeutic agents.

HORMONAL ASSAYS
Hormonal assays can be performed on serum or heparinised plasma samples, usually by radio-immunoassay. Single base-line meaurements of hormone concentrations are non-diagnostic and dynamic response or suppression tests should be performed to confirm the diagnosis of an endocrinopathy (Chapter 12).

Hypothyroidism
The routine haematological and biochemical abnormalities which may be found in cases of canine hypothyroidism are shown in Table 2.

Table 2
Laboratory findings in canine hypothyroidism

Mild, normocytic, normochromic anaemia (25% of cases, 35% low normal)
Hypercholesterolaemia (33-75% of cases)
Increased plasma lipids
Mild to marked elevation of liver enzymes (ALT in 25%, AP & AST in 20% of cases)
Elevation of CPK (10% of cases)

Although single baseline measurements of total triiodothyronine (T3) or thyroxine (T4) are usually non-diagnostic, a total T4 concentration of <8.5 nmol/l is suggestive of hypothyroidism. Results in the upper normal range (30-52 nmol/l) rule out hypothyroidism. Measurement of free T4 has been found to be no more useful than total T4 assay (Feldman and Nelson, 1987). If basal T3/T4 concentrations are unusually elevated when clinical signs are consistent with hypothyroidism, the presence of anti T3/T4 antibodies should be considered.

The best diagnostic test for confirmation of hypothyroidism is the **thyroid stimulating hormone (TSH) response test** which is performed as follows:

(i)   collect blood for baseline total T4
(ii)   inject 0.1 iu/kg TSH intravenously
(iii)   collect second blood sample 6 hours later.

Normal (euthyroid) dogs should show a 1.5-fold increase over their baseline concentration of total T4 and the concentration of T4 in the second specimen should fall within the normal range (20-52 nmol/l).

An alternative to the above test, since TSH can be difficult and expensive to obtain, is the **thyrotropin releasing hormone (TRH) response test**. Several protocols are described in the literature, but the work of Henfrey and Thoday (1991) shows the following method to be optimal:

(i)   blood sample collected for baseline total T4
(ii)   0.02 mg/kg TRH (Roche), injected <u>slowly</u> intravenously
(iii)   second blood sample collected 4 hours later.

Most normal (euthyroid) dogs show a 1.2-fold increase in total T4 concentration over basal value and the results of the second sample fall within normal range. It is the general opinion that this is a less reliable test for the detection of hypothyroid animals.

The routine availability of an assay of canine TSH would greatly facilitate the investigation and diagnosis of thyroid disorders and obviate the need for dynamic testing.

Hyperadrenocorticism (HAC)
The typical routine haematological and biochemical changes found in cases of canine HAC are shown in Table 3.

Table 3
Laboratory findings in canine hyperadrenocorticalism

Eosinopaenia <0.2 x 10^9/l (84% of cases)
Lymphopaenia < 1.5 x 10^9/l,
Neutrophilia, monocytosis.
Elevated AP, often marked, fairly consistent finding
Mild to moderate increased ALT
Increased bile salts
Hypercholesterolaemia, lipaemia
Fasting glucose high normal or elevated (overt diabetic)
Urea often low normal

Measurement of single resting cortisol concentration is non-diagnostic and dynamic testing is essential. Two screening tests are described

1. Adrenocorticotropin hormone (ACTH) stimulation test

The test should be performed in the morning to coincide with peak physiological cortisol concentrations. Several protocols have been published. The author's preferred method is as follows:

(i)   Collect blood sample collected for baseline cortisol estimation
(ii)   Inject tetracosactrin (Synacthen, Ciba) intravenously - dose 250 mg for dogs >10 kg, 125 mg if <10kg bodyweight
(iii)   Collect second blood sample 1 hour (0.5 - 2 hours) later

Normal ranges: baseline cortisol 50-250 nmol/l, post ACTH cortisol <500 nmol/l
Abnormal results: normal to elevated baseline with post ACTH value above 600 nmol/l

The ACTH stimulation test detects 85-90% of pituitary-dependent (PD)-HAC cases and about 50% of adrenal-dependent (AD)-HAC, but does not reliably distinguish between the two. It is the only test appropriate for the diagnosis of iatrogenic HAC, indicated by low to zero baseline cortisol and absent or minimal response to ACTH.

2. Low dose dexamethasone suppression test

This is a more sensitive screening test for HAC, detecting all adrenal and 90-95% of PD-HAC. It is performed as follows:

(i)   Collect blood sample for baseline cortisol estimation
(ii)   Inject 0.01 mg/kg dexamethasone i/v
(iii)   Collect second blood sample taken 8 hours later

Normal dogs show suppression of cortisol concentration to less than 40 nmol/l; dogs with HAC fail to suppress to this degree. An extra blood sample at 3 hours may give an indication of aetiology, since PD-HAC may suppress to 50% of baseline at this time.

If an individual dog with HAC is not detected by one of the screening tests, it should be by the other (Feldman, 1983a). In the occasional animal which gives borderline results the dynamic test(s) should be repeated after one month.

3. High dose dexamethasone suppression test

This may be helpful in the differentiation of PD-HAC and adrenal tumours, but is only appropriate after a positive screening test result has been obtained. The method is as follows:

(i)   Collect blood sample for baseline cortisol estimation
(ii)   Inject 0.1 mg/kg dexamethasone i/v
(iii)   Collect further blood samples 3 and 8 hours later

Interpretation: cases with PD-HAC suppress to <50% of baseline at 3 hours, although some may be >50% at 8 hours; cases with adrenal tumour show cortisol concentrations >50% of baseline at 3 and 8 hours. However, the test is not a completely reliable method of differentiation. The measurement of plasma ACTH concentration offers a better method for differentiation (Feldman, 1983b), if this assay is available. However, even this test is not totally reliable, non-diagnostic results occuring in 5% of cases. Where abdominal radiography, ultrasonography and the measurement of endogenous ACTH have been compared no one method was completely reliable in discriminating adrenal tumours from PD-HAC (Reusch and Feldman, 1991). If possible, all three investigations should be undertaken to confirm the presence of an adrenal tumour.

Sex hormone assays are available, but the normal ranges which have been established are wide and single, baseline estimations are often unhelpful in the investigation of cases with suspected sex hormone imbalance. An assay for canine growth hormone is available in some countries and growth hormone reserve can be assessed by use of either the xylazine or clonidine response test. It should be noted that there is considerable overlap between growth hormone responsive and castration responsive dermatoses and the distinction between the two conditions is far from clear at present (Chapter 12).

Faecal Examination

Examination of faeces is indicated where allergy to endoparasites is suspected, or cutaneous larval migrans in cases of hookworm infestation. It may also be useful if diarrhoea is an intercurrent feature, to identify forage mites (hypersensitivity reactions to these free living mites may result in cutaneous and/or enteric symptoms) or the presence of undigested food in malabsorption syndromes.

REFERENCES AND FURTHER READING

DOXEY, D.L. and NATHAN, M.B.F. (Editors) (1989) Manual of Laboratory Techniques. BSAVA Publications.

FELDMAN, E.C. (1983a) Comparison of ACTH response and dexamethasone suppression as screening tests in canine hyperadrenocorticism. *Journal of the American Veterinary Medical Association* **182,** 506.

FELDMAN, E.C. (1983b) Distinguishing dogs with functioning adrenocortical tumors from dogs with pituitary-dependent hyperadrenocorticism. *Journal of the American Veterinary Medical Association* **183,** 195.

FELDMAN, E.C. and NELSON, R.W. (1987) *Canine and Feline Endocrinology and Reproduction,,* W.B. Saunders Company, Philadelphia.

FERGUSON, E.A. (1992) A review of intradermal skin testing in the UK. *Veterinary Dermatology Newsletter* **14,** 13.

FREY, D., OLDFIELD, R.J. and BRIDGER, R.C. (1985) *A Colour Atlas of Pathogenic Fungi.* Wolfe Medical Publications Ltd., London

FUDGE, A.M. (1991) Parasites of pet and aviary birds. In: *Diagnostic Parasitology for Veterinary Technicians* (ed J Colville), pp239 American Veterinary Publications, Inc.

GEORGI, J.R. and GEORGI, M.E. (1990) *Parasitology for Veterinarians.* 5th Ed. W.B. Saunders Company, Philadelphia.

HALLIWELL, R.E.W. and KUNKLE, G.A. (1978) The radioallergosorbent test in the diagnosis of canine atopic disease. *Journal of Allergy and Clinical Immunology* **62,** 236.

HENFREY, J.I. and THODAY, K.L. (1991) Optimisation of the TSH and TRH stimulation tests for the diagnosis of canine hypothyroidism. *Proceedings of the BSAVA Congress 1991* p121.

HERRTAGE, M.E. (1990) The adrenal glands. In: *Manual of Small Animal Endocrinology* (ed M. Hutchison) pp 73-104. BSAVA Publications.

MINISTRY OF AGRICULTURE, FISHERIES and FOOD (1984) Bacteriology and Mycology In: *Manual of Veterinary Investigaion Laboratory Techniques* Vol. 1, Reference Book 389 3rd ed. 46 Her Majesty's Stationery Office, London.

MINISTRY OF AGRICULTURE, FISHERIES and FOOD (1986) Entomology In: *Manual of Veterinary Parasitological Laboratory Techniques* , Reference Book 418, 103. Her Majesty's Stationery Office, London.

McDOUGAL, B.J. (1987) Correlation of results of the radioallergosorbent test and provocative testing in 20 dogs with food allergy. *Proceedings of the Annual AAVD and ACVD* p42.

MILLER, W.H., SCOTT, D.W. and SCARLETT, J.M. (1992) Evaluation of an allergy screening test for use in atopic dogs. *J. Am. vet. med. Ass.,* **200,** 931.

MULLER, G.H., KIRK, R.W. and SCOTT, D.W. (1989) *Small Animal Dermatology ,* 4th ed.pp126-149 and 454-459. W. B. Saunders Company, Philadelphia

REEDY, L.M. and MILLER, W.H. (1989) *Allergic skin diseases of dogs and cats..* W.B. Saunders Company, Philadelphia.

REUSCH, C.E. and FELDMAN, E.C. (1991) Canine hyperadrenocorticism due to adrenocortical neoplasia. *Journal of Veterinary Internal Medicine* **5,** 3.

SCHMEITZEL, L.P. and IHRKE, P.J. (1991) Diagnosis of parasitism of the skin. In: *Diagnostic Parasitology for Veterinary Technicians* (Ed J Colville), pp85. American Veterinary Publications, Inc.

SCHMEITZEL, L.P. and IHRKE, P.J. (1991) External parasites of dogs and cats. In: *Diagnostic Parasitology for Veterinary Technicians* (Ed J Colville), pp46. American Veterinary Publications, Inc.

SHAFFER, D.A. and WAGNER, J.E. (1991) Parasites of rabbits and rodents. In: *Diagnostic Parasitology for Veterinary Technicians* (Ed J Colville), pp185 American Veterinary Publications, Inc.

SHIRK, M.E. (1986) The canine RAST: a diagnostic procedure for allegic inhalant dermatitis. *Proceedings of the Annual AAVD and ACVD* p32.

THODAY, K.L. (1990) The thyroid gland. In: *Manual of Small Animal Endocrinology* (Ed M. Hutchison) pp 25-57. BSAVA Publications.

WADE, W.F. and GAAFAR, S.M. (1991) Diagnosis of parasitism of miscellaneous body systems In: *Diagnostic Parasitology for Veterinary Technicians* (Ed J Colville), p49. American Veterinary Publications, Inc.

WILLEMSE, A., NOORDZIJ, A., VAN DEN BROM, W.E. and RUTTEN, V.P.M.G. (1985) Allergen specific IgGd antibodies in dogs with atopic dermatitis as determined by the enzyme linked immunosorbent assay (ELISA). *Clinical and Experimental Immunology* **59,** 359.

PRURITUS IN THE DOG

Craig E Griffin

INTRODUCTION

Pruritus (itch) is an unpleasant sensation within the skin that produces the desire to scratch. It is a primary sensation caused by the stimulation of free, unmyelinated, nerve endings associated with the epidermis. Pruritus can be stimulated by heat, electrical stimuli and a variety of chemicals, the most notable being histamine. Histamine induced pruritus results from stimulation of H_1 receptors. Other chemical mediators of itch include serotonin and a variety of peptide and proteolytic enzymes. Bacteria, fungi, leucocytes, mast cells and damaged epidermal cells are all sources of these stimuli (Denman, 1986; Halliwell, 1974).

Besides the stimuli for pruritus other factors are known to modulate the sensation. Prostaglandins (PGs) may alter the threshold for itch in different ways, according to the class of PG which predominates at any one time. Thus, they may either potentiate the effects of some stimuli or reduce the response to others. Many inflammatory mediators, such as leukotrienes (which are an end product of arachidonic acid metabolism), modulate or contribute to pruritus but do not directly induce it. Other factors such as dry skin (xerosis) will also lower the pruritic threshold. In humans boredom, stress and anxiety have all been shown to aggravate pruritus.

It is important for the clinician and client treating pruritus to understand the concepts of pruritic threshold and the summation effect. The pruritic threshold is the level of stimuli that will result in pruritus. This level will vary from patient to patient. Once reached, the addition of more stimuli will only enhance the sensation of pruritus and is referred to as the summation of effect. Additional stimuli can be totally unrelated to the primary disease.

Recent work in allergic dogs has shown that percutaneous absorption of staphylococcal antigen is increased in inflamed skin (Mason and Lloyd, 1990). These antigens can also increase inflammation and contribute to pruritus. Atopic dog corneocytes have been shown to have increased adherence for *Staphylococcus intermedius* (McEwan, 1990). This may make more antigen accessible for absorption. Chronic pruritus and inflammation both contribute to epidermal acanthosis and hyperkeratosis which clinically manifests as xerosis (dry skin). Therefore the condition of any pruritic dog with inflammation may be worsened by both increased bacterial antigen penetration and the dry skin which results from inflammation.

Pruritus is a non-specific sensation associated with a number of diseases. Appropriate therapy for pruritus can only be determined after a specific diagnosis is made. The most common causes are listed in Table 1. This is not a complete list but will allow the clinician to handle the majority of the pruritic cases seen in practice.

Table 1
Common pruritic diseases

DISEASE	METHOD TO RULE IN OR OUT
Allergy	
Atopy	Intradermal skin test
Insect	Intradermal skin test
Flea	Response to flea control or intradermal skin test
Food	Hypoallergenic diet trial and provocative exposure
Contact	Patch test, response to avoidance and challenge
Ectoparasites	
Sarcoptes scabiei	Microscopy of skin scrapings or response to trial therapy
Demodex canis	Microscopy of skin scrapings
Cheyletiella spp.	Flea comb and flotation of debris, microscopy of skin scrapings and mite identification or trial therapy
Pyoderma	Cytology, culture, trial antibiotic therapy
***Malassezia pachydermatis* dermatitis**	Cytology
Dermatophytosis	Microscopy of skin and hair samples or fungal culture
Xerosis	Physical examination, response to moisturisers

APPROACH TO THE CASE

A successful outcome to the approach of the pruritic dog is most likely to be realised if the following questions are answered:

1. What is the specific diagnosis or diagnoses? It is important to be aware that many cases may have more than one diagnosis.

2. What other factors are present that may add to the pruritic load or lower the pruritic threshold?

3. Will topical therapy be beneficial? Is it practical and feasible?

4. What will the diagnostic and management plan involve?

5. Has the client been educated about the plan and are they willing to follow it through? Client compliance and observations are critical to the success of managing most pruritic dogs.

To answer the preceding questions the clinician must have taken a complete history and made a complete physical examination, developed a differential diagnosis, looked for coexisting factors that may affect the pruritic load or threshold, formulated a diagnostic and/or treatment plan, discussed the plan with the client and received their agreement to proceed.

Taking the history

The initial approach, which helps to determine which of the many pruritic diseases may be present, is the acquisition of a thorough history (Chapter 2). The age and breed of the dog may be helpful in ranking the differentials. Pruritus that develops prior to six months age is likely to be related to ecto- or endo-parasites or food allergy. Dogs that develop their first symptoms of pruritus after 7 years of age are much less likely to be atopic.

The breed of the affected animal can also be helpful in suggesting a diagnosis since some of the common diseases have a genetic basis or breed predispositions. Breeds prone to atopic disease include: terriers (West Highland white, cairn, Scottish, wire haired fox, Boston); dalmatian; golden and labrador retriever; Chinese shar pei and boxer (Plates 17-21). Breeds prone to food allergy include: Chinese shar pei; cocker spaniel, labrador retriever and German shepherd dog. The basset hound, dachshund and possibly the cocker spaniel and West Highland white terrier breeds are at increased risk for the development of *Malassezia pachydermatis* dermatitis. The clinician must also be careful not to be misled by breed associations. Though the West Highland white terrier is very prone to atopic disease, not all have it; demodicosis, scabies or *Malassezia pachydermatis* dermatitis also occur in this breed.

Very important questions that need to be answered relate to the seasonality and duration of symptoms. In cases with seasonal pruritus the differential diagnosis is usually limited to atopic disease and seasonal ectoparasites. In cases that are perennial but have seasonal exacerbations the same differential plus the possibility of coexisting diseases must be considered.

There are a number of pitfalls to be aware of when questioning clients about their animal's pruritus. Many clients will respond to a question about itching very literally and only refer to where the dog scratches with its paws. However, pruritus may be manifested by licking, chewing, rolling, rubbing, biting, and shaking the head. Often, foot or flexor elbow licking will not be reported by the client because they believe that this behaviour is normal and that their dog "grooms like a cat" or "cleans his feet". Unless specifically questioned for these behaviours the client may not supply information which may suggest that the dog has atopic disease. Some clients will only report that their dog is pruritic wherever they see gross skin disease or alopecia. Other clients actually may not observe their dog scratch and just hear the scratching and tell the dog to stop it. This may even train the dog to leave the client's presence when it scratches so that the client may not be aware of all the information needed to make a complete differential diagnosis.

The first abnormality that develops should be determined. This often helps to rank the differential diagnoses based on the typical pattern of involvement for the diseases being considered. For example, of the major causes of pruritus, food allergy, atopic disease and *Malassezia pachydermatis* dermatitis are likely to involve otitis externa from the onset. Disease initially confined to the dorsal trunk is more likely to occur with flea allergy dermatitis, cheyletiellosis, demodicosis and pyoderma. Just as the initial pattern of pruritus helps establish the differential diagnosis, the progression of a disease and the final pattern of involvement are very important in ranking the differential diagnoses. It is also important to determine whether the disease is contagious to other animals or humans. If compatible lesions are present then a history of contagion suggests that fleas, scabies, cheyletiellosis or dermatophytosis is present. Papular lesions of the lower legs of humans may indicate that fleas are present while papular lesions involving the arms and trunk are more typical of scabies or cheyletiellosis. Though it may be difficult to obtain, the index of suspicion for these diagnoses increases if a history of a possible source of exposure to these parasites is determined.

Many clients will not really know if a rash preceded the development of pruritus but when this information is available and reliable it is very helpful. Pruritus without any obvious skin disease is more commonly associated with atopic disease (which may be accompanied by xerosis), cheyletiellosis and food allergy. A primary eruption is usually present in cases with scabies, flea allergy, contact allergy, pyoderma and demodicosis.

The presence of diarrhoea or vomiting raises the index of suspicion for food allergy. The number of bowel movements per day should be ascertained as dogs with food allergy often have an abnormally high number (3 or greater) (Frick, 1991). Weight loss is seen in some dogs with scabies or severely pruritic dogs. If other systemic signs are present then another disease or a disease coexisting with the cause of the pruritus should be suspected.

PHYSICAL EXAMINATION

A complete physical examination with close inspection of the entire body and hair coat is essential in accurately establishing the most likely differential diagnoses. The type and extent of primary and secondary lesions should be recorded. The pattern and type of lesions should also be compared with the historical description in order to determine how accurate and observant the clients are. This information helps the clinician decide how reliable the history is and is then used to help train the client on what they need to observe, especially following trial therapies.

The primary lesions present may aid in establishing the differential diagnosis (Table 2). As mentioned previously with the history, a helpful finding is determining whether the pruritus is associated with either a primary eruption or with lesion-free skin. Although this may not be determined at the initial examination it may be possible to do so on a subsequent examination. During the initial management phase the client can be instructed in what to look for and when to return the dog for follow-up examination. During the first examination the areas that historically were pruritic should be closely observed for a primary eruption; if none are found in some of these areas then the possibility of a disease that causes pruritus without a rash is more likely to be involved.

Secondary lesions may also be observed and often are evidence of pruritus. These include alopecia, broken hairs or whiskers, excoriations, lichenification and salivary staining.

Table 2
Primary lesions and diseases most commonly associated in pruritic dogs

PRIMARY LESIONS	MOST COMMON CAUSES	COMMON CAUSES
Papules	Pyoderma Scabies Flea allergy dermatitis	
		Contact allergy Yeast infection (Malassezia pachydermatis) Cheyletiellosis
Pustules	Pyoderma	
		Demodicosis Contact allergy Cheyletiellosis
Crusted/Papules	Flea allergy dermatitis Pyoderma Scabies	
		Demodicosis Yeast infection (Malassezia pachydermatis) Contact allergy Dermatophyte
Follicular Casts	Demodicosis Dermatophyte	
		Yeast infection (Malassezia pachydermatis)
No Primary Lesions	Atopic disease Food allergy	
		+/- Insect allergy
Vesicles	Contact allergy	

The pattern of lesions is helpful in establishing a diagnosis. Pinnal disease and otitis externa rarely are associated with flea allergy dermatitis and usually indicate that the dog has atopic disease, food allergy, scabies or *Malassezia pachydermatis* infection. Flea allergy dermatitis (FAD) classically affects the dorsal sacral lumbar area most severely but food allergy may also do so. In addition, cheyletiellosis should be considered as a possible cause of lesions with a distribution that is predominantly along the dorsal trunk. Pruritus of the ventral trunk and distal extremities is more typical of atopic disease, insect hypersensitivity, scabies and contact allergy. Foot and face pruritus most often occur from atopic disease. Ventral cervical, interdigital and axillary disease are suggestive of *Malassezia pachydermatis* dermatitis or atopic disease. Lesions confined to sparsely haired areas, ventral paws, and inguinal disease raises the index of suspicion for allergic contact or primary irritant dermatitis. Axillary and inguinal crusted, papular or pustular dermatitis is common with pyoderma while lesions confined to the ventral pinna are rarely seen with pyoderma and usually suggest another problem is present. A pattern of fold or frictional disease is suggestive of pyoderma or *Malassezia pachydermatis* dermatitis. Most allergic diseases tend to be associated with a symmetrical distribution of lesions and pruritus whereas the lesions of dermatophytosis and demodicosis are often asymmetrical.

It is often necessary to determine how much of the skin disease relates to secondary pyoderma. In many atopic and food allergic dogs the majority of the primary lesions seen will be associated with pyoderma and, following antibiotic therapy, the dog may remain pruritic but no longer have a primary rash.

ESTABLISHING THE DIAGNOSIS

The history and physical examination are utilised to determine the most likely differentials. Although patterns, lesions and histories allow a clinician to rank the probability that certain diseases are present we must also remember that exceptions exist. Few dogs read and follow textbook descriptions. Based on the ranking, initial laboratory tests can be recommended (Table 1). Cytology and microscopy of skin scrapings will rapidly help determine, or tentatively rule out, the presence of *Malassezia pachydermatis*, pyoderma, *Demodex canis*, and *Cheyletiella* spp. Cytology is the most common diagnostic procedure used in the author's practice, even exceeding skin scrapes. Scabies and cheyletiellosis cannot be ruled out with negative scrapings and, if still at the top of the differential diagnosis then trial therapy is warranted. Trial therapy with ivermectin (250ug/kg) subcutaneously every 7-10 days for 3-4 treatments will effectively rule out scabies or cheyletiellosis (Editors note: Ivermectin is not licenced for use in the dog or cat in the U.K.). All dogs in contact with the affected animal should be treated if scabies is to be ruled out. Cats and rabbits must also be treated to rule out *Cheyletiella spp*. If allergic diseases (FAD, atopy, food) are highest on the list of differential diagnoses initially, or following cytology and scrapes, then intradermal skin testing will rapidly help to determine whether atopy is present. If the clinician does not perform intradermal testing then trial therapy with either flea control (if FAD is suspected) or antihistamines and fatty acids (if atopy is suspected) and a hypoallergenic diet can be recommended. An alternative is to do a limited intradermal test with flea and housedust mite *(Dermatophagoides farinae)* antigens. Immediate or delayed reactions to flea allergen will be seen in most dogs with FAD and about 50% of dogs perennially affected with atopy will be housedust mite positive. A better screen would consist of these injections plus 2 or 3 of the most common weed, tree and grass antigens for that local area. If abnormal gastro-intestinal signs are present or food allergy is still high on the differential following the basic tests (as outlined above) then a hypoallergenic diet may be recommended. However, since it often takes a hypoallergenic diet trial 4-8 weeks to have a beneficial effect other trial therapies may be tried during the first four to six weeks of the diet. Often these trial therapies are utilised to help establish a diagnosis especially if clients are unwilling or reluctant to spend the money needed for more specific tests. The diagnosis of pyoderma and *Malassezia pachydermatis* is often secondary to another cause which should be pursued.

Many clients are not willing to try one diagnostic approach at a time. If only one differential is pursued at a time by trial therapy, two major consequences may result. First, it may take up to 5 months to determine what problems are present: 2-4 weeks on antibiotics, then 8 weeks spent on a hypoallergenic diet followed by 3-6 weeks trying antihistamines, 4-8 weeks trying fatty acid supplements and finally 3-4 weeks ruling out scabies. Most clients are interested in relief for their dog and if none is seen they may move on to another veterinarian or give up on the trial therapy approach.

The second problem is that many dogs have more than one disease present. Therefore, trying one therapy at a time can result in failure to eliminate the pruritus. This most commonly occurs when pyoderma or flea allergy is present with another disease. Without controlling the pyoderma, a diet change or antihistamines may seem ineffective when, in reality, without the pyoderma present they would have controlled the pruritus.

For these reasons the author's approach is a combination and sequential use of trial therapies. Generally this approach is utilised after fleas are controlled and scabies and dermatophytosis are ruled out or very low on the differential list. Table 3 is an example of the typical approach utilised. One problem with this approach is it may be confusing to the client. The client should keep a diary of changes each week so results can be interpreted. In addition, interpretation must be confirmed by challenge and repeat treatment with apparently effective therapies. In some situations it will also be determined that a combination was effective but a single agent was not. It is important the client and pet return at the end of the trial therapies to determine what occurred while on the various treatments. Besides helping to determine or rule out various disease, this approach also helps to establish which therapies may be effective. If there is no response then allergy testing, patch testing or biopsy sampling and dermatopathology are indicated. In some cases at this point the clinician and client may also decide that long term systemic glucocorticosteroids are indicated. It is crucial that the client understands the intent and what may be learned from the diagnostic tests as well as trial therapies. Only with the effort and help of the client may the clinician successfully approach the pruritic dog without the use of non-specific glucocorticosteroid therapy. By combining a thorough history, physical examination, limited diagnostic tests and trial therapies a successful outcome is most often achieved.

Table 3
Suggested approach to canine pruritus

WEEK	THERAPY
1	Antihistamine 1 (hydroxyzine)
2	Antihistamine 2 (diphenhydramine)
3	Antihistamine 3 (amitriptyline)
1-3	Antibiotic (Chapter 25)
1-4	Fatty acid supplement (Derm Caps, D.V.M.; Efavet, Efamol Vet)
1-4	Hypoallergenic diet
End 4	Re-evaluate - if pruritus was controlled during any week repeat that therapy without others while looking for recurrence after stopping therapy. If pruritus remains controlled without therapy, food allergy or pruritic pyoderma is likely: challenge with old diet. If pruritus still present end of week 4 consider doing intradermal or *in vivo* allergy test, patch test, continuing diet for 4 more weeks or biopsy and dermatopathology.

This protocol is utilised when allergic diseases and pyoderma are considered most likely. Demodicosis, dermatophytosis, scabies, cheyletiellosis, *Malassezia pachydermatis* infection and FAD should be ruled out or very low on the differential list.

REFERENCES

DENMAN, S. T. (1986). A review of pruritus. *Journal of The American Academy of Dermatology* **14**: 375.

FRICK, O.L. (1991). Pathogenesis of chronic allergic reactions using the atopic dog as a model. *Proceedings of the Academy of Veterinary Allergy 31st annual meeting.* Scottsdale, Arizona. p.7.

HALLIWELL, R.E.W. (1974). Pathogenesis and treatment of pruritus. *Journal of The American Veterinary Medical Association* **164**: 793.

MASON, I.S. and LLOYD, D.H. (1990). Factors influencing the penetration of bacterial antigens through canine skin. In: *Advances in Veterinary Dermatology. vol 1* (Eds. C.von Tscharner and R.E.W. Halliwell) p370 Baillière Tindall, London.

McEWAN, N.A. (1990). Bacterial adherence to canine corneocytes. In: *Advances in Veterinary Dermatology. vol 1* (Eds. C.von Tscharner and R.E.W. Halliwell) p454 Baillière Tindall, London.

CUTANEOUS SCALING DISORDERS IN THE DOG

Kenneth W Kwochka

INTRODUCTION

One of the most common clinical presentations to the small animal practitioner is a dog with scaly skin (Plates 34-37, 39). This was the fourth most common cutaneous abnormality in North American dogs in a study conducted during 1983 (Sischo et al., 1989). The frequency of occurrence is at least comparable in other parts of the world.

The major challenge facing the veterinarian is to determine whether the scaling is secondary to another underlying dermatosis or associated with a primary keratinisation defect. At least 80% of cutaneous scaling cases seen in general practice are secondary. A primary keratinisation disorder should never be diagnosed until secondary causes of scaling have first been considered.

Dermatoses causing secondary scaling (Table 1) are usually classified as pruritic or non-pruritic although some variability in level of pruritus may exist. Primary disorders of keratinisation (Table 2) are those dermatoses usually manifested clinically by excess scale formation in which the primary pathophysiology involves a defect in the keratinising epithelium or cutaneous glandular function. There may be important implications for breeders since most of these conditions are hereditary and breeding of affected animals should be discouraged.

To differentiate between secondary scaling and a primary keratinisation disorder requires a complete well-organized diagnostic plan, a knowledgeable cooperative owner, good client communication, and adequate finances. A complete diagnostic plan usually results in a definitive diagnosis allowing a more accurate prognosis and a better decision on specific treatment.

Secondary scaling usually has an excellent prognosis for complete cure or control when the underlying dermatosis is identified and treated. Scaling associated with primary keratinisation defects is more difficult to control and requires a lifelong clinical management program with topical and systemic therapy.

Cutaneous scaling in dogs has often been referred to as "seborrhoea". This erroneous terminology has lead to much confusion. It is not always clear if the term is being used in a general sense (i.e. scaling regardless of the cause) or more specifically to refer to a primary keratinisation disorder (eg. primary seborrhoea of spaniels). For clarity, the term will be used in this chapter only in the latter sense.

This chapter details the general clinical approach to cutaneous scaling of dogs and presents an organised plan to differentiate scaling secondary to other dermatological diseases versus that due to true primary keratinisation disorders. A full discussion of each of the primary keratinisation disorders is beyond the scope of this chapter but is found elsewhere (Kwochka, 1993a).

Table 1
Dermatoses with common diagnostic criteria which cause secondary scaling in dogs

Level of Pruritus	Disease	Common Diagnostic Evaluations
Pruritic	Flea allergy dermatitis	Examination, skin test, response to flea control
	Pyoderma	Examination, cytology, culture and sensitivity, response to antibiotics
	Atopy	Skin test, *in vitro* test
	Scabies	Skin scrapings, response to ivermectin[1]
	Food allergy dermatitis	Hypoallergenic dietary trial
	Cheyletiellosis*	Skin scrapings, combing, acetate tape preparations, response to ivermectin[1]
	Malassezia dermatitis	Skin swabs
Non-pruritic	Demodicosis*	Skin scrapings
	Dermatophytosis	Wood's lamp, KOH preparation, fungal culture
	Hypothyroidism*	Baseline T4, TSH stimulation test
	Hyperadrenocorticism	Low dose dexamethasone suppression test
	Sex hormone abnormality	Assay hormone levels, skin biopsy, neuter
	Metabolic disease	Haematology, serum biochemical profile, urinalysis
	Pemphigus foliaceus*	Skin biopsy
	Mycosis fungoides*	Skin biopsy
	Environment with low humidity*	Response to topical moisturisers
	Endoparasitism	Faecal examination

* Level of pruritus variable depending on chronicity, secondary changes in the skin, and presence of secondary pyoderma.

1 Not licenced for dogs and cats in the U.K.

APPROACH TO THE CASE

Signalment

The signalment provides some useful information in distinguishing between primary and secondary scaling. Generally, the primary keratinisation disorders are hereditary and will appear during the first two years of life. This is especially true of primary idiopathic seborrhoea, epidermal dysplasia, follicular dystrophy, schnauzer comedo syndrome, canine ichthyosis and canine acne. Infectious (pyoderma, dermatophytosis), parasitic (scabies, demodicosis, cheyletiellosis, endoparasitism), and allergic (flea allergy dermatitis, atopy, food allergy dermatitis) dermatoses are the most common causes of secondary scaling in this age range.

Middle aged animals are less likely to have primary keratinisation defects. They are more likely to have secondary scaling due to pyoderma, endocrinopathies (hypothyroidism, hyperadrenocorticism), allergies (as above) and autoimmune diseases (especially pemphigus foliaceous). For older animals, cutaneous neoplasms such as mycosis fungoides and metabolic diseases (especially liver disease) should also be considered.

There is no characteristic sex predilection for the primary scaling disorders. Breed, along with the early age of onset, is the most important part of the signalment in considering differentials for the primary keratinisation disorders (Table 2).

Table 2
Primary keratinization disorders in dogs with breed incidence

Disease	Breed(s)
Primary idiopathic seborrhea	Cocker spaniel
	English springer spaniel
	Basset hound
	West Highland white terrier
	Doberman pinscher
	Labrador retriever
	Irish setter
	Chinese Shar Pei
Follicular dystrophy	Doberman pinscher
	Rottweiler
	Yorkshire Terrier
	Irish setter
	Dachshund
	Chow chow
	Standard poodle
	Great Dane
	Italian greyhound
	Whippet
Epidermal dysplasia	West Highland white terrier
Ichthyosis	West Highland white terrier
Vitamin A responsive dermatosis	Cocker spaniel
	Miniature schnauzer
	Labrador retriever
Zinc responsive dermatosis	Alaskan malamute
	Siberian husky
Sebaceous adenitis	Standard poodle
	Akita
	Vizsla
	Samoyed
Nasodigital hyperkeratosis	Cocker spaniel
Lichenoid psoriasiform dermatosis	English springer spaniel
Schnauzer comedo syndrome	Miniature schnauzer
Ear margin dermatosis	Dachshund
Acne	English bulldog
	Boxer
	Doberman pinscher
	Great Dane

From Kwochka, K.W. (1993) Overview of normal keratinization and cutaneous scaling disorders of dogs. In: *Current Veterinary Dermatology: The Science and Art of Therapy*, (Eds. C.E. Griffin, K.W. Kwochka & J.M. MacDonald) p. 167, Mosby Year Book, St. Louis.

History

A complete history will reveal that the scaling started at a young age in dogs with primary keratinisation disorders. However, as stated above, infectious, parasitic and allergic dermatoses may cause secondary scaling in this age range.

With primary keratinisation disorders, an observant owner will indicate that the scaling or comedones were present prior to the development of secondary signs such as pruritus, pyoderma, inflammation and alopecia. Conversely, if these signs were observed before the scaling, then the scaling is secondary and a primary keratinisation disorder is unlikely.

Another extremely important aspect of the history is response to previous therapy. Both the primary keratinisation disorders and secondary causes of scaling are often complicated by pyoderma and some degree of pruritus associated with that pyoderma. If the scaling resolves completely by treatment of the pyoderma with antibiotics and topical antibacterial therapy, then it is unlikely that a primary keratinisation defect is present. Some degree of scaling, comedones or follicular casts would still be present. The presence of these lesions after antibiotics without pruritus or cutaneous inflammation would suggest a primary keratinisation defect, an endocrine dermatosis (hypothyroidism, hyperadrenocorticism), or environmental factors (low humidity). Scale remaining after antibiotics with significant pruritus and inflammation would be more indicative of parasitic (scabies, cheyletiellosis) and allergic (flea allergy dermatitis, atopy, food allergy dermatitis) dermatoses.

There are other aspects of the history which are important in establishing a diagnosis of the specific cause of secondary scaling. Exposure to an infested animal or environment prior to development of acute scaling suggests a parasitic dermatosis (especially scabies and cheyletiellosis) or dermatophytosis. Seasonal pruritus associated with scaling suggests atopy, flea allergy dermatitis, or other insect hypersensitivities such as those due to biting flies, mosquitoes or ants. Concurrent systemic signs with scaling such as polyuria, polydipsia, lethargy, cold intolerance and abnormalities in oestrus cycle or sexual behaviour may suggest an endocrinopathy. Endocrine dermatoses are usually associated with minimal pruritus unless complicated by pyoderma or severe xerosis.

PHYSICAL EXAMINATION

Dogs with cutaneous scaling are characterised clinically by mild to severe, dry, waxy, or greasy scales. There may also be some degree of "seborrhoeic odour" associated with the skin condition. In fact, the severe "rancid fat odour" in dogs with greasy scale and secondary bacterial or yeast infections is often the owner's primary complaint.

Since hair follicles and glandular structures may also be involved, especially with the primary keratinisation defects, it is not unusual to see comedones and follicular casts. Comedones are blackheads resulting from dilation of hair follicles with keratin plugs. Follicular casts are tightly adherent scale around hair shafts.

Common secondary findings include alopecia, inflammation, crusts, pruritus with secondary excoriations and pyoderma. Unfortunately, these secondary findings are common to see with virtually any dermatosis. Secondary *Malassezia* colonisation may also be associated with primary and secondary causes of scaling, especially with greasy scale. Presence of these yeasts should always be evaluated by skin swabs and cytologic examination.

The most difficult task for the practitioner is to determine if a primary keratinisation defect is present or if the scaling and other signs are simply secondary to an underlying dermatosis. The latter is a much more common occurrence so should be considered first when formulating a diagnostic plan. Important diseases causing secondary scaling are listed in Table 1.

Character of scale

There are some important observations to be made during the physical examination which may help differentiate some of these conditions which cause secondary scaling. The first is the character of the scale. Dry scale with minimal inflammation and pruritus is most often associated with endocrinopathies, dermatophytosis, low humidity, endoparasitism, cheyletiellosis and some cases of demodicosis and pyoderma. Waxy or greasy scales with inflammation and pruritus are more commonly seen with allergic disease, scabies and some cases of pyoderma.

Distribution of scale

How the scale is distributed is another important observation. With flea allergy dermatitis and cheyletiellosis the scale is usually confined to the caudal dorsal portion of the body. Of course, a thorough examination for these parasites should be undertaken during the examination. Dogs with atopy and scabies are most severely involved on the face, pinnae, ventrum and extremities. Scale associated with food allergy dermatitis has a variable distribution. Pyoderma involves the trunk in a diffuse fashion but usually spares the head and distal extremities. Pemphigus foliaceus has a generalized distribution, including the head and ears, with frequent severe scaling of the footpads (footpad hyperkeratosis). A generalised distribution of scaling is also seen with generalised demodicosis, generalised dermatophytosis and endocrine dermatoses.

Primary lesions

Another observation during the physical examination should be whether primary lesions are present along with the scaling. Follicular papules and pustules are indicative of pyoderma, demodicosis or dermatophytosis. Non-follicular papules suggest flea allergy dermatitis, other insect hypersensitivity reactions or scabies. Follicular and non-follicular papules and pustules are seen with pemphigus foliaceus and when allergic dermatoses are complicated by a secondary pyoderma.

ESTABLISHING THE DIAGNOSIS

Initial Diagnostics

A scaling dermatosis, especially if involving large areas of skin, should never be diagnosed as a primary keratinisation defect without a complete diagnostic plan to first rule out secondary causes of scaling (Table 1). In addition to the complete history and physical examination, certain diagnostic tests should be utilised at the first visit. These include skin scrapings, flea combings and acetate tape preparations for ectoparasites; skin swabs for *Malassezia*; Wood's lamp examination, KOH preparation and fungal culture for dermatophytosis; faecal examination for parasites and cytology of any exudative lesions for pyoderma (Chapter 3). These diagnostic tests should be sufficient to eliminate demodicosis, dermatophytosis, *Malassezia* dermatitis and endoparasitism from the list of differentials. They will also be helpful, but not definitively rule out, flea allergy dermatitis, cheyletiellosis and scabies. If the former is suspected, but fleas cannot be found, a control programme should be instituted with topical and environmental flea control products with re-evaluation after four weeks. If the latter two are suspected, but mites cannot be found, a trial with ivermectin is recommended using a 1% aqueous solution at a dose of 0.2 mg/kg, s/c, administered three times with two week intervals between injections. This should not be used in collie or collie related breeds. It is not licenced for dogs and cats in the UK.

Secondary Pyoderma

At the first visit it is also necessary to determine if a pyoderma is present. Pyoderma is a very common secondary problem because of barrier abrogation associated with cutaneous scaling. A diagnosis is usually established by examination (follicular papules and pustules) and cytology (Gram-positive cocci). Culture and sensitivity are usually not needed but are recommended if the pyoderma is chronic or has been treated previously. The recommendation is that if a pyoderma is suspected for any reason - TREAT FOR IT! The patient should be discharged with systemic antibiotics and an antibacterial shampoo with re-evaluation in three to four weeks (Chapter 25). At that time the status of the pyoderma, amount of scaling and amount of pruritus should be assessed. This step may be skipped if there is only scaling with no evidence of pyoderma.

INITIAL MANAGEMENT

Pruritic Scaling

At the time of revaluation the pyoderma should be under good control if appropriate therapy has been prescribed. If scaling and pruritus remain then allergic and ectoparasitic dermatoses should next be considered. Skin scrapings, flea combings and acetate tape preparations should be repeated to again check for scabies and cheyletiellosis. If these tests are negative, but one of these ectoparasites is still suspected, then a therapeutic trial using ivermectin is recommended if this was not employed at the first visit. If these ectoparasites have been eliminated from consideration then intradermal or *in vitro* allergy testing should be considered for flea allergy dermatitis, other insect hypersensitivities and atopy. Finally, a four to six week hypoallergenic dietary trial should be utilised for a food allergy dermatitis. This diagnosis can be more definitively confirmed by recurrence of symptoms following food provocation.

Non-pruritic Scaling

If scaling without pruritus remains after control of the pyoderma then non-pruritic causes of scaling are considered. Skin scrapings should be repeated for demodicosis. A complete blood count (CBC), serum biochemical profile, urinalysis and baseline T4 should be obtained to determine general health and the possibility of hypothyroidism. If the T4 is equivocal then a TSH stimulation test is recommended to further evaluate the condition. Clinical signs (polyuria/polydipsia, lack of hair regrowth, muscle wasting, excessive panting, bullous impetigo, poor wound healing, hepatomegaly) and laboratory abnormalities (eosinopaenia, lymphopaenia, increased serum alkaline phosphatase, elevated serum cholesterol) suggesting hyperadrenocorticism warrant further evaluation with a low dose dexamethasone suppression test or ACTH stimulation test. Tests for sex hormone abnormalities will depend on the specific syndrome under consideration. Biopsies are also indicated to screen for pemphigus foliaceus, mycosis fungoides and any changes which may be consistent with one of the primary keratinisation disorders.

Primary Keratinisation Defects

After elimination of secondary causes of scaling following the above guidelines, it can still be difficult and frustrating to make a definitive diagnosis of a primary keratinisation disorder (Table 2) because there is no one specific laboratory test for these diseases. A combination of factors is considered including the signalment (especially age and breed) and history as described above, findings on histopathological examination of skin biopsies and response to appropriate therapy based on the histologic findings.

Lichenoid-psoriasiform dermatosis, canine ichthyosis, nasodigital hyperkeratosis, ear margin dermatosis and canine acne are primary keratinisation disorders so characteristic, either clinically or histologically, that often the diagnosis can be made using skin biopsy and minimal additional diagnostics.

Skin Biopsy

Skin biopsy is the most important diagnostic tool for primary keratinisation disorders. Histological changes will either be diagnostic for (sebaceous adenitis, follicular dystrophy, schnauzer comedo syndrome, lichenoid-psoriasiform dermatosis, canine ichthyosis, canine acne), compatible with (vitamin A responsive dermatosis, zinc responsive dermatosis) or suggestive of (primary idiopathic seborrhoea, epidermal dysplasia, nasodigital hyperkeratosis, ear margin dermatosis) a primary keratinisation disorder. Additionally, histological changes may suggest or help rule out dermatoses associated with secondary scaling.

As indicated above, the best time to take the skin biopsy is after secondary pyoderma has been controlled with antibiotics and topical therapy. Histological changes associated with pyoderma make evaluation of the biopsy difficult.

It is important to take at least three biopsies from lesions of various ages to maximise the chance of a definitive diagnosis. The diagnosis is usually best made from biopsies of early lesions uncomplicated by chronic changes. Multiple biopsies also allow the pathologist to determine stage of the disease which may affect choice of therapy and prognosis. For example, early stages of sebaceous adenitis show inflammation centered on sebaceous glands while chronic changes are often associated with complete absence of sebaceous glands. The latter carries a poorer prognosis for successful clinical management.

Skin biopsies should be sent to a veterinary pathologist specialising in dermatopathology. The primary keratinisation disorders are unique enough that a general pathologist may not be able to make the diagnosis.

Some patients will have more than one underlying disease which needs to be controlled. An example would be a dog with secondary scaling due to atopy and food allergy. Some patients may also have a primary keratinisation disorder which is further complicated by another skin disease which together make the condition of the skin especially bad. An example of this is the West Highland white terrier with idiopathic seborrhoea or epidermal dysplasia complicated by severe atopy.

General Treatment Guidelines

Treatment of scaling usually starts before a specific diagnosis is made. In fact treatment starts even before it is clear if the scaling is secondary or due to a primary keratinisation defect. This is due to the desire of the owner and veterinarian to make the patient look and feel as good as possible as quickly as possible.

Since many dogs with scale have secondary pyoderma, initial treatment consists of antibiotics (Chapter 25) and a topical antibacterial/keratolytic shampoo for three to four weeks (Chapter 26). Not only does this improve the condition of the skin and hair coat but allows assessment of the role of infection in scaling when the patient is re-evaluated.

During the course of the diagnostic evaluation steroids should not be administered. First, steroids may affect the ability to control any concurrent pyoderma. Second, it is important to determine how much pruritus remains after the pyoderma is controlled. This information will help determine if parasites and allergies (pruritus remains) or endocrine and primary keratinisation disorders (pruritus resolved) are considered as major differentials. Concurrent use of steroids masks signs and does not allow such an assessment. Third, use of topical or systemic steroids before a definitive diagnosis is made may make the condition worse by adverse effects on sebaceous secretions, keratinisation and hair production.

Secondary scaling is best treated by management of the underlying disease. However, symptomatic topical therapy is helpful in controlling scale formation until the disease is treated with more specific therapy. Symptomatic topical therapy with shampoo formulations is the major form of treatment used to manage most of the generalised primary keratinisation defects. The active ingredients in these shampoos are moisturisers, keratolytics, keratoplastics, antibacterials, degreasers and follicular flushers. These ingredients are also incorporated into ointments, gels, creams, lotions and pads for some of the more localised keratinisation abnormalities. The proper agent depends on the specific condition. Specific treatments are covered Chapter 26.

When topical therapy fails to adequately control a primary keratinisation defect, or if topical therapy is too time consuming for the owner, system agents can be utilised. Most work has been done with three retinoids (Kwochka, 1993b; Power and Ihrke, 1990); retinol, isotretinoin (Accutane), and etretinate (Tegison). These have been used for idiopathic seborrhoea, vitamin A responsive dermatosis, sebaceous adenitis, schnauzer comedo syndrome, canine ichthyosis, nasodigital hyperkeratosis and acne.

Oral zinc is used for zinc responsive dermatosis. Steroids may be helpful for epidermal dysplasia and sebaceous adenitis. Cyclosporine A has also been used for sebaceous adenitis. Antibiotics are often needed to control secondary pyoderma associated with many of the primary keratinisation disorders.

REFERENCES AND FURTHER READING

KUNKLE, G.A. (1983) Managing canine seborrhea. In: *Current Veterinary Therapy VIII*, (Ed. R.W. Kirk) W.B. Saunders, Philadelphia.

KWOCHKA, K.W. (1993a) Primary keratinization disorders of dogs. In: *Current Veterinary Dermatology: The Science and Art of Therapy*, (Eds. C.E. Griffin, K.W. Kwochka & J.M. MacDonald) p. 176, Mosby Year Book, St. Louis.

KWOCHKA, K.W. (1993b) Retinoids and vitamin-A therapy. In: *Current Veterinary Dermatology: The Science and Art of Therapy*, (Eds. C.E. Griffin, K.W. Kwochka & J.M. MacDonald) p. 203, Mosby Year Book, St. Louis.

MULLER, G.H., KIRK, R.W., and SCOTT, D.W. (1989) Keratinization defects. In: *Small Animal Dermatology, Fourth Edn*, W.B. Saunders, Philadelphia.

POWER, H.T. and IHRKE, P.J. (1990) Synthetic retinoids in veterinary dermatology. *Veterinary Clinics of North America.* **20**, 1525.

SISCHO, W.M., IHRKE, P.J. and PRANTI, C.E. (1989) Regional distribution of ten common skin diseases in dogs. *Journal of the American Veterinary Medical Association.* **195**, 752.

CHAPTER SIX

PUSTULES AND CRUSTING PAPULES

Ian S Mason ———————————————————————

INTRODUCTION

Definitions and Mechanisms of Lesion Development

Papules are defined as small solid elevations of the skin which are up to 1 cm in diameter. They are usually palpable and erythematous and result from infiltration of inflammatory cells into the dermis or from epidermal oedema or hypertrophy. Where papules coalesce to form lesions that are larger than 1 cm in diameter or where large elevations of the skin are present, they are described as plaques. Papules may or may not be adjacent to hair follicle infundibula. Crust formation arises as a result of a cutaneous exudate such as serum, pus or blood drying on the skin surface.

Pustules are also small (< 1 cm diameter) circumscribed elevations of the epidermis but are filled with pus. They are small abscesses either within the inter-follicular epidermis or, more commonly, associated with hair follicle infundibula. Pustules may develop from papules as a result of exocytosis of inflammatory cells into the epidermis. Often, crust formation follows rupture of pustules. Pustule formation requires breakdown of adhesion between epidermal cells; this can result from physical separation by oedema and the influx of inflammatory cells. However, intercellular bonds may also be broken down by epidermolytic toxins from bacteria, as seen in pyoderma, or by autoimmune mechanisms as in the pemphigus group of diseases. Pustules usually contain micro-organisms such as bacteria but may occasionally be sterile.

Clinical Significance of Papules and Pustules

Table 1 lists examples of dermatoses which may lead to pustule and papule formation in the skin of cats and dogs. Some of the immune mediated and autoimmune disorders are included although they may present with bullae and vesicles (see glossary in Chapter 2) as well as with crusts and crusted papules. Sub-corneal pustular dermatosis is a rare disorder in which sterile pustules occur within the interfollicular epidermis. It is a variably pruritic disease and it has been a number of years since a case was last reported in the veterinary literature. Sterile eosinophilic pustular dermatitis is an uncommon, highly pruritic disorder which has been recently reported in the UK (Scarff, D.H. personal communication, 1992).

Dogs and cats do not usually present with solely papular lesions or solely pustular lesions. More likely the lesions represent the whole chronological spectrum from papules to pustules, with or without overlying crusts, to epidermal collarettes and patchy hyperpigmentation.

Papular dermatoses are commonly seen in canine and feline practice. However, pustules are a much less frequently encountered phenomenon. This is partly because, in dogs, the epidermis is rather thin and so pustules rupture rapidly and are therefore rather transient. One of the most important causes of pustule formation is bacterial skin disease; pyoderma is uncommon in cats and this is the major reason for the scarcity with which pustules are seen in the skin of this species. Canine pyoderma is covered later in this chapter.

Table 1

Examples of causes of papules and pustules in canine and feline skin

CANINE DERMATOSES:

Staphylococcal pyoderma
- acne
- impetigo
- folliculitis

Sarcoptic mange and other ectoparasitic infestations

Immune mediated/autoimmune disorders
- pemphigus foliaceus
- pemphigus erythematosus
- pemphigus vulgaris
- pemphigus vegetans
- bullous pemphigoid

Hypersensitivity
- flea hypersensitivity
- atopy
- dietary intolerance/hypersensitivity
- contact hypersensitivity

Sub-corneal pustular dermatosis

Sterile eosinophilic pustular dermatitis

Drug-eruptions

Contact irritant dermatitis

FELINE DERMATOSES:

Miliary dermatitis complex*

Pemphigus foliaceus

Superficial pyoderma
- acne
- folliculitis

*Readers are referred to Chapter 16 for an account of the causes of miliary dermatitis.

APPROACH TO THE CASE

In common with all dermatoses, the approach to papular and pustular disorders should follow the logical principles discussed in Chapter 2. A full history should be taken followed by a thorough clinical examination. These should lead to the establishment of a list of possible causes which can then be narrowed by the application of appropriate diagnostic tests (Chapter 3).

Pyoderma should be suspected in all cases in which papules, pustules, epidermal collarettes and crusts are present. It is a secondary disorder and may follow virtually any dermatosis. It is essential in all cases of pyoderma that a meticulous search for the underlying cause is made. For example, hypersensitivities often lead to secondary bacterial folliculitis and it has been suggested that there is not a primary papular eruption in atopy until secondary bacterial infection supervenes. Metabolic and endocrine disorders such as hypothyroidism can lead to pyoderma with the formation of papules and pustules. There are many other causes of pyoderma; these will be covered separately later in this chapter.

Taking the History

A suggested list of questions designed to obtain a concise and accurate history is given in Chapter 2. By using this list a number of salient points will emerge while talking with the owner.

The presence or absence of pruritus may suggest to the clinician that certain of the disorders given in Table 1 are more likely than others. For example, in ectoparasitic disorders, pruritus is often intense and may be refractory to even high doses of glucocorticoids. This is particularly the case in sarcoptic mange. Hypersensitivity disorders are pruritic and, in cases of dietary intolerance, pruritus is also said to be rather refractory to glucocorticoid therapy. However, using assessment of the degree of pruritus to narrow the list of differential diagnoses may be misleading as secondary bacterial infection of a primary non-pruritic disorder may lead to pruritus following the production of pro-inflammatory substances by the bacteria. Questions about response to previous therapy are particularly relevant. For example, a response to appropriate antimicrobial therapy (see Chapter 25) might lead a clinician to suspect that staphylococci have complicated the clinical picture. Ectoparasitic disorders are often zoonotic and so owners should be asked whether any human skin lesions have developed since the pet started to scratch. Pruritus in in-contact animals may also suggest that an ectoparasitic disorder is present. A seasonal problem suggests that atopy, flea allergy or another, seasonally limited, ectoparasite, such as *Neotrombicula autumnalis*, is present.

PHYSICAL EXAMINATION

A thorough physical examination may indicate that a systemic disease is present which predisposes the skin to pyoderma. Occasionally dogs with hepatic and renal disease may present with a papular and pustular dermatosis secondary to such internal disorders.

The distribution and spread of lesions may be helpful. In sarcoptic mange the elbows and pinnae are often affected. In superficial folliculitis, secondary to atopic dermatitis, papules and pustules are present on the ventral abdomen and pedal and facial pruritus is also a feature. The nature of the lesions might narrow the possible list of possible causes. For example, pemphigus foliaceus generally presents with papular, pustular or vesicular lesions with extensive crust formation.

ESTABLISHING THE DIAGNOSIS

The most important question to ask oneself when confronted with a dog with a papular and pustular dermatosis is "is this a case of pyoderma?". Pyodermas are among the most common of the skin diseases in canine practice but may be difficult to recognise clinically. Table 2 lists some of the primary conditions that should be considered in cases of staphylococcal pyoderma associated with papule and pustule formation. Cases of pyoderma are usually classified by both aetiology and by depth of infection. The identification of the underlying cause is very important in the management of cases of pyoderma as it enables specific therapy to be administered. However, recognition of the depth of the disease is also important as it may narrow the list of differential diagnoses and will also influence the type and duration of antibacterial therapy and the prognosis. The deeper the infection the poorer the prognosis and the more prolonged and aggressive the treatment required.

Superficial pyoderma is defined as bacterial skin disease involving the superficial portion of hair follicles (folliculitis) or the interfollicular epidermis immediately below the stratum corneum (impetigo).

Impetigo is a benign condition in which lesions form in the inguinal and axillary regions of sexually immature dogs. It may be mildly pruritic or asymptomatic with lesions noted as an incidental finding during routine physical examination. Although poor management of pups has been suggested as an underlying cause the condition may occur in well managed litters. Recovery may be spontaneous and most cases will respond to topical antimicrobial therapy (see Chapter 25). Occasionally short term systemic antibacterial therapy is required. Glucocorticoids must not be used as they may lead to worsening of the condition.

Table 2

Primary causes of canine pyoderma
associated with papules and pustules

SUPERFICIAL PYODERMA:

Folliculitis	Hypersensitivity:	atopy, flea, contact, dietary intolerance
	Endocrinopathy:	hypothyroidism, hyperadrenocorticism
	Ectoparasitism:	demodicosis, sarcoptic mange
	Idiopathic:	immune incompetence or defective barrier function
Impetigo		may be idiopathic sometimes associated with management factors (endo- or ectoparasites, viral infections, poor nutrition, dirty environment)

DEEP PYODERMA:

demodicosis, hypothyroidism, hypersensitivity, idiopathic

Most cases of superficial folliculitis are secondary to an underlying condition and so, although they respond to antimicrobial therapy, recurrence is a common problem. Management of these disorders is based on identification and correction of the underlying cause in association with topical and systemic therapy.

Deep pyodermas are serious and, in some instances, life-threatening conditions which occur when bacterial infections involve not only the hair follicles but also the dermis or even the subcutis. The follicular wall may rupture to release hair shaft keratin, bacteria and bacterial products into the dermis resulting in furunculosis or a foreign body reaction. The prognosis for deep pyoderma is worse than in the other forms and requires prolonged antimicrobial therapy along with a determined investigation of possible underlying causes.

INITIAL MANAGEMENT

Examination of smears of the contents of pustules is a valuable initial diagnostic test. In cases of superficial pyoderma it will often reveal significant numbers of neutrophils and coccoid bacilli along with smaller numbers of other inflammatory cells such as macrophages and eosinophils. It may allow a limited assessment of the immune response if, for example, neutrophils are seen to contain bacteria that have been phagocytosed. However, such an assessment may be unreliable; effective phagocytosis does not imply that intracellular killing of bacteria can occur.

It is important that smears are taken for examination on the first occasion that the animal is seen, before any medication is given, as treatment may alter the results obtained. For example, antibacterial therapy will reduce bacterial populations. If smears are taken after antimicrobial therapy has been administered to a dog with pyoderma, then this may give the erroneous impression that a sterile pustular disorder is present. Similarly, glucocorticoid therapy inhibits the immune response and so the numbers and types of inflammatory cells present in the smear may be affected by the administration of such drugs. In most instances bacterial culture is less useful than the microscopical examination of smears from pustules. Culture will often lead to the isolation of staphylococci but as these are often part of the normal cutaneous microflora their significance can be difficult to assess. A discussion of the indications for bacterial culture and antimicrobial sensitivity testing is given in Chapter 3.

In all cases skin scrapings should be taken and examined microscopically. This will enable the identification of ectoparasitic or, in some cases, fungal causes. Many ectoparasitic diseases are characterised by papule and pustule formation and in the case of *Demodex canis* infestation, may be a cause of pyoderma.

These two simple laboratory tests will readily enable the identification of pyoderma, ectoparasites and possibly fungi at the first presentation of the animal. In the case of the pemphigus group of diseases, evidence of acantholysis (or breakdown of intercellular cohesion) will be present. Acantholysis might indicate that autoimmune disease is present but histopathology of skin samples taken using biopsy techniques will be required to confirm this diagnosis. This is because breakdown of intercellular bonds could occur as a result of the action of bacterial toxins in some cases of pyoderma or following the epidermal oedema which occurs in some cases of primary irritant dermatitis. Following the principles outlined in this chapter, it should be possible to definitively diagnose the cause of the problem or to narrow down the list of differential diagnoses so that rational therapy can be implemented.

The plan can be summarised as follows:

Take a detailed history and make a full physical examination.

Draw up a list of differential diagnoses and a diagnostic/therapeutic plan.

Undertake preliminary tests such as microscopical examination of skin scrapings and of stained smears from pustules.

If there are no signs of ectoparasites and no definitive diagnosis has been made then assess response to systemic and topical antimicrobial therapy as detailed in Chapter 25.

Undertake specific diagnostic tests such as a trial with an hypoallergenic diet, skin biopsy or assessment of thyroid function as appropriate.

FURTHER READING

IHRKE, P.J. (1987) An overview of bacterial skin disease in the dog. *British Veterinary Journal* **143**, 112.

MASON, I.S. (1991) Canine pyoderma. *Journal of Small Animal Practice* **32**, 381.

WHITE, S.D and IHRKE, P.J. (1987) Pyoderma. In: *Dermatology. Contemporary issues in small animal practice, volume 8.* (Ed. G.H. Nesbitt) New York, Churchill Livingstone.

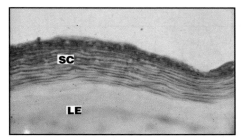

Photo: David Lloyd

Plate 1
Frozen section of bovine skin after treatment with alkaline buffer swelling the stratum corneum. Red-staining lipid (Sudan IV stain) can be seen in the distal intercellular layers of the corneum. The blue-staining nuclei of the living epidermis can just be seen in a different plane of focus below the stratum corneum. In the more compact canine stratum corneum, Sudanophilic intercellular lipid can also be demonstrated but the layers are thinner. SC, stratum corneum; LE, living epidermis

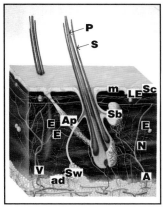

Diagram: SmithKline Beecham Animal Health

Plate 2
Diagram of canine skin: Sb, sebaceous gland; Sw, epitrichial sweat gland; Ap, arrector pili muscle; Sc, stratum corneum; LE, living epidermis; m melanocyte; A, artery; V, vein; N, nerve; E, specialised endorgan; Ad, adipose tissue; P, primary hair; S, secondary hair
(Diagram courtesy of SmithKline Beecham Animal Health)

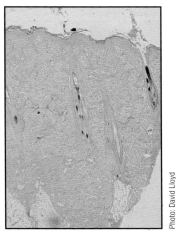

Photo: David Lloyd

Plate 3a
Canine skin, illustrating the dermal connective tissue structure. Gomori's aldehyde fuchsin with light green stain. Low power view of epidermis and dermis, stained to show collagen (green) and elastin fibres (mauve)

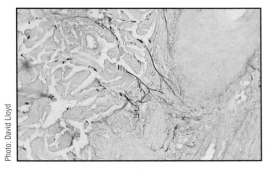

Photo: David Lloyd

Plate 3b
Canine skin, illustrating the dermal connective tissue structure. Gomori's aldehyde fuchsin with light green stain. High power view showing the elastin fibres surrounding the hair follicle

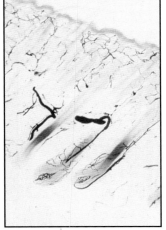

Photo: David Lloyd

Plate 4
Cutaneous blood supply. A section of bovine skin following arterial perfusion with Indian ink. Note that the thin superficial epidermal tissue stained with haematoxolin is avascular. Indian ink couterstained with haematoxolin

Ectoparasites

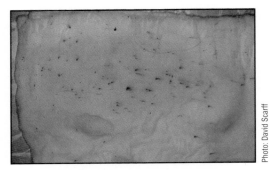

Plate 5
Appearance of flea faeces when placed on wet cotton wool

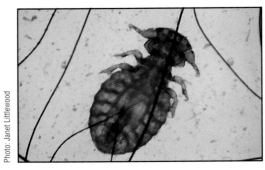

Plate 6
Trichodectes canis

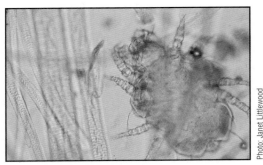

Plate 7
Cheyletiella parasitivorax

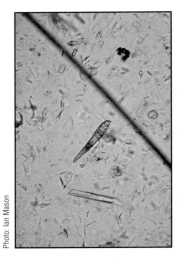

Plate 8
Demodex canis

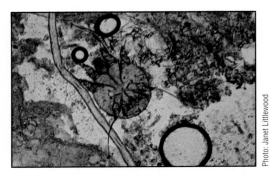

Plate 9
Sarcoptes scabiei var *canis*

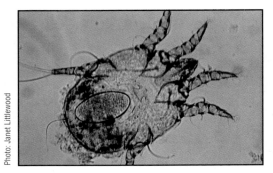

Plate 10
Otodectes cynotis

Pyoderma and conditions resembling pyoderma

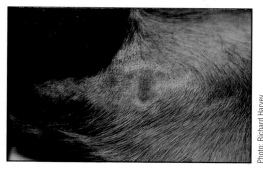

Photo: Richard Harvey

Plate 11
Superficial folliculitis (ventral abdomen).
Annular lesions with central hyperpigmentation and
peripheral erosion and erythema

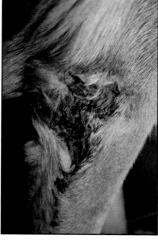

Photo: Ian Mason

Plate 12
Deep cellulitis of German shepherd dog
(right elbow)

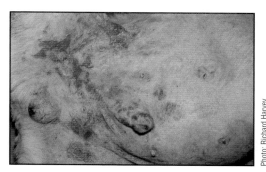

Photo: Richard Harvey

Plate 13
Hyperadrenocorticism with mildly inflamed lesions
of pyoderma. The ulcerated areas are lesions of
calciuosis cutis

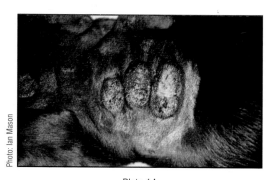

Photo: Ian Mason

Plate 14
Fenbendazole drug reaction (dorsal neck)

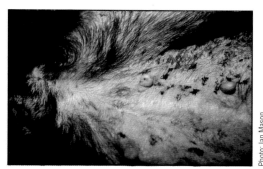

Photo: Ian Mason

Plate 15
Lymphoreticular neoplasia

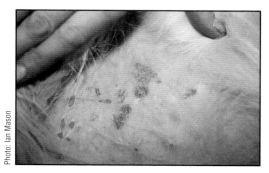

Photo: Ian Mason

Plate 16
Panniculitis and ulceration associated with renal disease

Atopic dermatitis
(Figures 17-20 are of the same English setter)

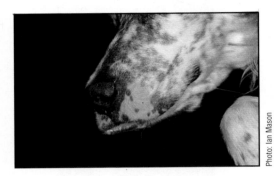

Plate 17
Erythema and alopecia of muzzle

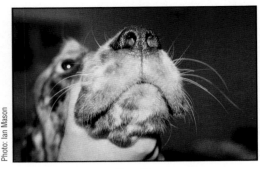

Plate 18
Erythema and alopecia of chin and muzzle

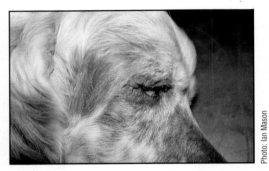

Plate 19
Periorbital alopecia, scarring and hyperpigmentation

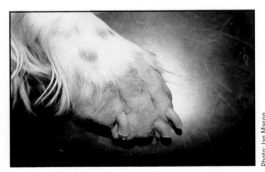

Plate 20
Pedal erythema and alopecia

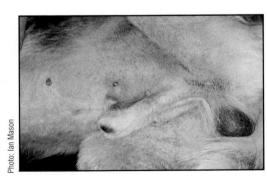

Plate 21
Superficial folliculitis (papules, erythema and alopecia)

CHAPTER SEVEN

NODULAR LESIONS

David H Scarff

INTRODUCTION

The presence of nodules (masses greater than 1 cm diameter) on the skin of cats and dogs is a common reason for their presentation to the veterinary surgeon (Plates 57-62). Obviously the presence or absence of neoplasia is the first question to be addressed; however, inflammatory lesions may also be difficult to manage.

Nodular lesions in the skin can be classified under three headings;

Developmental
Inflammatory
Neoplastic

The importance of a diagnostic approach to nodular skin diseases cannot be over emphasised. Firstly, the decision whether to treat a nodule with surgical, medical or other modalities cannot be made without a diagnosis. Secondly, the best opportunity to cure malignancies such as mast cell tumours is on the first surgical intervention. If initial treatment is inadequate, as may occur if removal of such a mass is not sufficiently pre-planned, a second opportunity may not occur. Finally, accurate diagnosis is also essential for the provision of a prognosis to the owner. Treatment planning is essential in neoplastic disease, and the treatment of nodular inflammatory diseases can be prolonged. The involvement of the owner in decision making cannot take place if a diagnosis has not been made, neither can the owner be reassured that neoplasia is not present.

APPROACH TO THE CASE

As in any skin disease, diagnosis depends upon the history, clinical examination, formation of a list of differential diagnoses and confirmation by diagnostic tests (Chapter 2).

History

The breed, age and sex of the animal may be of importance. Breed predilections for neoplastic diseases are listed in Table 1.

The age of the animal may be a factor in assessing the likelihood of lesions being neoplastic. It may help also in deciding on the type of tumour present, for example histiocytomata (Langerhans cell tumours) are more common in younger animals whilst mast cell tumours usually occur in older dogs. These generalisations do not always apply however, as the author can testify having just been presented with a twelve year old collie with a histiocytoma!

Very few nodular diseases have a sex bias. Possible exceptions to this would be metastases from mammary neoplasms and the inflammatory nodules seen on the dorsum of dogs with Sertoli cell tumours. Knowledge of the rate of growth and the time taken for the owner to recognise the presence of a nodule may be valuable. For example, histiocytomata are often well into the stage

Table 1
Some skin neoplasms with a breed predilection

NEOPLASM	BREED
Canine Langerhans cell tumour (hystiocytoma)	Boxer, dachshund, great Dane, Shetland sheepdog.
Haemangiopericytoma	Boxer, German sheperd dog.
Haemangiosarcoma	Bernese mountain dog, corgi, German sheperd dog.
Histiocytoma	Boxer, dachshund, great Dane, Shetland sheepdog.
Lymphoma	Beagle, German shepherd dog, golden retriever, cocker and springer spaniels, Scottish terrier.
Melanoma	Airedale, cocker and springer spaniels, Scottish terrier.
Pilomatricoma	Poodle, Kerry blue terrier.
Squamous cell carcinoma	Boxer, bull terrier, dalmation, Pekinese, poodle, Scottish terrier.

of lymphocytic infiltration and starting to resolve when first noticed by the owners and presented to the veterinarian. The reason for this is that these lesions have a far more "angry" appearance to owners at this time and may be suffering from a degree of self-trauma from the dog.

The degree of self attention by the animal may be indicative of the type of lesion present. Pruritus is often a feature of inflammatory disease, but may be present in mastocytomata, especially once traumatised, due to the release of inflammatory mediators. Neoplastic lesions such as rapidly progressing lymphoma may be painful, again leading to self-trauma. The space occupying nature of some lesions may be troublesome to the dog or cat, particularly if associated with a distal limb or interdigital space.

Pigmentary changes may be of some help in the diagnostic process, particularly if erythema was present in the early development of the lesions. This would suggest inflammatory involvement. Later in the course of inflammatory lesions hyperpigmentation may be a feature.

The change in appearance of the lesions and rate of increase in size can give useful information with regard to the biological behaviour of neoplastic masses. Mast cell tumours that have slowly progressed over months are unlikely to be highly aggressive in their biological behaviour. The appearance of many lesions at the same time may suggest systemic involvement as in the haematogenous spread of lymphoma metastases.

Other historical details of value are the presence of other cutaneous or systemic signs.

PHYSICAL EXAMINATION

General examination

A full clinical examination is necessary for a number of reasons. Firstly this allows evaluation of potential anaesthetic risk prior to further examination or diagnostic tests. Secondly the presence of systemic disease may be an indication of neoplastic disease elsewhere. Inflammatory skin disease associated with infection may also result in systemic signs and some dermatoses are indicative of systemic disease.

Examination of the nodules

Examination of the mass(es) must be painstaking and carefully recorded, especially if non-surgical treatment is decided upon. Factors of importance include the depth of the lesion, mobility, degree of circumscription and presence of ulceration or pain.

Depth of lesion: Lesions may be epidermal, dermal, subcutaneous of a mixture of all these. The position within the skin can help to identify the origin of the tissue mass. Most developmental defects such as dermoid cysts are dermal or epidermal, whereas lipomata are subcutaneous.

Mobility: The degree of fixation to underlying tissues is important when assessing the degree of malignancy, ie. whether spread has occurred across a tissue boundary. Nodular inflammatory diseases are diffuse, involving all the layers of the skin but seldom fix to underlying tissues.

Ulceration: Ulceration may occur due to two differing mechanisms. Firstly, the neoplasm or inflammatory lesion may destroy the overlying epithelium due to necrosis following ischaemia or infiltration. Secondly, the dog or cat may remove the epithelium by self trauma if the mass is pruritic or painful. Ulceration can be helpful in a diagnostic sense however, allowing access to the stroma of the mass for exfoliative cytology.

Pain: The degree of pain associated with any nodular disease can be difficult to assess and is generally an indicator of inflammatory or malignant neoplastic nodules. Examples of the latter include lymphoma and skin metastases from mammary neoplasia.

Examination of local lymph nodes

Grading of malignancy can be assessed by the tumour, node and metastasis (TNM) system. It is therefore important to examine the local lymph nodes. It must be realised however that enlargement of nodes may be due to either metastasis or reactive change. Inflammatory skin diseases, especially when associated with infection, will often result in enlargement of local nodes. Fine needle aspirates may help in the differentiation between these reactions, but the absence of neoplastic cells in an aspirate does not rule out neoplasia.

Examination of distant sites

If malignant neoplasia is suspected, examination of distant sites such as the lungs is mandatory. Treatment options may be limited if the chest is already full of metastases.

ESTABLISHING THE DIAGNOSIS

Two methods are available to the dermatologist for the diagnosis of nodular skin disease - exfoliative cytology and histopathology. Advantages and disadvantages exist for both techniques and these will be discussed below.

EXFOLIATIVE CYTOLOGY

In no other field is the technique of exfoliative cytology of greater value; the skin is readily available for the collection of samples and many skin nodules are amenable to cytological diagnosis. Two techniques for harvesting cells are of value - direct smears and fine needle aspirate biopsy (FNAB).

Direct smears: Cells can be collected either from the cut surface of an excised nodule, or from scrapings taken from the surface of ulcerated masses. Slides are gently dabbed onto the wiped surface of the mass or small amounts of scraping are spread between two slides prior to fixation and staining in the normal way.

FNAB: A 10 ml syringe is attached to either a 23g or 25g hypodermic needle. With the mass stabilised in one hand the needle is pushed into the stroma of the nodule. Several aspirations are then made in different directions, prior to releasing the suction and withdrawing the needle. The material in the needle is then expressed onto a slide and treated as for the direct smear.

Advantages of cytological examination:

1. Technique is quick, easy and cheap to perform.
2. Anaesthesia is rarely required.
3. "In-house" examination of samples is possible.
4. Samples may provide a definitive diagnosis.
5. Identification of aetiology possible in inflammatory nodules - this may be difficult in histopathology.

Disadvantages of exfoliative cytology:

1. Some masses do not exfoliate and so little information is gathered about the type of neoplasm.
2. Skill is needed in examination.
3. No information is gathered about biological behaviour of neoplasms.
4. Margins of excision and degree of malignancy are difficult to assess.

HISTOPATHOLOGY

Three techniques for obtaining material for histopathology are appropriate in nodular skin diseases; incisional biopsy, excisional biopsy and Tru-cut needle biopsy. Of these three, only the first two will be covered; Tru-cut needle techniques are difficult to perform and yield samples too small to be of diagnostic value in many cases.

Incisional biopsy

A small piece of the mass is removed by sharp incision with either a scalpel, electrosurgery unit (set to cut only) or a skin biopsy punch.

Advantages: The treatment may still be planned with the maximum information about diagnosis and prognosis available.

Disadvantages: Neoplastic masses may change in behaviour following biopsy, as surgery may increase the active growth fraction of the tumour. Histopathology is relatively expensive and slow compared with cytology. General anaesthesia is normally required. Wound repair may be difficult in solid masses.

Excisional biopsy

The whole mass is removed for examination.

Advantages: Treatment and diagnosis are achieved on one occasion: only one anaesthetic is needed; the maximum information is gathered for diagnosis and prognosis and costs are minimised.

Disadvantages: Margins of excision are difficult to assess and excision may be inadequate if a malignancy is present. Excision may be difficult in inflammatory nodules.

Obviously cytology is no replacement for histopathology when assessing biological behaviour and malignancy of masses. In many instances a combination of the two techniques may be necessary.

TREATMENT OF NODULAR SKIN DISEASES

Treatment regimes for the different types of nodules found in the skin rely upon diagnosis, prognosis and treatment planning to involve the owner.

For inflammatory masses the treatment often depends upon control of the inflammatory response together with identification and removal of the inciting cause.

Treatment of neoplastic masses has advanced considerably in recent years - the reader is referred to the BSAVA manual of Small Animal Oncology for a fuller description of possible treatment choices (See Further Reading).

CLASSIFICATION OF NODULAR DISEASES

DEVELOPMENTAL ABNORMALITIES

Although associated with developmental faults, these conditions are often not present until maturity or even old age. Some lesions are subject to breed predisposition. There are two major groups of developmental abnormalities; cysts and naevi. Of the two, cysts are far more common.

Cysts

Epidermoid cysts are very superficial, containing either fluid or keratinaceous debris. Fine needle aspirates are diagnostic, and surgical excision is curative. Many of these lesions are asymptomatic and once identified may be left.

Dermoid cysts are dermal in location, but may involve adnexal structures. For this reason contents often include hair and glandular secretions. If traumatised, release of their contents into the dermis is possible, resulting in a foreign body reaction. For this reason surgical excision may be advisable. Dermoid cysts are often found on the midline, and setter breeds are predisposed.

Apocrine hydrocystomata are similar to epidermoid cysts. These are very superficial and fluid-filled. No treatment is required in many cases, but excision is curative.

Pilar cysts (also known as sebaceous cysts) are common lesions which tend to occur from middle age. The lesions often present with a central pore from which a pseudohorn may arise. Again disruption of the cysts may lead to a severe inflammatory reaction which may be difficult to control. Excision is curative, but lesions may be numerous and recur continuously at different sites.

Naevi

The term naevus (pl. naevi) is used to describe several types of non-cystic cutaneous developmental abnormalities. Naevi are generally of little significance in the dog and cat, as these species do not suffer from neoplastic transformation of pigmented lesions which is an important problem in man. Some breeds e.g. great Danes develop many of these lesions which may be subject to self trauma and haemorrhage.

It may be difficult to obtain characteristic cells from these lesions by aspiration techniques. In the cat they must be differentiated from fibrous neoplasms and basal cell tumours.

INFLAMMATORY DISEASES

Almost any severe inflammatory disease of the skin may result in nodule formation. Inflammatory lesions are often pruritic and may be ulcerated. As a general rule, aspiration cytology and the examination of impression smears are helpful in their diagnosis.

Classes of inflammatory reactions often associated with a nodular pattern include:-

Folliculitis and furunculosis
Granulomatous diseases
Panniculitis
Abscesses

Folliculitis and furunculosis often present with a nodular pattern. This is due to the intensity of the dermal inflammatory reaction which may be so profound as to be termed granulomatous. Demonstration of the causal organisms (which may include bacteria, fungi and parasites such as *Demodex spp.*) is often easiest using cytology (Chapter 3).

Dermal granulomatous diseases are among the most difficult to investigate and manage, with many different antigens being responsible for their initiation. Causal antigens include hair and keratin, micro-organisms, foreign material and auto-antigens. Of these hair and keratin are most commonly involved. The release of hair and other keratin from disrupted follicles and cysts can be a potent initiator of granulomatous reactions. In particular "short-coat" folliculitis in contact areas of dobermans, boxers and bull terriers commonly presents in a nodular form.

Although staphylococci associated with pyoderma may be found in granulomata as a result of furunculosis, other organisms can be involved in granulomatous disease. The isolation of fungal organisms or opportunist bacteria from granulomata may imply immunosuppression. Some of the organisms may be difficult to culture and so staining of smears and sections from granulomata is mandatory. However some of the causative agents are also difficult to demonstrate with conventional stains!

"Feline leprosy" is caused by organisms such as *Mycobacterium lepraemurium* and is characterised by draining nodules. Other mycobacteria, including those associated with tuberculosis may be recovered uncommonly. The work-up of such cats requires assessment for feline leukaemia virus and feline immunosuppressive virus.

With the exception of keratin, foreign material is uncommonly demonstrated in granulomata. However the identification of such material is difficult, even with experience, and so if it is suspected this should be highlighted on laboratory request forms. Aluminium silicate crystals are sometimes found and recently it has been suggested that they are novel biocrystals, which cause granulomata in skin and lymph nodes.

Dogs with chronic pododermatitis should always be assessed for the presence of foreign material. Grass awns may cause nodular and granulomatous disease if migration is slow.

One other foreign material of significance is the persistence of parasitic mouthparts, particularly those of ticks. Inadequate removal of ticks by owners (and veterinary surgeons) may leave remnants of mouth-parts buried deeply in the skin resulting in granuloma formation. Of course, reactions to buried suture material also cause dermal nodules.

Antigen associated with autoimmune diseases may be the cause of granulomatous disease in the skin. These diseases are often difficult to diagnose, due to the difficulty in demonstration of auto-antigen, the diagnosis relies heavily upon the failure to identify infectious agents and as previously mentioned, this can be very difficult. Canine sterile granulomata, whether eosinophilic or neutrophilic in the dog may need immunosuppressive treatment for successful management.

Panniculitis in the dog may be associated with bacterial or fungal pathogens, autoimmunity, foreign bodies, vasculitis or dietary vitamin E deficiency. Clinically one or more draining nodules develop deep in the dermis and exude an oily, haemorrhagic discharge.

The investigation of panniculitis must include a thorough search for underlying causes, although the great majority of cases are idiopathic. In this case the cautious use of systemic glucocorticoid therapy may be warranted.

Abscesses are a common reason for which dogs, and more particularly cats, are presented to the veterinary surgeon. Abscesses may be associated with a variety of underlying aetiologies. The bacterial content of these lesions varies considerably, with both aerobic and anaerobic organisms being isolated. The overwhelming majority in the cat result from cat bites, hence the majority of feline abscesses are associated with the feline oral flora, particularly *Pasteurella spp.*

Abscesses found on the feet of dogs must be carefully investigated to rule out the presence of foreign bodies, commonly grass awns.

Neoplastic nodules

One of the first objectives of the diagnosis of nodular skin diseases is the assessment of the nodule(s) for the presence of neoplasia.

Neoplastic nodules may present arising from several different cell types within the skin; the following groups of cells of origin will be discussed here:

Epithelial
Adnexal
Melanocytic
Mesenchymal
Round cell

Again the reader is referred to the BSAVA Manual of Small Animal Oncology and other oncology texts for a more in-depth description of the various skin neoplasms.

Epithelial tumours

Basal cell tumours: arise from the epidermal or hair follicle basal cells and are relatively common in the dog and more so in the cat. They are often highly pigmented and have a different appearance in the dog and cat. In the dog these neoplasms are often circular and solitary with the suggestion of a central pore. They are classified as carcinomata but although some degree of local infiltration may occur they rarely metastasise. In the cat, the basal cell tumour is often highly pigmented and cystic. It is also benign in behaviour and in dogs and cats local excision is usually curative.

Papillomata: The commonest skin neoplasm in the dog is the humble papilloma. Whilst these masses may be associated with a viral aetiology when present in or around the oral cavity of young animals, the vast majority are the papillomata of old age. There is some breed predilection for these neoplasms, with cocker spaniels and miniature poodles commonly affected with large numbers of these "warts".

Papillomata are best left untreated unless they are inconveniently situated, for example on the eyelid. Treatment options include sharp surgery, cryosurgery and ligation. Recurrence at the same site is common, and new lesions frequently occur elsewhere. Viral papillomata are often self limiting and therefore rarely require attention.

Squamous cell carcinomata: As with basal cell tumours, distinction must be made between the behaviour of these tumours in the cat and dog (Plates 60 and 61).

In the cat, squamous cell carcinoma has been recorded as a congenital problem affecting multiple digits. However, most commonly this neoplasm is actinic (sunlight induced) in origin. This explains the distribution of lesions in depigmented sites such as the pinna, nasal planum and eyelid. Long standing self trauma may also induce neoplastic transformation, particularly as a sequel to eosinophilic ulcer of the lip.

Treatment of these masses involves sharp excision, which must be radical due to their locally invasive nature, or cryosurgery if superficial. These tumours are radiosensitive, and such therapy may be useful, especially in those tumours involving the nasal septum.

In the dog, squamous cell carcinoma is less common, and may occur at a variety of sites. The one area to be particularly aware of is the nail bed, where these masses may resemble paronychia. At this site considerable local invasion may be present, necessitating amputation of the digit. Following excision of any squamous cell carcinoma, histopathological assessment of the adequacy of excision is mandatory.

Adnexal tumours

Neoplasms arising from the adnexae may be benign or malignant and may be difficult to assess clinically as they are poorly exfoliative. Such masses may become quite large, and may calcify in the case of pilomatricomata. Intracutaneous cornifying epitheliomata (keratoacanthomata) may be multiple in the elkhound and other breeds and there is some evidence for response to medical (retinoid) therapy. Otherwise surgical excision is the treatment of choice with adequate margins allowed in cases of carcinomata.

Melanocytic tumours

Benign melanomata: are relatively common in the dog and cat, usually appearing as solitary tumours at any site. Local excision is curative.

Malignant melanomata: are less common, being found most often in the oral cavity and nail bed of the dog. Radical surgical treatment is necessary, although metastasis to local and regional lymph nodes is rapid and may precede diagnosis.

Mesenchymal tumours

Arising from fibrous, adipose or vascular tissues, these classes of neoplasm may present as benign variants or sarcomata.

Fibrosarcomata: are not uncommon in the dog or cat and are amongst the most aggressive of cutaneous neoplasms. Again radical therapy is necessary, but careful assessment for metastasis is important.

Lipomata: are amongst the more common of cutaneous neoplasms. These lesions may be hyperplastic rather than truly neoplastic. The diagnosis of these masses, unlike the other mesenchymal tumours, is easily achieved with fine-needle aspirate biopsy.

Round cell tumours

This group contains some of the most clinically important nodular neoplasms. These include lymphoma, Langerhans cell tumours and mast cell tumours. The early identification and management of mast cell tumours is essential. However although the diagnosis of round cell tumours may often be made cytologically, rather than histologically, the histological assessment of cell differentiation is important in the planning of the treatment of mast cell tumours.

Mast cell tumours: although these do occur as solitary tumours, they are often widespread and in some cases may be considered systemic (Plate 62). For this reason surgery of multiple masses, or the inadequate excision of the solitary mass may not only be unhelpful but may reduce the prospects of long term cure. The appearance of these tumours is very variable, from alopecic nodules to eosinophilic plaques.

It is beyond the scope of this chapter to discuss the management of mast cell tumours in detail, but the following algorithm represents an overview of the clinical approach:

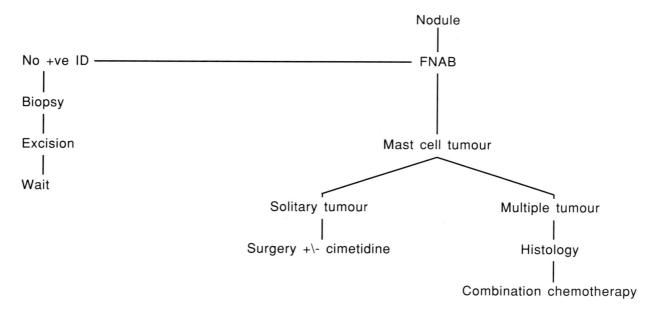

Canine Langerhans cell tumours: these masses, previously known as canine cutaneous histiocytomata, have now been demonstrated to arise from Langerhans cells (Plate 59). These tumours are fascinating, having all the histological markers of malignancy but being self-limiting in most cases. The masses present as raised hairless nodules, which have a red and inflamed appearance in the resolution phase. These neoplasms are generally found on the head and limbs of young animals, and are often noticed by the owners after resolution has already commenced.

The histological appearance may be confusing to pathologists experienced only in human pathology, as they resemble malignant histiocytoma in man.

Should treatment be deemed necessary, either cryosurgery or local excision is curative.

Lymphomata

Cutaneous lymphoma in the dog can arise in three distinct forms; epitheliotropic lymphoma (mycosis fungoides), primary cutaneous B-cell lymphoma and cutaneous metastases arising from a primary lymphoma elsewhere. In the cat, mycosis fungoides is very rare, but the other types occur more frequently.

Mycosis fungoides: Epitheliotropic (T-cell) lymphoma is an uncommon cutaneous neoplasm presenting as an exfoliative dermatosis with plaques and nodules (Plate 37). Lesions may occur anywhere on the body, although the face and muco-cutaneous junctions are commonly affected. Depigmentation of affected areas is a common feature of this disease, which may have a fluctuating course.

Treatment is difficult, with no really successful regime being reported.

Primary B-cell lymphomata: B-cell lymphomata usually present as solitary masses. They are often aggressive in behaviour, as they increase in size rapidly and may be associated with intense pain. Other presentations include diffuse dermal infiltrates with some degree of epitheliotropism. Surgical therapy is often inadequate and medical therapy, even aggressive chemotherapy, may not be helpful.

Occasionally dogs may present with a benign form of lymphoma presenting as multiple nodules in aged individuals.

Metastatic disease: Unlike primary lymphoma, metastatic B-cell lymphoma may present as multiple nodules in the skin. Young dogs are often represented as with any B-cell lymphoma. Successful treatment requires control of the primary tumour, usually with combination chemotherapy.

CONCLUSIONS

In cases of nodular skin diseases, whether singular or multiple, a logical diagnostic approach is essential for successful planning of treatment. Using the techniques discussed here, the presence or absence of neoplasia may be demonstrated and appropriate action taken.

FURTHER READING

GORMAN, N.T. and DOBSON, J.M. (1991). The Skin and Associated Tissues. In: *Manual of Small Animal Oncology.* (Ed. R.A.S. White) B.S.A.V.A., Cheltenham.

MACY, D.W. and MACEWEN, E.G. (1989). Mast Cell Tumors. In: *Clinical Veterinary Oncology.* (Eds. S.J Withrow and E.G. MacEwen) Lippincott, Philadelphia.

OWEN, L.N. (1980). TNM *Classification of Tumours in Domestic Animals.* Published by World Health Organisation, Geneva.

SUSANECK, S.J. and WITHROW, S.J. (1989). Tumors of the Skin and Subcutaneous Tissues. In: *Clinical Veterinary Oncology.* (Eds. S.J. Withrow and E.G. MacEwen) Lippincott, Philadelphia.

THE DISCHARGING SINUS

David H Shearer

INTRODUCTION

The discharging sinus is a common presenting sign in small animal clinical practice. The underlying cause can be common, as in the case of a cat bite abscess, or extremely rare, as in the case of a subcutaneous mycosis. The draining sinus tract represents the body's attempt to reject material within the dermis or subcutis. Material can enter the skin by traumatic penetration, via the hair follicles or by systemic routes. Foreign bodies, necrotic tissue, bacteria, fungi, or parasites can all lead to a draining sinus.

A logical approach to diagnosis is important, especially in cases that do not respond to initial treatment.

APPROACH TO THE CASE

A careful history and examination should be performed as detailed in Chapter 2. Breeds commonly affected with dermatoses presenting as discharging sinuses include German shepherd dogs and English bull terriers which can suffer from a severe folliculitis, furunculosis and cellulitis syndrome.

Long-haired breeds of dogs are prone to developing discharging sinuses in the summer months due to grass awn migration; the awn is initially trapped in the coat and then moves towards, and penetrates, the skin. In cats, bite wound abscesses are the commonest cause of a discharging sinus. Entire male cats are predisposed to cat bite abscesses because they are more likely to fight.

PHYSICAL EXAMINATION

As with all dermatoses a general clinical examination should be performed for evidence of systemic disease e.g. pyrexia, anorexia, anaemia, lymphadenopathy and weight loss. The skin should be examined and particular attention should be paid to the appearance, progression and distribution of lesions.

The clinical diseases that present with discharging sinus formation can be usefully divided into four groups, ie.

1. Folliculitis / furunculosis
2. Cellulitis
3. Pyogranuloma / panniculitis
4. Neoplasms

It is useful to use this classification when considering the differential diagnoses in an individual case as the dermatosis should fit one of these groups. Once the animal's dermatosis has been classified, the underlying aetiology is considered and a list of differential diagnoses created. Investigations based on the differential diagnoses are then performed.

Differential Diagnosis

The infectious causes and non-infectious causes of discharging sinuses are classified in tables 1 and 2 respectively.

Table 1
Infectious causes of discharging sinuses

Bacterial.
  1. Subcutaneous abscesses/cellulitis
      Aerobic bacteria eg. *Pasteurella multocida*, ß-haemolytic *Streptococci*
      Anaerobic bacteria eg. *Bacteroides* spp., Fusiform bacilli
  2. Bacterial pseudomycetoma (Botryomycosis)
      Staphylococcus spp.
  3. Actinomyces
      A. viscosus
  4. Nocardiosis
      N. asteroides
      N. brasiliensis
      N. cavia
  5. Mycobacterial granulomas
      a. Cutaneous tuberculosis
          M. tuberculosis
          M. bovis
      b. Feline leprosy
          M. lepraemurium
      c. Atypical mycobacterial infections
          M. fortuitum
          M. chelonei
          M. phlei
  6. Feline plague
      Yersinia pestis

Fungal.
  1. Pseudomycetoma
      M. canis
      T. mentagrophytes
  2. Subcutaneous mycoses
      a. Eumycotic mycetomas
          Pseudoallescheria spp.
          Curvularia spp.
          Helminthosporium speciferum
          Allescheria boydii
          Maduralla spp.
      b. Phaeohyphomycosis
          Drechslera spp.
          Moniella spp.
          Cladosporium spp.
      c. Pythiosis
          Pythium spp.
      d. Protecosis
          Prototheca wickerhamii
      e. Sporotrichosis
          Sporothrix schenkii
      f. Zygomycosis
          Mucor spp.
          Rhizopus spp.
          Absidia spp.

Table 1 (Cont.)

3. Deep / Systemic mycoses
    a. Cryptococcosis
       Cryptococcus neoformans
    b. Histoplasmosis
    c. Coccidioidomycosis
    d. Blastomycosis
    e. Paecilomycosis

Parasitic.

1. Demodicosis
       Demodex canis
2. Cuterebriasis
       Cuterebra spp.
3. Dracunculosis
       Dracuncula spp.

Table 2
Non-infectious causes of discharging sinuses

Neoplastic.

1. Cutaneous or subcutaneous masses with necrotic centres

Physical causes

1. Foreign bodies
       Hair
       Keratin
       Bone sequestrae
       Plant material
       Wood (Splinters)
2. Iatrogenic material
       Sutures
       Implants
       Swabs
3. Pressure point and callus formation

Miscellaneous causes

1. Panniculitis
       Immune mediated / nutritional / infectious / idiopathic
2. Idiopathic sterile pyogranuloma

ESTABLISHING THE DIAGNOSIS

The following investigations should be performed to establish a specific diagnosis:

1. Skin scrapings to establish the presence, or otherwise, of ectoparasites such as *Demodex canis*.

2. Microscopical examination of exudate to identify fungal or bacterial organisms. A stain such as "Diff Quik" may be useful for routine examination of exudates (see Chapter 3).

3. Culture of the sinus exudate for aerobic bacteria, anaerobic bacteria and fungi.

If there is no improvement after the initial management then surgical exploration of the sinus tract(s) combined with biopsy of the lesion(s) should be performed. The biopsy can divided, one half of the tissue used for histopathology and the other half for bacterial or fungal culture. Further investigations that should be performed in cases not responding to treatment include radiography (fistulograms), complete blood count, serum biochemistry and serology for FeLV / FIV as appropriate.

INITIAL MANAGEMENT

In the dog, the commonest cause of a discharging sinus is a foreign body such as a grass seed, whilst in the cat it is a cat bite abscess. The animal should be sedated or anaesthetised and the sinus opened to allow drainage and/or to remove the foreign body. Systemic antibacterial treatment is usually provided. The animal should be examined 5-7 days later and further investigations performed if there is no evidence of improvement or if there has been spread locally or elsewhere on the body.

Diseases

FOLLICULITIS/FURUNCULOSIS SYNDROMES

Folliculitis is inflammation of the hair follicle which, if severe, leads to follicle rupture and inflammation of the dermis; furunculosis. The inflammatory reaction to the follicular contents (hair, sweat, sebum, bacteria) within the dermis results in sinus formation. Syndromes characterised by furunculosis can be usefully divided into local and generalised conditions when considering the differential diagnosis.

Localised Furunculosis

Facial furunculosis - Canine and feline acne are common conditions seen in general practice. Young, usually male short coated dogs are affected up to the end of puberty. The condition may resolve once the dog is sexually mature although residual scarring may occur. The pathogenesis is thought to involve hypertrophy and hyperplasia of sebaceous glands with excess secretion leading to blocking of hair follicles and subsequent bacterial infection. Lesions associated with canine acne are pustules, papules and comedones on the lower chin and muzzle. In severe cases this may progress to furunculosis and multiple discharging sinuses on the chin and lateral aspect of the muzzle. Treatment involves benzoyl peroxide gel applied topically once daily and systemic antibiotics for four to six weeks in severe cases. All animals with chin acne should be checked for demodicosis by microscopical examination of skin scrapings.

In cats the condition has no age, sex or breed predisposition and although an inability to groom the chin has been proposed the condition may reflect a defect in keratinisation. Treatment with benzoyl peroxide gel or shampoo may be helpful and is applied until remission is achieved and then once weekly, or as necessary, for control.

(Editors note: Benzoyl peroxide gel is not licenced for use in cats in the U.K.)

Nasal furunculosis - This condition affects doliocephalic breeds such as rough collies, German shepherd dogs and pointers. The differential diagnosis includes discoid or systemic lupus erythematosus, pemphigus foliaceus, demodicosis, dermatophytosis, drug eruptions, dermatomyositis, insect bite hypersensitivity, trauma and solar dermatitis. In addition to the microscopical examination of skin scrapings for the identification of *Demodex canis*, fungal culture should be performed for dermatophytes. Skin biopsy should also be performed. Histopathology is particularly useful in the diagnosis of some of the underlying causes such as immune mediated disease and insect bite hypersensitivity. Treatment should be aimed at the underlying cause. Systemic antibacterial agents for three to six weeks (based on culture results) and twice daily, gentle topical chlorhexidine washes should be used if no underlying cause is found.

Interdigital furunculosis (interdigital "cysts") - This is an extremely frustrating condition or group of diseases to deal with; the lesions are not cysts. The following factors should be considered:

1. Trauma. Large, obese, working or racing dogs are more likely to suffer traumatic damage followed by infection and with chronicity, permanent scarring. The environment should be carefully considered eg. bedding, hygiene and the frequency and intensity of grooming or clipping. Obesity may predispose to the development of interdigital furunculosis. Excessive exercise or work may lead to trauma and subsequent furunculosis.

2. Poor foot conformation. Some breeds have poor foot conformation with excessive or abnormal weight distribution and abnormal interdigital anatomy. The English bull terrier, Staffordshire bull terrier and bulldog appear to be particularly prone to conjoined pads and recurrent interdigital furunculosis. It is thought that feet that accumulate soil and sand are predisposed to this condition.

3. Contact allergic or contact irritant dermatitis should be considered. Plants, building materials, chemicals on paths or lawns, in ponds or in the home or kennel may cause an interdigital dermatitis and furunculosis.

4. Parasite migration may be the underlying cause eg. *Uncinaria* sp. or *Ancyclostoma* sp. Skin scraping or biopsy may reveal the parasites.

5. Foreign body. A grass seed is the commonest cause of an interdigital discharging sinus in dogs during the summer and autumn.

6. Secondary bacterial infection should always be considered when dealing with a chronic recurrent pedal pyoderma.

In addition to the microscopical examination of skin scrapings and the submission of swabs for bacterial culture, surgery should be considered to search for any suspected foreign body. Biopsy of the lesions should be performed at the time of surgery. Treatment should be directed at both the underlying cause and the secondary staphylococcal infection and advice given to the owner on how to prevent recurrence if necessary. An example of the latter would be clipping of long hair around the toes and checking the feet after walks to prevent grass seed penetration and abscessation.

Anal Furunculosis - This is a furunculosis affecting the perianal skin. The German shepherd dog is most commonly affected although the condition is seen in Irish setters and other breeds. The underlying aetiology is unknown although conformation, anal sac disease, an immunological abnormality and diarrhoea have all been suggested as possible causes (Muller *et al*, 1989).

Generalised Furunculosis

The English bull terrier, German shepherd dog, doberman pinscher, weimaraner, boxer, Irish setter and rottweiler appear to be predisposed to developing a generalised furunculosis. The cause of the condition is unknown although infection with *Staphylococcus intermedius* is thought to be a secondary feature. Some of the affected animals may respond poorly to systemic antibiotic therapy. It is important to look for underlying causes such as demodicosis, flea allergic dermatitis, atopy, food allergy, hypothyroidism, immunological abnormalities or underlying genetic abnormalities.

Treatment should be directed at the underlying cause and the secondary infection. The animal should be clipped and the whole body soaked in dilute chlorhexidine or povidone-iodine each day. Systemic antibacterial therapy (based on culture and sensitivity results) should be continued for at least two weeks beyond clinical cure (Chapter 25). This may incur several months of treatment and the owner should be advised of both the cost and the guarded prognosis in these cases.

CELLULITIS

Abscess and cellulitis

Cellulitis is a deep, suppurative infection with poorly defined margins. The infection usually tracks along the tissue planes. Bacteria are inoculated into the deep dermis and subcutis by traumatic injury and there is subsequent abscess formation within 48-96 hours. The commonest cause is cat fight injuries: however any penetrating wound can lead to abscess formation or cellulitis. Affected animals develop localised swellings which are painful on palpation and there is often anorexia, pyrexia and lethargy. Anaerobic bacteria can be isolated from wounds. *Pasteurella multocida*, fusiform bacilli, ß-haemolytic *streptococci* and *Bacteroides* sp. are the most commonly encountered within a cat bite abscess. Carro *et al.* (1989) reported subcutaneous abscesses in a household of cats and incriminated a bacterial L-form; these can be treated with tetracyclines but are not responsive to penicillin-based antibiotics. Treatment of abscesses is by surgical drainage and systemic antibiotics if considered appropriate. Cellulitis lesions should be poulticed with hot, wet dressings and systemic antibiotics prescribed. Synthetic penicillins for seven to ten days are usually effective.

Juvenile cellulitis (puppy strangles, juvenile pyoderma)

This condition occurs in pups between three weeks and four months old. It tends to occur in short-coated breeds such as the labrador retriever, weimeraner, German shorthaired pointer and Gordon setter. One or more puppies in a litter may be affected. The lesions are mainly around the mucocutaneous junctions of the head with oedema, cellulitis, alopecia and seropurulent exudation from follicles and, in some cases, sinus tracts. The inflammation is so severe that some hair follicles are permanently destroyed and scarring often occurs. The puppy may develop anorexia, pyrexia and generalised lymphadenopathy.

The aetiology is unknown although it is thought that there is a primary pyogranulomatous lymphadenitis with a secondary pyoderma. Appropriate antibiotics should be used to treat the staphylococcal pyoderma along with immunosuppressive doses of prednisolone to control the pyogranulomatous lymphadenitis. Topical therapy with daily wet soaks of chlorhexidine are also indicated. Response to treatment is usually rapid but therapy should be continued for at least three weeks. The owner should be warned that scarring is likely to occur.

PYOGRANULOMAS/PANNICULITIS

Non Infectious Causes

Foreign body - This is a common cause of draining sinus formation in dogs and a migrating grass seed is the usual cause during the summer months. However, other foreign bodies such as hair, keratin, mineral crystals and iatrogenic material such as sutures may cause pyogranulomas or panniculitis. The sinus tract should be explored and any macroscopic material removed. Inflammatory tissue should be removed and sent for histology to detect microscopic material e.g. mineral crystals. This may lead to rational advice on means of avoiding recurrence in the future.

Decubital callus formation - Pressure sores develop as the result of prolonged excessive pressure or trauma over bony prominences such as the elbows, hocks or the sternum. Excessive body weight and hard sleeping areas are contributing factors. Lesions often become infected leading to ulceration and sinus formation. Treatment should be aimed at reducing the trauma in addition to treating the infection. Soft bedding, padded bandages and sometimes surgical excision all play a role in the treatment of this condition. Topical soaks, two to three times daily in chlorhexidine and systemic antibiotics should be prescribed.

Nodular panniculitis - Panniculitus is inflammation of the subcutaneous fat. Nodular panniculitus (a sign rather than a specific disease) can occur in cases of nutritional imbalance, bacterial infection (see bacterial pseudomycetoma, actinomycetes), immune mediated diseases (systemic lupus erythematosus, erythema nodosum) and idiopathic disease. The clinical case presents with single or multiple subcutaneous nodules which progress, in some cases, to discharging sinus with an oily, yellow-brown discharge. Investigation should be directed toward isolating one of the known causes by examination of a direct smear of the exudate. Bacterial and fungal culture and histology of excised lesions are used to confirm the diagnosis. Once all known underlying causes have been eliminated then a diagnosis of sterile idiopathic panniculitus can be made. Treatment should be directed at the underlying cause or, in the case of sterile idiopathic disease, systemic glucocorticoids at immunosuppressive doses are indicated (prednisolone; dogs 2 mg/kg daily; cats 4 mg/kg daily). Therapy should be stopped once the lesions have resolved. If recurrence occurs then long term alternate day prednisolone may be necessary.

Infectious Causes

Bacterial infections

Diagnosis of bacterial causes of discharging sinuses is confirmed by cytological examination of the exudate, histopathology and bacterial culture.

Botryomycosis is a suppurative, granulomatous disease caused by *Staphylococcus* sp. or Gram-negative bacteria forming compact colonies or grains within an area of pyogranulomatous inflammation (Walton *et al*, 1983). The organisms are introduced by trauma or with a penetrating foreign body. Clinically the patient presents with draining nodular lesions producing small white granules. Treatment is by surgical excision and systemic antibacterial therapy.

Actinomycosis is a rare cause of pyogranulomatous or subcutaneous abscesses which tends to affect the face or neck. They are characterised by a reddish brown exudate often described as a "tomato soup" exudate. The *Actinomyces* spp. are commensal organisms in the oral cavity and gastrointestinal tract and cutaneous infection follows inoculation by trauma, usually a bite wound. Cytological examination of the exudate will reveal Gram-positive branching filamentous rods and cocci. Therapy is by surgical excision or drainage and high doses of penicillin (100,00 U/kg/day) for at least one month.

Nocardiosis presents clinically as discharging nodules and cellulitis and follows the introduction of the causal organism along with a penetrating foreign body or trauma. The exudate is brownish red and cytological examination will reveal acid-fast, Gram-positive filamentous rods and cocci. Diagnosis is confirmed by aerobic culture (at both 25° and 37° Centigrade), cytology and histopathology. Treatment should be continued for several weeks or months with potentiated sulphonamides (Hardie and Barsanti, 1982).

Mycobacterial Infections (cutaneous tuberculosis) due to *Mycobacterium tuberculosis* or *M. bovis*, is a rare cause of multiple nodules, abscesses or ulcers in small animals. Diagnosis is confirmed by inoculation of guinea pigs. Bacille Calmette-Guerin (BCG) has been used for confirmation of the diagnosis in dogs (Parodie *et al*, 1965). This condition is a public health hazard and euthanasia is indicated.

Feline leprosy presents clinically as single or multiple cutaneous nodules, with or without abscessation, sinus formation and lymphadenopathy. The cause is thought to be *Mycobacterium lepraemurium* or *Mycobacterium leprae*. Diagnosis is confirmed by the presence of acid-fast organisms on cytological examination, histopathology and guinea pig inoculation to rule out tuberculosis. Treatment is by surgical excision of solitary lesions and/or dapsone at a dose of one to 50 mg/kg bid for several weeks (Muller *et al*, 1989).

Atypical Mycobacterial infections are caused by opportunistic mycobacteria such as *M. fortuitum*, *M.chelonei*, *M.phlei*, and *M. smegmatis*. The clinical disease presents as chronic subcutaneous abscesses, ulcerations and discharging sinuses. Diagnosis is confirmed by cytological examination (revealing acid-fast bacteria), culture of the exudate and histopathology of a lesion showing a pyogranulomatous panniculitis and acid-fast bacteria.

Fungal infections

It is important to have some appreciation of the likely cause in each individual case when collecting material for fungal culture since organisms vary in their requirements for growth and identification *in vitro*. It is vital that a clinician asks the diagnostic laboratory to culture for specific organisms and not just "fungi"!

Subcutaneous mycoses

These develop at the site of inoculation following a bite or trauma. The infection may remain localised or may spread via the lymphatic system. The diagnosis of these conditions is based on cytological examination of the exudate, fungal culture and histopathological examination of biopsy material.

Dermatophytosis (pseudomycetoma) presents with one or more draining nodules and is due to infection by *Microsporum canis* or *Trichophyton* spp. Longhaired cats are thought more likely to develop a deep dermatophyte infection and underlying immunological abnormalities should always be considered e.g. FeLV and FIV infection. Diagnosis is confirmed by histopathological examination and fungal culture of biopsy material. Treatment is by surgical excision of large lesions and systemic griseofulvin.

Eumycotic mycetomas may be caused by numerous fungi including *Pseudoallescheria* spp., *Curvularia* spp., *Helminthosporium speciferum*, *Allescheria boydii*, and *Maduralla* spp. Clinical presentation is swelling with draining sinuses producing an exudate with granules. Treatment is by surgical excision.

Phaeohyphomycosis is caused by brown pigmented (dematiaceous), septated-hyphal fungi such as *Drechslera* spp., *Moniella* spp., *Cladosporium* spp., *Phialophora* spp. and *Alternaria* spp. The condition is more often seen in cats and presents as nodules producing a pink to yellow exudate. The cytology and histopathology reveal pigmented, septate, branching hyphae and chlamydospores. Surgical excision is the first line of treatment, however combinations of amphotericin B / flucytosine or ketoconazole / itraconazole may be effective (Sousa and Ihrke,1984).

Pythiosis is a rare disease caused by a fungus of the genus *Pythium*. It has been reported in dogs in South Eastern USA. The lesions are usually poorly defined, ulcerating nodules but some lesions present with discharging sinuses. Treatment involves surgical excision as these lesions do not respond to medical treatment (Pavletic and MacIntire, 1982)

Prototothecosis is a rare cause of nodular lesions with a discharging sinus and is due to an alga, *Prototheca wickerhamii*. Treatment is by surgical excision.

Sporotrichosis is caused by *Sporothrix schenkii*, a soil organism which enters the skin by inoculation, or as a sequel to trauma, puncture or wound contamination. Lesions may be ulcerated or draining nodules and located on any part of the body. Sporotrichosis is a public health hazard and, if suspected, all personnel should wear protective clothing and masks. Treatments available include inorganic iodides with or without ketoconazole and amphotericin B (Muller *et al*, 1989).

Zygomycosis may be caused by a number of water and soil-borne fungi of the class Zygomycetes including *Mucor* spp., *Rhizopus* spp. and *Absidia* spp. The subcutaneous form presents as pruritic, granulomatous nodules with discharging sinuses producing a purulent exudate. There can be a lymphadenopathy and systemic or visceral involvement. Amphotericin B or ketoconazole are used for treatment.

Deep / Systemic Mycoses

In the deep and systemic mycoses the cutaneous lesions are accompanied by internal disease and frequently occur as an extension of this internal disease.

Cryptococcosis is caused by *Cryptococcus neoformans*, a soil saprophyte which may also be found in pigeon droppings. In dogs, the central nervous system (CNS) and eyes are usually affected. Cutaneous nodules with discharging sinuses occur in a minority of canine cases. Cats are more often affected than dogs and the respiratory system, CNS, eyes and skin can all be involved. Solitary or multiple cutaneous nodules with draining sinuses, nasal discharge, sneezing and lymphadenopathy can occur in cats. Cytological examination should reveal the presence of large, round, encapsulated yeasts. Serology is available and may be useful for the diagnosis and monitoring of treatment. Treatment is possible with amphotericin B, flucytosine, ketoconazole and itraconazole. The infection is zoonotic and gloves should be worn when handling the patients.

Histoplasmosis is caused by *Histoplasma capsatum*, a dimorphic fungus growing as a yeast in animal tissue and as a mould in soil. The organism usually affects the respiratory system, however subcutaneous nodules and discharging sinuses have been seen in cats.

Coccidioidomyosis usually affects the respiratory system and not the skin. Diagnosis is by cytology, serology, histopathology and treatment with amphotericin B and ketoconazole.

Blastomycosis infection in dogs causes a benign pulmonary disease initially. Resolution may follow or the organism may disseminate to affect the skin, eyes, and bones. Affected dogs are anorexic, pyrexic and have nasal and ocular discharges, draining lymph nodes, skin lesions and a cough. Skin lesions may be single or multiple discharging sinuses producing a purulent or blood tinged exudate. Diagnosis is confirmed by cytological examination, immunohistopathology, and radiology. Treatment is with amphotericin B and ketoconazole or itraconazole.

Aspergillosis is thought to be due to opportunistic infection of an immunosuppressed patient with a fungus of the genus *Aspergillus*. The usual clinical signs are associated with infection of the nasal cavity or frontal sinuses i.e. a chronic nasal discharge. Cutaneous granulomas, diarrhoea, weight loss and ocular lesions may also be seen. Diagnosis is by cytology, culture, histopathology and serology. Treatment by surgical excision and itraconazole therapy.

Neoplasms

Cutaneous or subcutaneous neoplasms with necrotic centres can present with a discharging sinus. Examples are haemangiosarcoma and liposarcoma. Diagnosis is by histopathology of biopsy material, taken before complete surgical excision so that other methods of treatment can be prescribed, if indicated.

REFERENCES

CARRO, T., PEDERSON, N.C., BEAMAN, B.L. & MUNN R. (1989). Subcutaneous abscesses and arthritis caused by a probable bacterial L-form in cats. *Journal of the American Veterinary Medical Association* **194**; 1583.

HARDIE, E.M. & BARSANTI, J.A. (1982). Treatment of Actinomycosis. *Journal of the American Veterinary Medical Association* **180**; 537.

MULLER, G.H., KIRK, R.W. & SCOTT, D.W. (1989). Eds. *Small Animal Dermatology* 4th edn. W. B. Saunders, Philadelphia.

PAVLETIC, M.M. & MACINTIRE, D. (1982). Phycomycosis of the axilla and inner brachium in the dog : Surgical excision and reconstruction with a thoracodorsal axial pattern flap. *Journal of the American Veterinary Medical Association* **180**; 1197.

PARODIE, A., FONTAINE, M., BRION, A., TISSEUR, H. & GORET.,P. (1965). Mycobacterioses in the Domestic Carnivora - Present-Day Epidemiology of Tuberculosis in the Cat and Dog. *Journal of Small Animal Practice* **6**; 309.

SOUSA, C.A. & IHRKE, P.J .(1984). Subcutaneous phaeohyphomycosis (*Stemphyllium sp.* and *Cladosporium sp.* infections) in the cat. *Journal of the American Veterinary Medical Association* **185**; 673.

WALTON, D.K., SCOTT, D.W. & MANNING, T.O. (1983). Cutaneous bacterial granuloma (Botryomycosis) in the dog and cat. *Journal of the American Veterinary Medical Association* **19**; 537.

DISORDERS OF PIGMENTATION

David H Scarff ————————————————————

INTRODUCTION

The pigmentation of the skin and coat of mammalian species is of great importance in camouflage, in reproductive behaviour and in social hierarchy. In household pets it is less important to the animals than to their owners. For example, success in the show ring is partly dependent on "correct" pigmentation. Pigmentary disorders, even when of no clinical significance, are often a source of great distress to dog and cat owners (Plates 52-56).

The pigmentary system

Normal pigmentation of skin and hair stems from the inclusion of melanin pigments in the keratinocytes of epidermis or hair matrix. The proportion and amounts of the differing types of pigment (or no pigment at all) determine the shade and density of pigment. Two distinct types of melanin are found in skin: the eumelanins, which are brownish-black in colour, and the phaeomelanins which range from yellow to reddish-brown. A third group found in man in yellow and red hair are called trichochromes.

Melanin granules are derived from the oxidation of tyrosine and polymerisation of dihydroxyphenylalanine (dopa) in intracellular organelles (melanosomes) within specialised, dendritic, melanin forming cells, melanocytes. These cells are of neural crest origin, and are principally found in the basal layer of the epidermis and the hair matrix. Melanin granules are incorporated into keratinocytes by pinocytosis. With the exception of skin depigmented by a destructive process directed at the melanocytes, the numbers of these cells is similar in all shades of pigmented skin and hair.

Control mechanisms influencing the pigmentary system include pituitary hormones such as melanocyte stimulating hormone (MSH) and poorly understood local factors. Neurogenic influences on melanocytes may also be of importance. Pineal hormones such as melatonin are likely to have little or no influence on skin pigmentation.

Abnormalities of pigmentation may be congenital or acquired, and may involve only the pigmentary system or be polysystemic. In the latter case, disorders of skin pigmentation may act as early pointers towards the diagnosis of more serious internal illness, including neoplasia.

Terminology

There are a number of terms which are used in the description of the pigmentary diseases:

Macule -   An area of skin of noticeably different pigmentation with a diameter of less than 1 cm. A macule is neither raised nor depressed when compared with the surrounding skin surface.

Patch -   A macular area with a diameter greater than 1 cm.

Leukoderma -	Depigmentation of the skin.
Leukonychia -	Depigmentation of the nail(s).
Leukotrichia -	Depigmentation of the hair.
Melanoderma -	Increase in skin pigmentation.
Melanotrichia-	Increase in hair pigmentation.

APPROACH TO THE CASE

The diagnostic approach adopted for disorders of pigmentation is essentially the same as that for other dermatoses (Chapter 2). Steps include:-

1) History taking

2) Physical examination

3) Establishing a list of differential diagnoses

4) Diagnostic tests

Taking the history

It is important in cases of pigmentary disorders to rule out the presence of either inflammatory or systemic illnesses. To this end the clinician should pay particular importance to signs of involvement of other systems such as polyuria/polydipsia, joint disease or lethargy. These could indicate the presence of a multi system disease such as systemic lupus erythematosus.

The initial appearance, progression of lesions and presence or absence of pruritus are of great significance. Lesions may be modified by secondary inflammatory changes or infection, making diagnosis more difficult.

Physical examination

The examination should concentrate on ruling out both systemic diseases and neoplastic skin disease. If neoplasia is suspected a complete examination for metastasis to distant sites is appropriate.

When examining individual lesions the thickness of the skin should be assessed, together with examination for surface changes and evidence of self trauma. Assessment of epidermal pigmentation can be difficult and so care must be taken in assessment of these changes.

Establishing a list of differential diagnoses

Once a list of differential diagnoses has been drawn up, specific diagnostic tests may be used to narrow the list and arrive at a definitive diagnosis.

Diagnostic tests

There are several tests which may be particularly useful in cases of pigmentary disturbance:

a) Diascopy: Examination of skin through a glass slide pressed on the skin can differentiate between erythema and either pigment or haemorrhage.

b) Hair pluckings: Examination of epilated hairs can be helpful in the diagnosis of parasitic conditions such as demodicosis, as well as in identifying diseases with pigmentary change in the hair shaft. Examples of these conditions include colour dilution alopecia and Chediak-Higashi syndrome where macro-melanosomes are to be found in the hair shaft and bulb.

c) Skin scrapings: Microscopical examination of skin scrapings in either liquid paraffin or potassium hydroxide can provide evidence of inflammatory skin disease or endocrinopathies in the form of follicular casts. In colour dilution alopecia and black hair follicle dysplasia the contents of follicles are in the form of hyper-pigmented casts with macro-melanosomes. Scrapings are also indicated in all cases where ectoparasitism is suspected.

d) Skin biopsy: Biopsy specimens may be the only way to diagnose pigmentary disorders. It must be remembered, however, that both depigmented and heavily pigmented skin can be normal physiologically. For this reason the use of an elliptical biopsy taken from the edge of a lesion may be useful, as this allows examination of the developing edge of the lesion. Biopsy samples are also mandatory if immune mediated or neoplastic diseases are suspected.

INITIAL MANAGEMENT

Diseases characterised by increase in pigmentation

Acromelanism

Cats with pigmented points such as the Siamese, Balinese, Himalayan and Burmese breeds have been selected for this feature. Kittens are born without points, developing pigmented extremities as a response to the lower temperature of the extremities. For the same reason these breeds will develop pigmented patches at sites of alopecia (including clipped surgical sites!). Lesions acquired later in life are often present only for one hair cycle but can be permanent.

Canine lentigo

This condition is a common disorder of mature dogs. One or more deeply pigmented macules are found on the trunk or legs and may be found in clusters. Both the number of lesions and intensity of pigmentation may increase with age. Affected dogs are unaware of the lesions. Many breeds may be affected by lentigo lesions (plural lentigines) although an hereditary form of lentigo (lentiginosis profusa) has been described in pugs.

Clinical examination reveals no evidence of systemic disease. The presence of intensely pigmented macules and patches is diagnostic.

Histological examination of biopsy specimens from affected areas will reveal the presence of areas of mild acanthosis associated with increases in melanocyte and basal cell melanosis. Lesions are often sharply demarcated.

No treatment is indicated, and there is no evidence of neoplastic transformation in these lesions in the dog.

Lentigo simplex in the ginger cat

This condition (analogous to human lentigo simplex) is characterised by the presence of intensely pigmented macules on the facial muco-cutaneous junctions of ginger (or orange) cats.

The history in unremarkable and again the problem is only cosmetic.

Lesions may be numerous, increasing with age. Histopathology is similar to that of canine lentigo and no treatment is necessary.

Acanthosis nigricans

This term has been used to describe any dog with a ventral pattern of skin disease involving acanthosis, lichenification and hyperpigmentation. It is important however to distinguish between secondary acanthosis nigricans, a reaction pattern seen with many inflammatory dermatoses (Plate 53), and primary acanthosis nigricans (Plate 52), a disease restricted in the dog to the dachshund breed.

Primary acanthosis nigricans: Clinically this disease is somewhat similar to that found in man. Although histologically the canine disease demonstrates both acanthosis and hyperpigmentation, neither of these changes are found in human patients. These changes make the primary disease indistinguishable from other inflammatory dermatoses on examination of skin biopsy specimens.

The disease affects dachshunds of either sex below one year of age. Initially lesions are restricted to bilateral hyperpigmentation, alopecia and acanthosis of axillary skin. Lesions develop to include all ventral surfaces in some dogs, leading to extensive lichenification and secondary seborrhoeic change.

The diagnosis is based upon a suitable history and appearance, together with the ruling out of other inflammatory (especially allergic) dermatoses. *Malassezia* dermatitis may closely resemble this condition in both dachshunds and basset hounds.

Treatment involves either topical glucocorticoids or Vitamin E given orally at 400 IU daily.

Secondary Acanthosis Nigricans: Any ventral inflammatory reaction involving acanthosis and hyperpigmentation can be described in this fashion, although this terminology is unhelpful on diagnostic and management grounds and should be avoided.

Treatment of dogs with this pattern **must** involve identification of underlying factors such as endocrine disease or hypersensitivity disorders and their management. In humans acanthosis nigricans is associated with malignancies in a proportion of patients - this has also been reported in the dog. Symptomatic therapy is not acceptable and is rarely effective.

Post-inflammatory hyperpigmentation

Hyperpigmentation is a common sequel to any inflammatory skin lesion in the dog or cat, being most marked in healing lesions of pyoderma or dermatophytosis. This can result in the characteristic "bulls-eye" lesion of so-called "bacterial hypersensitivity".

No specific action is required to treat the pigmentary changes associated with such lesions, although the prolonged period before resolution of these changes may be a cause of concern to some owners.

Pigmented neoplasms

Two neoplasms of clinical significance are commonly pigmented in the dog and cat. Basal cell tumours, which often have a crater-like appearance in the dog but are cystic in the cat, may be highly pigmented. Melanomata are often benign in the skin unless found in the nail bed. These neoplasms may be difficult to diagnose clinically as they are often amelanotic when poorly differentiated.

Non-neoplastic masses such as epidermoid or dermoid cysts can be heavily pigmented, as may aggregates of fibrous tissue secondary to chronic self trauma. For this reason it is always wise to submit material from pigmented masses for histopathology.

Diseases characterised by lack of pigment

Albinism

The occurrence of albinism in dogs and cats is extremely rare compared to other small domestic animals such as the rabbit and mouse.

Albinism is caused by an inherited lack of tyrosinase enzyme with a subsequent inability to produce melanin pigment. True albino animals have a lack of pigment in both the skin and iris, in contrast to animals selected for a white coat.

Albinism is generally inherited as a recessive trait.

Tyrosinase deficiency in the chow chow

A depigmenting problem affecting the hair coat and buccal mucous membranes of chow chow puppies has been reported. Affected puppies spontaneously recover however, without treatment. The course of the problem is between two and four months from development of disease to resolution.

Vitiligo

This condition is characterised by varying degrees of leukoderma and leukotrichia and may be found in both dogs and cats. The history is usually of a mature animal with progressive depigmentation of skin, hair and mucous membranes over months to years (Plate 56). The footpads and nails may also be affected. In the dog lesions often start around the nasal planum and face in a symmetrical pattern, whereas in the cat a more generalised distribution may be seen.

Affected breeds include the rottweiler, German shepherd dog, Belgian tervuren and doberman pinscher. Siamese cats are also affected, as may be crossbred dogs and cats.

Examination reveals no evidence of systemic disease in most cases. In humans vitiligo may be associated with systemic disease including neoplasia, pernicious anaemia and diabetes mellitus, but this has not been reported in the dog or cat. Depigmentation at the site of previous trauma is relatively common in these species.

Affected skin is of normal thickness and, similarly, hairs appear structurally normal. The distribution of depigmented hairs may be either clumped, possibly representing the contents of single compound follicles, or individually distributed within the coat.

Diagnosis is made on the basis of history, clinical signs and skin biopsy, if appropriate. Histological signs are confined to the pigmentary apparatus, with a complete absence of melanocytes and melanin pigment. The histological diagnosis of vitiligo when only leukotrichia is present is more difficult.

Suggested pathogeneses of vitiligo includes heredity and auto-immunity. Evidence for the latter has been produced in the detection of anti-melanocyte antibody in the Belgian tervuren.

There is no effective treatment for vitiligo, and the problem is only a cosmetic one.

Nasal depigmentation

A localised form of depigmentation in the dog is not uncommonly found in several large breeds including the German shepherd dog, labrador and golden retrievers. Again a problem of young, mature dogs, affected individuals are presented for progressive depigmentation affecting the nasal planum only. No other clinical signs are present and again there is no effective treatment. Show dogs may be considered at fault for this abnormality, and hence are presented to veterinary surgeons by their owners.

Periocular leukotrichia

In acromelanic breeds of cat such as the Siamese, metabolic stress, systemic disease or the administration of some drugs (e.g. beta-lactam antibiotics) can result in the appearance of periocular depigmentation of hairs. This can present either as localised bands of periocular depigmentation (goggles) or the more generalised appearance of a speckled mask. These changes usually resolve at the next hair cycle if the source of stress has been removed.

Unilateral periocular leukotrichia has been reported associated with Horner's syndrome, corneal necrosis and upper respiratory infection in Siamese cats.

Diseases associated with macro-melanosomes

A number of dermatological and systemic diseases have been reported which are characterised by the presence of abnormally large melanin granules in hairs. These are not always associated with clinical skin disease however, and so this finding alone on histopathology or examination of hair pluckings must be interpreted with care.

Chediak-Higashi syndrome

An autosomal recessive disorder of "blue smoke" longhair cats with yellow eyes, this syndrome is associated with large granules in many cells including melanocytes and neutrophils. Resultant systemic disorders in this disease include susceptibility to infection and a bleeding disorder. There is no effective treatment. As with all inherited disorders, affected cats should not be used for breeding.

Colour-dilution alopecia

This condition, known variously as blue doberman disease, colour mutant alopecia and fawn Irish setter syndrome, is an inheritable follicular dysplasia (Plates 54 and 55). The history in affected dogs, which may be of any colour dilute breed, is typified by the gradual loss of coat from the trunk and proximal limbs. In dogs with tan points, these remain unaffected. Blue doberman pinschers are almost invariably affected with this disease.

Examination reveals the coat to be harsh, of moth eaten appearance and often scaly and dry. Close examination with a hand lens may demonstrate poor quality hairs with broken shafts. Lesions of secondary pyoderma are commonly found and the author has seen several affected dobermans with concurrent demodicosis. The diagnosis is based on the history, clinical examination, examination of skin scrapings and hair plucks and histopathology. Examination of hairs taken from affected areas show variable quantities of large pigment granules within the hair shaft and attached to the root. Hairs may have shaft fractures and be contorted at the root. Microscopy of skin scrapings often reveal large numbers of highly pigmented comedones, with or without damaged hair remnants. Histopathology is characterised by the presence of abnormal follicles containing variable numbers of macro-melanosomes. Pigmentary incontinence and the presence of macro-melanosomes within dermal melanocytes may be seen. Hairs may be missing entirely or obviously dysplastic.

The management of this disease is based on ameliorating the keratinisation disorder and pyoderma associated with the follicular changes. The alopecia cannot be treated and tends to be progressive. Topical anti-seborrhoeic shampoos may be used (Chapter 26), together with essential fatty acid supplementation. Concurrent demodicosis should be managed in the usual way (Chapter 29).

Black hair follicle dysplasia

An identical syndrome to that found in colour dilute dogs may be seen in dogs with a black coat. This includes crossbred dogs and Gordon setters. The history is similar, with gradual coat loss and thinning in affected areas, although changes are confined to the black areas of the coat. Again there is no specific treatment.

Depigmentation associated with autoimmunity

Loss of pigment may be associated with autoimmunity in diseases other than vitiligo.

Alopecia areata

This condition is a cell mediated inflammatory disorder directed at hair bulb melanocytes. Clinical signs include focal alopecia, with hairs regrowing white. Spontaneous resolution may occur, but this is variable.

Diagnosis depends upon the finding of characteristic peribulbar aggregates of mononuclear cells on histopathology. The demonstration of such lesions may be very difficult, but is most likely in biopsy specimens taken from the advancing edge of lesions.

No specific treatment is possible and the course may be long.

The author has seen one Bernese mountain dog with concurrent alopecia areata and vitiligo. This is not surprising bearing in mind the antimelanocytic nature of both conditions.

Canine nasal dermatitis

This is a group of conditions which are often exacerbated by sunlight exposure. The mechanism in these conditions appears to be related to damage to the basement membrane. Signs include alopecia, crusting and ulceration of the nasal planum and dorsal nasal skin. Depigmentation of affected areas is common and may make the area more prone to actinic (sunlight induced) damage.

Many of these cases are either discoid lupus erythematosus or pemphigus erythematosus. The management of these conditions is discussed in Chapter 32. Para-amino benzoic acid sun blocks may have some effect in limiting actinic damage, but are rapidly removed from the nasal planum by licking.

Vogt-Koyanagi-Harada like syndrome

This disease, characterised by progressive depigmentation and concurrent uveitis, is a rare disorder of Japanese akitas, Siberian huskies and samoyeds. Diagnosis is made by appropriate history, clinical signs and skin biopsies. Treatment with glucocorticoids may be successful for the dermal component of the disease, but owners should be warned that the uveitis is of greater significance and referral to an ophthalmologist should be considered.

Systemic lupus erythematosus

Depigmenting or alopecic skin disease may be features of this polysystemic disease.

Depigmentation associated with physical and chemical insults

Depigmentation may occur as a sequel to many chemical and physical insults including contact reaction to plasticisers in bowls or toys, actinic damage and as a sequel to irradiation for the treatment of neoplasia. Such lack of pigment is sometimes reversed by the removal of the inciting cause, but may be permanent.

Depigmentation associated with neoplasia

Leukotrichia may be a feature of epitheliotropic lymphoma (mycosis fungoides). This condition can be an exfoliative dermatosis, but may present in the same way as alopecia areata, i.e. involving alopecia and localised leukotrichia.

As discussed earlier, neoplasia may be an underlying feature in vitiligo.

FURTHER READING

BRIGGS, O. M., (1985) Lentiginosis profusa in the pug: three case reports. *Journal of Small Animal Practice.* **26**, 675.

HARGIS, A. M., BRIGNAC, M. M., KAREEM AL-BAGDADI, F. A., MUGGLI, F. AND MUNDELL, A. (1991) Black hair follicular dysplasia in black and white saluki dogs: differentiation from color mutant alopecia in the doberman pinscher by microscopic examination of hairs. *Veterinary Dermatology,* **2**, 69.

MILLER JR., W. H., (1990) Colour dilution alopecia in doberman pinschers with fawn or blue coat colours: a study on the incidence and histopathology of this disorder. *Veterinary Dermatology,* **1**, 113.

CHAPTER TEN

FOCAL ALOPECIA IN THE DOG

David I Grant

INTRODUCTION

Focal alopecia in the dog is a common diagnostic problem in small animal practice. The alopecia may consist of one circular patch on any part of the body, or may be multifocal with a moth eaten appearance. Pruritus may be present or absent, or the condition may have started as non-pruritic with the development of pruritus subsequently. There are a number of potential causes, some common and others quite rare (Table 1) and the clinician will need to adopt a painstaking approach to the problem, allied to a knowledge of the typical signs of each disease, in order to formulate a diagnostic plan.

Table 1

Some possible conditions causing focal alopecia in the dog

> Dermatophytosis eg. *M.canis, T.mentagrophytes*
> Folliculitis — *S.intermedius*
> Demodicosis — *D.canis*
> Circular wounds, abrasions
> Flea-bite hypersensitivity
> Contact hypersensitivity
> Food hypersensitivity
> Atopy
> Autoimmune and immune mediated disease
> Alopecia areata
> Dermatomyositis
> Follicular dysplasia
> Colour dilution alopecia
> Infection with *Malassezia pachydermatis*
> Scabies — *Sarcoptes scabiei* (in early stages)
> Infestation with *Cheyletiella* spp.
> Hypersensitivity to *Otodectes cynotis*
> Zinc responsive dermatosis
> Mycosis fungoides

APPROACH TO THE CASE

As many of the diseases listed in Table 1 cannot be differentiated by physical examination alone, it will be necessary to formulate a diagnostic plan. Time must be allocated, so that a logical approach described in Chapter 2 may be followed.

Much of the diagnostic information is derived from the first essential procedures – the history and physical examination. Subsequent examinations will need less time if a meticulous and logical plan has been followed right from the outset.

Taking the history

The author usually takes the history without looking at the dog – this avoids distractions, the temptation to jump to conclusions and also helps to concentrate the mind of the owner who will be listening to the questions and not having to restrain the dog.

The age, breed and sex of the dog is noted.

AGE

In general diseases such as dermatophytosis, staphylococcal folliculitis (Plate 25), demodicosis, atopy and dermatomyositis will occur more frequently in younger dogs. For example, atopic dogs usually show symptoms for the first time between the ages of 1 to 3 years. Demodicosis is mainly seen in dogs less than a year old, the adult form of the disease being very much rarer. Most cases of dermatomyositis are recognised by 6 months of age.

BREED

Several breeds of dog are predisposed to conditions listed in Table 1. Dermatomyositis is seen in rough collies and Shetland sheepdogs. Demodicosis is commonly a disease of short-coated breeds such as the doberman pinscher, English bulldog, Chinese shar pei, beagle, and Staffordshire bull terrier, although some long-haired breeds are also susceptible, eg. the old English sheepdog, collie, Afghan hound, West Highland white terrier and German shepherd dog. Atopy affects many breeds such as the boxer, cairn terrier, English setter and West Highland white terrier. Black hair follicular dysplasia has been recognised in the bearded collie, dachshund, basset hound, schipperke and papillon. Colour dilution alopecia is described particularly in blue dobermans, but also in the fawn Irish setter, red and fawn doberman pinscher, blue dachshund, blue chow, blue standard poodle, blue great Dane, blue Italian greyhound and the blue whippet. The Alaskan malamute and the Siberian husky are susceptible to zinc responsive dermatosis.

SEX

Conditions such as Sertoli's cell tumour or ovarian imbalances are restricted to males or females respectively and will be considered in the differential diagnosis accordingly.

The clinician will need to know when the problem began and what treatment if any has been given. If the patient has been treated previously, although symptoms may have been masked, the response to treatment may give useful diagnostic clues. For example, a good response to glucocorticoids is seen initially in atopy, but not always in food hypersensitivity. Lack of response or deterioration may suggest drug eruption. A deterioration following the use of glucocorticoids may suggest demodicosis or staphylococcal folliculitis. Are other animals kept in the same environment? Is the condition contagious to animals? Are there zoonotic lesions? Dermatophytosis, fleas or scabies should be considered if there is evidence of contagion.

It is essential to ascertain whether the condition is pruritic. A useful procedure is to teach the owner to score the level of pruritus. For example, a dog without skin lesions and which hardly ever scratches would be allocated 0/10. A dog with severe generalised scabies which constantly scratches day and night is given 10/10. Although this is subjective, many cases of atopy will be around 5/10. If these cases are complicated by secondary pyoderma the level will rise to 7/10 or higher. Such information is useful as base line data to be compared following therapy. It is also useful as a means of educating the owner about the pathogenesis of pruritus, and gradual improvement following therapy may be appreciated more easily. In some pruritic conditions, the owner will be able to describe particularly favoured sites for the dog to scratch or lick, for example the face, feet and ventrum in atopy, the pinnae, elbows, limbs and brisket in scabies, the posterior dorsal lumbar region in flea bite hypersensitivity.

Conditions may be non-pruritic at first, only to become pruritic with the advent of secondary pyoderma. Demodicosis is a prime example. If staphylococcal folliculitis is inadequately treated, or mismanaged with glucocorticoids, the history will usually be one of a gradual increasing level of pruritus, extension of lesions and an increasing requirement for glucocorticoids. In these cases subsequent effective management of the folliculitis with long term appropriate antibacterial therapy will diminish or eliminate the pruritus – depending on the underlying cause.

Note should be made of the diet. Dogs fed on good quality canned food are unlikely to suffer from diet related dermatological conditions. Zinc responsive dermatosis in the United Kingdom. has been mainly associated with the feeding of dry cereal based food. The incidence of this condition has been lessened due to the manufacturers adding extra zinc to such diets. Cases are still seen, however, associated with some dry dog food, or in association with malabsorption. A note of the components of the dog's diet is made. Such information is essential if food hypersensitivity is suspected, as in subsequent investigations a diet unfamiliar to the dog will need to be fed.

An assessment of the dog's ability to digest and absorb food can be made from the history. Dogs which regularly vomit or have persistent diarrhoea may be suffering from a maldigestion or malabsorption problem which could be responsible for the cutaneous signs under investigation. While questioning about the diet, note of water intake is made. Although owners are often vague about the exact quantity drunk it should be possible to establish whether this appears abnormal or not, and if doubt exists precise measurement can be made either by the owner or during hospitalisation. Polydipsia is an important sign with hyperadrenocorticism.

Are the problems seasonal - or were they seasonal initially? These are important questions when evaluating possible hypersensitivity disorders. Seasonality suggests atopy and/or flea bite hypersensitivity which in turn may both be possible underlying causes of staphylococcal folliculitis. Seasonality may also be a feature of contact hypersensitivity to grass pollen. Assessment of the dog's environment is useful here. Where does it go for walks? What does it come into contact with? The owner should be asked about the dog's exercise tolerance at this stage. Poor exercise tolerance is often noted with hypothyroidism and hyperadrenocorticism, the former being an important underlying cause of staphylococcal folliculitis.

Following a careful history, a good assessment should have been made of the problem, including some ideas as to possible causes, and a appreciation of the dog's general health will have been obtained. The next step is to build on this information by means of the physical examination, which will include a separate dermatological examination.

THE PHYSICAL EXAMINATION

The purpose of the physical examination is to find evidence of conditions which may be the cause of the skin problem, but also to find out if concurrent disorders exist. For example, it is helpful to be aware of the existence of cardiac valvular disease prior to treating a hypothyroid dog, as high levels of thyroxine too quickly introduced may precipitate cardiac insufficiency.

The examination is performed systematically starting at the head and working backwards. Particular note is made of the lymph nodes, (which may be enlarged in demodicosis and folliculitis), and muscle mass (atrophied in hyperadrenocorticism). The heart and lungs are auscultated and the abdomen is palpated. Hepatomegaly is often a feature of hyperadrenocorticism.

Specific points in the dermatological examination are:

a)   **The site of the lesions**. In dermatomyositis, a newly described condition affecting rough collies, these are initially seen around the lips, nose and face, and the tips of the ears. In demodicosis, the lesions will be found on the face and feet. Occasionally, cases of demodicosis present with solitary patches of alopecia anywhere on the body. Hypersensitivity disorders tend to have lesions in well defined areas. For example in flea bite hypersensitivity, the lesions occur especially on the posterior dorsum. In atopy they are seen on the face, feet and ventrum or combinations thereof. Cases of plastic dish dermatitis or hypersensitivity to toys will tend to have lesions on the mouth and lips.

b) **The nature of the lesions.** The alopecic patches may be non-inflammatory or there may be obvious self-trauma inducing the lesions. Is there obvious inflammatory pathological change, eg. generalised erythema, which might suggest an underlying pruritic cause? Are there any pustules or papules – suggesting pyoderma?

c) **The symmetry of the lesions.** Bilaterally symmetrical alopecia suggests a hormonal cause, for example a patch of alopecia on each flank is typically seen in hypothyroidism.

d) **Evidence of ectoparasites.** A careful search is made for fleas or flea dirt. Even if the lesions are not caused by fleas, there is the possibility that folliculitis could be secondary to flea bite hypersensitivity. Any pruritus caused by fleas will in any case add to the clinical signs due to self trauma from scratching and resultant skin changes.

e) **The texture and elasticity of the coat.** Endocrine diseases are noted for a preponderance of hairs in the telogen phase, which are easy to epilate. The skin is thin and inelastic in cases of hyperadrenocorticism, and may feel thickened and cool to the touch in hypothyroidism. In early cases of scabies with alopecic areas localised to the pinnae, a useful test is to rub the ear with the finger and thumb. This usually provokes a pronounced scratch reflex which is highly suggestive although not pathognomonic.

ESTABLISHING THE DIAGNOSIS

It is important to recognise and to explain to the owner that in many cases even after the most careful history and physical examination, the diagnosis is not yet possible. There will inevitably, however, be several possibilities. A period of five minutes spent thinking about these possibilities is most valuable at this stage. Much information both from the owner and from the clinician's own observations will have been amassed. It is necessary to consider other aspects. For example, the lesion may look like ringworm, but this is a rare disease in the dog. Staphylococcal folliculitis is more likely. Demodicosis (Plate 32) should always be suspected in focal alopecia, but if the dog is five years old and the condition has only just begun it is less likely. Atopy, hypothyroidism, staphylococcal folliculitis and demodicosis are all fairly common. Dermatophytosis, contact hypersensitivity, autoimmune disorders and food hypersensitivity are all rare, although there is some controversy about the prevalence of the latter. During the five minute thinking time a list of the possible diseases can be made, starting with the most likely and ending with the least likely according to the clinician's judgement in the particular case.

Having made the list, the priority of the investigative techniques can now be established. This is important because in practice many owners are unwilling to pay for a large number of investigations all performed at the same time. There are nonetheless some procedures which will be necessary in virtually all cases. These are skin scrapings, tape strips and hair pluckings for subsequent microscopical examination. These procedures are discussed in detail in Chapter 3.

Further investigations will depend on the findings to date in an individual case. A pustule with a hair protruding from it is highly suggestive of staphylococcal folliculitis. A pustule can be pricked with a sterile 25 gauge needle, the contents smeared on a slide, air dried and stained. The presence of large numbers of micrococci confirms pyoderma and antibacterial therapy is often initiated on an empirical basis. Alternatively in recurrent or deep pyodermas culture and antibacterial sensitivity may be undertaken.

INITIAL MANAGEMENT

It can be difficult to distinguish clinically between dermatophytosis and staphylococcal folliculitis. In such cases mycological culture is necessary. In the meantime while waiting for the results of the culture a 3 to 4 week course of systemic antibacterial therapy can be made empirically. Suitable antibacterial agents include erythromycin, lincomycin,and potentiated sulphonamides. Detail of antibacterial therapy is discussed in Chapter 25. Good response to such treatment is strong supportive evidence for the diagnosis of staphylococcal folliculitis.

There are many other diagnostic tests which may be necessary if there is still no conclusive diagnosis. These may include a basal assay of blood for thyroxine concentration, a thyroid stimulating hormone (TSH) response test, an adrenocorticotropic hormone (ACTH) response test, low and high dose dexamethasone response tests, trial "hypoallergenic" diets, elimination and provocative exposure procedures for contact hypersensitivity allied with patch testing, intradermal allergy testing, zinc administration, and haematology and biochemical profiles.

Finally the value of histopathology cannot be stressed enough. Valuable information is obtained in most of the conditions listed in Table 1. In some disorders, alopecia areata for example, or autoimmune diseases, the diagnosis cannot be made without a cutaneous biopsy, and if these conditions are suspected this procedure will be one of the first to be performed. Biopsy has often been the means of diagnosis in other conditions such as demodicosis and dermatophytosis. Methods of biopsy sampling are described in Chapter 3. The specimen should be sent to a veterinary histopathologist with an expertise in dermatology, and the clinician is advised to supply comprehensive case details to aid the pathologist.

Focal alopecia in the dog, like many other dermatological conditions can be diagnosed and managed successfully in many instances. Time, thought and planning are necessary and it is hoped that this chapter will have helped to suggest the principles that will lead to effective diagnosis and treatment.

FURTHER READING

BAKER, K.P. and THOMSETT L.R. (1990). *Canine and Feline Dermatology*. Blackwell Scientific Publications, Oxford.

MULLER, G.H., KIRK, R.W. and SCOTT, D.W. (1989). *Small Animal Dermatology* 4th. Edn. W.B. Saunders Co., Philadelphia.

NESBIT, G.H. and ACKERMANN, L.J. (1991). Eds. *Dermatology for the Small Animal Practitioner*, Veterinary Learning Systems Co. Inc.

FOCAL ALOPECIA IN THE CAT

Craig E Griffin ——————————————————————

INTRODUCTION

Alopecia can occur as a result of many diseases and is a common aspect of feline skin disease. In general, two basic mechanisms may occur; failure to grow hair (eg. genetically programmed endocrine, nutritional or metabolic alopecia) or abnormal loss of hair. The majority of feline alopecia cases present because of abnormal loss of hair. This may result from hair breaking off (eg., dermatophytosis, excessive licking/chewing/scratching) or hair falling out (eg., post inflammatory, telogen effluvium, folliculitis, hormonal, some drug reactions). Self trauma from licking or scratching is the commonest cause of alopecia. Some cases may result from a combination of the two mechanisms (eg., hormonal and some drug reactions).

The majority of skin diseases in the cat result in some degree of alopecia however, certain presentations are more common. Unless there is a finding suggesting a uncommon disease is present then the more common causes of focal alopecia should initially be pursued (Table 1). The initial approach is to determine if the alopecia is focal, multifocal, regional or generalised. There may be an overlap or progression from one to another of these patterns. This discussion will be directed at the diseases that often present with, or initially start as focal non-regional alopecia. The diseases that often present with small focal, non-regional alopecia are dermatophytosis, mosquito bite and idiopathic eosinophilic granulomas, solar dermatitis and squamous cell carcinomas, contact dermatitis, localised demodicosis, injection reactions, pyoderma and stud tail. Psychogenic alopecia and atopy often start with focal alopecia which usually spreads into a regional pattern. Flea allergy and food allergy usually start with a regional pattern although initially lesions may be relatively focal within the region.

APPROACH TO THE CASE

Initially the signalment (breed, age and sex) should be determined as it is helpful in ranking the differentials as predispositions may be present. Young cats are more likely to present with dermatophytosis or genetic alopecia. Allergic and psychogenic alopecia is seen more in the young adult to middle aged cats while neoplastic diseases occur more in old cats. Knowledge of the breed may also be helpful as dermatophytosis should always be high on the list of differential diagnoses for alopecia in the Persian or Himalayan cat (Plates 29 and 30). Coat colour is important as solar dermatitis occurs in white cats with a white nasal planum and pinnae. Psychogenic alopecia occurs in breeds that are more easily stressed such as with Siamese and Abyssinian cats.

After the signalment, a thorough history should be obtained. The major objectives of the history are to determine whether:
1. The alopecia is due to excessive loss of hair. This most often results from pruritus, but increased shedding or breaking of hair and failure of hair growth may also occur.
2. Pruritus is present.
3. Any previous medications or injections that may be associated with alopecia have been given. Especially important are glucocorticoids (oral, injectable or topical), progestagens (oral or injectable), vaccinations and worming injections.

4. The alopecia is associated with erythema, scaling, crusts, nodules, or plaques.
5. The lesion is enlarging. (The pattern of the lesion should be noted)
6. Any environmental factors are present that may be involved in lesion development (eg., outdoor cats are more frequently exposed to insects, fleas, contact irritants and other cats with contagious diseases)
7. The response to any previous therapies
8. Any psychological disturbances were associated with the onset of the alopecia
9. There is any seasonality to the disease. Seasonal problems strongly suggest an environmental problem - fleas, atopy.
10. There are any other abnormal signs or symptoms. Thus gastrointestinal symptoms may be seen in food allergic cats.

Determining pruritus can be difficult in the cat as many will hide while grooming excessively and owners may not be aware their cat is pruritic. In other cases, the owner may observe excessive grooming but consider it normal. Other historical information that may help determine whether pruritus is present include: vomiting of hair balls, hair in faeces noted when cleaning litter pans, tufts of hair in favourite resting or hiding areas or the cat hiding more frequently. Although the

Table 1
Common causes of focal alopecia in the cat

DISEASE	COMMON LOCATION	SHORT, STUBBY BROKEN HAIR
Dermatophytosis	Facial, pinna, anywhere	+
Cheyletiellosis	Dorsal thorax	+/-
Otodectic mange	Facial	+/-
Allergy		
Flea	Neck, Dorsal lumbar	+
Food	Periauricular, face	+
Atopy	Abdomen, groin	+
Mosquito	Nose, pinnae	-
Contact Dermatitis	Paws, abdomen, pinnae	-/+
Idiopathic eosinophilia	Neck, extremities	-/+
Psychogenic alopecia	Abdomen, groin	+
Solar dermatitis/ squamous cell carcin.	Nose, pinnae	-
Pemphigus foliaceous		-
Genetic	Face, head, anywhere	-
Localized demodicosis	Face, abdomen	-
Injection reaction	Dorsal cervical, shoulder	-
Pyoderma	Anywhere	+/-
Stud tail	Tail	-

96

client may not initially be aware of this information they should be instructed to investigate when returning home after the consultation. Contagion to humans or other pets as well as access to other pets, outdoor environments, kennels, catteries or cat shows should also be ascertained. If lesions affect other pets or humans, dermatophytosis, cheyletiellosis or flea infection are the most likely diagnosis. In contrast, infection of only one cat in a multi cat environment would make cheyletiellosis less likely and is somewhat uncommon with dermatophytosis.

PHYSICAL EXAMINATION

The physical examination is extremely valuable in helping determine the most likely differential diagnosis. The pattern of involvement and presence of short stubby hairs quickly allows the clinician to rank the most common differentials (Table 1). The presence or absence of inflammation characterized by erythema, papules, crusts or erosions is also helpful in determining which diseases to consider (Table 2). Gross inflammation may not be visible in some cats but may be present histologically if clinically non-inflammatory skin is biopsied. Alopecic areas should be closely inspected to determine if hair loss is complete or if short stubby hairs are still present. This may be ascertained by rubbing the fingertips against the normal direction of hair growth for that body region. Another helpful technique is to roll or fold the skin so the remaining hair will be elevated from the margin of the skin fold. A complete physical examination should also be made. Lymphadenopathy may be noted in cats with some allergic or neoplastic diseases.

ESTABLISHING THE DIAGNOSIS

The initial step in establishing the diagnosis is to develop a problem list and then a list of differential diagnoses which might result in these problems. This process is based on the historical and physical examination findings. This list should be organised so that the most likely diagnoses comprise the top two or three differentials. Unless there is compelling evidence, uncommon or rare diseases should not be high on this list. The diagnostic procedures or therapeutic recommendations will be determined from the differential diagnosis list. The client's willingness (or otherwise) to countenance diagnostic tests will often influence the approach and may result in trial therapy for the most likely differential. In practice, the approach to a cat with focal alopecia should include consideration of costs. In general, diagnostic tests and trial therapies should only be recommended for those diseases that are high on the differential list. Where an inexpensive test will diagnose or rule out a primary differential then that test should be recommended. It is not cost effective to run tests for diseases not high on the differential diagnosis list, nor is it cost effective to run inexpensive tests that will not address the likely differentials unless they are indicated. For example, consider a white cat with alopecia on the ear tip associated with erythema, scale and crust. Dermatophytosis and solar dermatitis are the most likely differentials. In this case, skin scrapes for ectoparasites and cytologic evaluation are not cost effective. Instead, a fungal culture and histopathological examination of biopsies are indicated. If squamous cell carcinoma is suspected and cost is a major factor to the client a biopsy should be performed before spending money on a fungal culture. A biopsy is required to diagnose squamous cell carcinoma and may add information about the possible presence of dermatophytosis as well. A positive fungal culture does not rule out underlying solar dermatitis.

The following tests and their indications are most commonly utilised as the initial diagnostic approach in cats with focal alopecia. The first five investigations are relatively inexpensive tests. These are recommended initially for any of the top few differentials. Tests 6, 7 and 8 are more expensive and are recommended only when they are likely to lead to a definitive diagnosis.

1. Examination of the hair shafts (Figure 1)
2. Microscopical examination of skin scrapings
3. Examination using a Wood's light
4. Fungal culture of hair and scale
5. Cytological evaluation of impression and aspiration samples
6. Allergy testing using restricted and provocative feeding trials and intradermal skin testing
7. Histopathological examination of biopsy specimens
8. Complete haematology, plasma biochemistry and ELISA assays for FeLV and FIV
9. Restriction or confinement of the cat to aid in the diagnosis of contact dermatitis, flea allergy dermatitis or mosquito hypersensitivity.

Table 2
Correlation of the more common causes of focal alopecia with the presence or absence of lesions

DISEASE	INFLAMMATION	DIAGNOSTIC TESTS	FREQUENCY OF OCCURENCE
Dermatophytosis	-/+	Fungal culture	High
Cheyletiellosis	+/-	Scrapings + response to therapy	High
Otodectic mange	+	Scrapings + response to therapy	High
Allergy - Flea	+/-	IDST, response to flea control	High
Food	+/-	Hypo diet trial	Moderate
Atopy	-/+	IDST	High
Mosq. bite hyp.	+	Avoidance, and exposure, ? IDST	Rare
Contact Dermatitis	+	Response to avoidance	Rare
Idiopathic eosinophilic granuloma	+	Biopsy	Rare
Psychogenic Alopecia	-	Biopsy	Moderate
Solar dermatitis/ squamous cell carcin.	+	Biopsy	Moderate
Pemphigus foliaceous	+	Biospy	Rare
Genetic	-	Biopsy	Rare
Localised demodicosis	-/+	Skin scrape	Rare
Injection reaction	-/+	History, biopsy	Rare
Pyoderma	+	Biopsy and response to therapy	Rare
Stud tail	+/-	Physical exam., biopsy	Rare

IDST = Intra dermal skin test

INITIAL MANAGEMENT

The examination of hair samples, skin scrapings and fungal cultures, the consideration of the results of allergy tests and the study of histopathological reports will allow the clinician to identify the cause in most cases of feline focal alopecia. However, in some cases, response to trial therapy is often needed to help make a diagnosis. In some cases trial therapy is undertaken because the client requests that it is employed either before, or instead of, definitive tests. In these cases trial therapies should be selected that have some specificity of effect in order to help establish the diagnosis.

Figure 1
Fractured hairs from licking
Can be demonstrated by microscopy of hair from affected regions

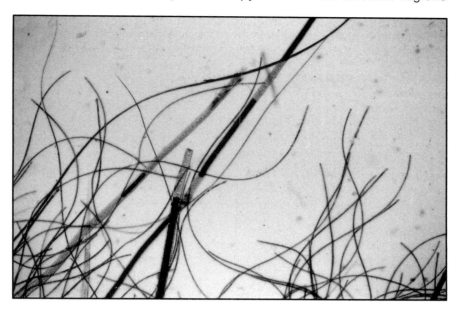

Trial therapies most commonly utilised by the author include antibiotics, antihistamines and the use of Elizabethan collars to determine if alopecia is self induced. In cases with inflammation, crusts or papules, trial therapy with flea control, antibiotics or the antihistamine chlorpheniramine (0.4 mg/kg/bid) may be tried. Antibiotics most commonly utilised by the author in cats are trimethoprim-sulfadiazine (30 mg/kg bid) and cefadroxil (22 mg/kg bid). Trimethoprim-sulfadiazine can cause excessive salivation which is not harmful but is very messy and disconcerting to the owner. It is usually self limiting within 30 minutes and will often only occur following the first couple of doses. Cefadroxil causes frequent problems with diarrhoea or soft stools.

Without an appropriate diagnosis which indicates their use, corticosteroids should be avoided until these other trial therapies have been utilised. Even in cases with a suspected diagnosis of eosinophilic granuloma, initial therapy with antibiotics is preferred as some cases will respond favourably.

Corticosteroids are helpful, at least temporarily, in many diseases but do not significantly add to the diagnostic information. In other cases glucocorticoids may aggravate the disease and are associated with more harm than the other trial therapies described. A temporary, favorable response to corticosteroids may be seen with pyoderma or dermatophytosis but it eventually results in progression of the disease.

In cases where dermatophytosis is suspected trial therapy should be greatly discouraged unless a lesion is focal and localised. Even in these cases it is only appropriate to use a topical antifungal lotion such as 1% miconazole. In dermatophytosis, early lesions may not be grossly apparent and will develop into active disease while the treated lesions respond. At this point a fungal culture, if not already done, should be obtained as systemic therapy may be required. Systemic therapy should not be prescribed until a definitive diagnosis of dermatophytosis is made.

In suspected cases of psychogenic alopecia, trial therapy with diazepam (0.2 mg/kg bid) is recommended initially. Phenobarbital (2-5 mg/kg sid-bid) may be recommended if diazepam is ineffective.

Suspected atopic or flea allergic cats may respond to trial therapy with fatty acids (Derm Caps, DVM; or Efavet, Efamol Vet) or antihistamines (chlorpheniramine 0.4 mg/kg bid or hydroxyzine 2 mg/kg bid). These types of trial therapies are preferable to glucocorticoids or progestagens because in addition to possibly controlling or eliminating the problem they will add to the diagnostic information. In contrast, trial therapy with glucocorticoids or progestagens will not add as much diagnostic information and are associated with more serious side effects. Once a specific diagnosis is made the appropriate therapy and/or preventative measures for that disease should be prescribed.

REFERENCES AND FURTHER READING

FOIL, C. (1993). Dermatophytosis. In: *Current Veterinary Dermatology*. (Eds. C.E. Griffin, K.W. Kwochka, and MacDonald) p. 22-33. Mosby Year Book

GRIFFEN, C. E. (1993). Approach to Feline Alopecia. *Proceedings Waltham Feline Symposium*, Orlando, FL. Veterinary Learning Systems. in press.

SCHMEITZAL, L. P. (1989). Alopecia. In: *Textbook of Veterinary Internal Medicine* (Ed. S. Ettinger) 3rd pp. 113-121.

WHITE, S. D. (1991). Pyoderma in Five Cats. *Journal of the American Animal Hospital Association*, **27**: 141-146.

SYMMETRICAL ALOPECIA IN THE DOG

Ewan A Ferguson

Dogs with non-pruritic, symmetrical alopecia are regularly encountered in both referral and first opinion clinics (Plates 22-27). It has been common practice to ascribe this clinical presentation to an endocrinopathy and in the majority of cases this assumption will be correct. However, there are a number of important dermatoses which may mimic the typical "endocrine pattern" and these should be eliminated from the list of differential diagnoses at an early stage. The mechanisms by which endocrinopathies affect the skin and hair follicles are, for the most part, still poorly defined but an increasing appreciation of the importance of adrenal sex hormones and improved understanding of the physiology of the gonads and peripheral target tissues has prompted the re-evaluation of several previously described endocrine dermatoses. The complex interplay that exists between the steroid hormones can make the interpretation of laboratory data difficult and the importance of a thorough history and physical examination cannot be over-emphasised.

The aim of this chapter is to provide the clinician with a guide towards the systematic investigation of the non-pruritic dog presenting with symmetrical alopecia. Aspects of the history and clinical examination which have particular relevance to this group of dermatoses are emphasised. The laboratory investigations that may be performed to aid or support diagnosis are discussed and their interpretation summarised. Practical aspects are stressed over detailed discussion and a recommended reading list is provided for those who wish to explore the subject further.

APPROACH TO THE CASE

On initial presentation, the first decision that will have to be made will focus upon whether or not the alopecia present is associated primarily with an endocrine disturbance or whether there are alternative or additional disease processes involved. Figure 1 outlines a diagnostic plan for the investigation of symmetrical alopecia.

HISTORY AND PHYSICAL EXAMINATION

A detailed history and clinical examination are mandatory and will provide valuable clues as to the nature of the disease process. The overall health and physique, exercise tolerance and physical condition of the animal should be assessed. Chest auscultation and abdominal palpation should be performed. Thirst and appetite may be altered. The age at onset is an important consideration; congenital alopecias, follicular dysplasias and other ectodermal defects will be apparent at or shortly after birth whilst pattern baldness may manifest only when the puppy coat is shed or at puberty. Endocrine related alopecias generally develop in previously normal adults. Congenital endocrinopathies such as pituitary dwarfism frequently involve more than one endocrine system and usually adversely affect growth and physique, As a result, diagnosis should not present a problem.

The sex and reproductive status are important considerations with the sex-hormone related dermatoses. If one or both testicles are absent from the scrotum, it must be determined whether this is the result of surgery or cryptorchidism. Some breeds are at greater risk of developing certain endocrinopathies and many of the non-endocrine alopecias are heritable or have strong breed predispositions. If any hair regrowth has occurred, it is important to ascertain whether this has been spontaneous or associated with oestrus, treatment or season. Rarely, dietary history may suggest a vitamin or mineral imbalance as the cause of non-pruritic hair loss.

Figure 1
Diagnostic plan for non-pruritic symmetrical alopecia in the dog

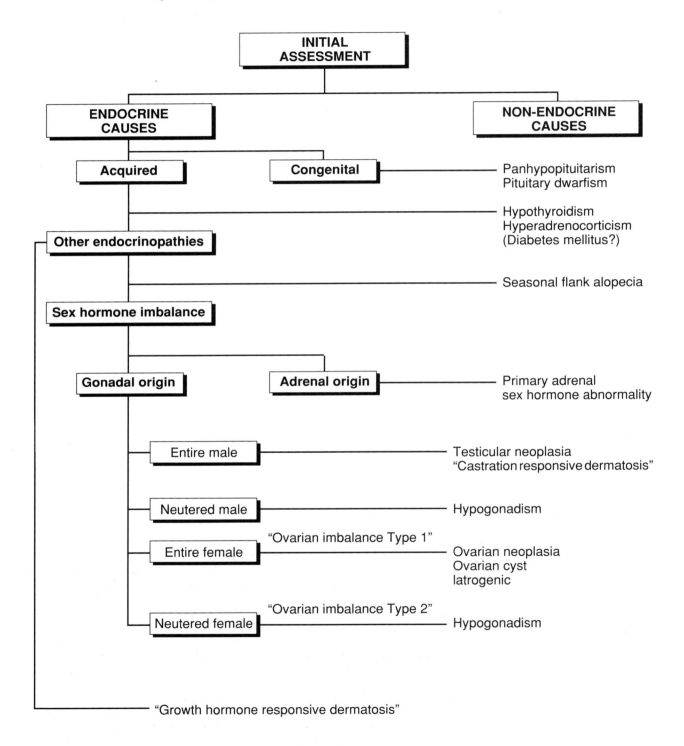

Examination of the skin

Close examination of alopecic skin can be particularly rewarding. The pathological changes which occur in the skin are not diagnostic of endocrine disease but consistent patterns do appear. The epidermis may be normal or show mild to moderate thickening. Epidermal and follicular hyperplasia are common as are changes in pigmentation. Clinically, these usually manifest as hyperpigmentation, lichenification and comedone formation, particularly around the nipples. Heavy scaling and flaking of the superficial epidermis are not normally seen although mild scaling and moderate to severe seborrhoea may be. However, in hyperadrenocorticism the epidermis may be atrophic, leading to increased cutaneous fragility and dermal telangectectasia.

Endocrine-associated alopecia occurs as the follicles undergo hair growth cycle arrest, entering a prolonged catagen or telogen phase. The hairs that are present are normal and have tapered points. Broken hairs strongly suggest self-trauma and this is normally indicative of pruritus. Unless there are also signs of secondary bacterial infection such as papules, pustules and collarettes or of erythema, lichenification and seborrhoea suggestive of a *Malassezia* dermatitis, the presence of pruritus would tend to direct attention away from the endocrinopathies. Hair pluckings may provide useful information. Telogen hairs epilate relatively easily so it is necessary to grasp the hair sample firmly or these will be over-represented in the plucking. The hair roots and shafts should be examined microscopically. Anagen hairs will be absent in most endocrinopathies and pigment clumping may be seen in the hair shaft in follicular dysplasias such as colour dilution alopecia. The presence of follicular casts around the lower hair shaft suggests follicular hyperkeratosis; this is a non-specific feature of atrophic and dysplastic follicular disease but may be particularly marked in sebaceous adenitis. It may also be seen in vitamin A and zinc responsive dermatoses, primary and secondary keratinisation disorders, dermatophytosis and demodicosis. Follicular plugging may also occur leading to the formation of comedones. This is often particularly marked with hyperadrenocorticism, demodicosis and primary seborrhoea.

The pattern of hair loss is often significant. Endocrine-associated alopecia tends to be broadly symmetrical and most marked over the flanks, dorsum, ventral abdomen and chest, medial and posterior thighs, tail and perineum. The precise distribution varies with the particular hormonal imbalance encountered and is likely to reflect the distribution of specific receptors in the skin. The alopecia varies from almost total to mild and diffuse but is confined to distinct regions of the body. The head and limbs are usually spared. Involvement of these areas or widespread, non-regional diffuse alopecia or multifocal patchy hair loss is less suggestive of endocrine disease. Such a pattern is often seen with folliculitis and follicular dysplasias. Dermatomyositis may produce patchy follicular atrophy and alopecia and complete alopecia is seen in alopecia areata but the distribution in these cases rarely mimics that of the endocrinopathies.

Erythroderma, inflammation and primary focal skin lesions are generally absent in endocrine diseases except where they are due to secondary problems such as pyoderma and *Malassezia* dermatitis. Erythroderma may be the principle clinical sign in epidermotrophic lymphoma which can cause widespread alopecia with minimal pruritus. Cutaneous hyperpigmentation develops early in the course of many endocrine dermatoses but more commonly is associated with long-standing hypersensitivity in which case the skin is frequently lichenified and the dog is invariably pruritic.

Clinical pathology

As part of the initial assessment, deep and superficial skin scrapings should always be collected and examined to check for ectoparasites, particularly *Demodex*. Dry scrapes or tape strips of the superficial epidermis should be stained and examined for the presence of *Malassezia* yeasts. Blood should be collected for routine haematology and biochemistry profiles following a 12 hour fast. Hair pluckings may be collected and examined microscopically for signs of damage, abnormal pigmentation and anagen activity. *Demodex* may be demonstrated or the egg cases of other ectoparasites may be found attached to the hair shafts. Pluckings may be examined in 10% aqueous potassium hydroxide for fungal spores. If dermatophytosis is suspected, samples must be submitted for fungal culture. Failure to demonstrate fluorescent hair shafts under Wood's lamp examination does not reliably rule out dermatophytosis in the dog. These procedures do not require expensive facilities or equipment and samples need not be examined during the consultation period. The investment of a few well-spent minutes at this stage may save a great deal of wasted time and effort later.

If these steps do not suggest a diagnosis and a non-endocrine aetiology or component is still suspected, multiple skin biopsies should be collected and submitted to a pathologist practised in veterinary dermatopathology. Early lesions should be selected for biopsy and clinically normal skin submitted for comparison. Biopsies of the transition zone between normal and affected skin may also be useful.

NON-ENDOCRINE ALOPECIA

The clinical signs that would direct attention away from the endocrine causes of non-pruritic, symmetrical alopecia in the dog are summarised in Table 1 whilst Table 2 summarises some of the differential diagnoses that should be considered. Biopsy will usually help to eliminate most of these possibilities, should categorise the pathogenic processes present and may provide a definitive diagnosis. Many of these dermatoses are difficult to treat or manage and early diagnosis allows clients to come to terms with the problem before patience and finances are exhausted.

Congenital

Congenital ectodermal defects are apparent from birth and should present few diagnostic dilemmas when a good history is available (Plate 27). Hypotrichosis varies in severity from the thin ventral pelage frequently encountered in dachshunds and bull terriers to the extensive alopecia seen in hairless breeds such as the Chinese crested dog. Pattern baldness usually develop gradually after puberty or following the loss of the puppy coat and may affect different regions in different breeds. Pinnal alopecia is seen in several breeds including the dachshund, chihuahua, whippet, miniature poodle and Italian greyhound. In Yorkshire terriers, alopecia of the dorsal muzzle may be accompanied by intense hyperpigmentation. A number of follicular dysplasias have now been described in dogs and can be considered as variants of a primary follicular keratinisation defect. Black hair follicular dysplasia and colour dilution alopecia are seen in a number of breeds. Some black and the majority of blue and fawn doberman pinschers exhibit varying degrees of this hereditary tardive alopecia. There are no effective treatments available for any of these genetically-determined dermatoses and symptomatic management is all that can be offered.

Table 1
Clinical signs distinguishing endocrine vs. non-endocrine alopecia

NON-ENDOCRINE	ENDOCRINE
Pruritus	No pruritus
Multifocal primary skin lesions	Lesions diffuse or regional
Pigmentation usually appears late in the course of the disease	Pigmentation may appear early
Involvement of atypical regions such as head, face and limbs	Alopecia generally confined to flanks, ventrum, perineum, thighs
Age of onset variable. Birth to adult	Onset usually in adult dogs
Progression variable	Progression usually slow

Congenital
    Ectodermal defects
    Follicular dysplasias
    Congenital hypotrichosis
    Melanoderma and alopecia
    Pattern baldness

Infective/parasitic
    Demodicosis
    Dermatophytosis
    Pyoderma (folliculitis)

Immune-mediated
    Pemphigus foliaceus
    Alopecia areata

Miscellaneous
    Sebaceous adenitis
    Epidermotrophic lymphoma
    Acanthosis nigricans
    "Post-clipping alopecia"
    Telogen and anagen defluxation
    Short-hair syndrome of Silky breeds

Infective/Parasitic

The treatment of demodicosis is covered in Chapter 29 and diagnosis is rarely a problem if skin scrapings are examined routinely. Dermatophytosis is a zoonosis and must always be eliminated from consideration at an early stage. Bacterial folliculitis is an extremely common secondary complication of many dermatoses and may give rise to widespread, non-pruritic hair loss. The hair is often lost in small clumps causing a moth eaten appearance and careful examination usually reveals the presence of primary lesions such as papules or pustules which are suggestive of pyoderma. This should be eliminated by treating with a systemic antimicrobial agent known to be effective against *Staphylococcus intermedius* for a minimum of three weeks and the case reassessed (Chapter 25). The underlying cause must be identified and controlled if the pyoderma is not to return.

Immune Mediated

Few immune mediated dermatoses will present with histories or clinical signs that are likely to be confused with the endocrinopathies. Marked exfoliation and alopecia are occasionally the principle feature of pemphigus foliaceus but it may rarely be confined to the hair follicle causing diffuse hair loss. Alopecia areata usually produces focal or multifocal patches of alopecia but these may coalesce to form a broadly symmetric pattern, often on the face. Biopsy is required to diagnose this disease and there is no effective treatment.

Miscellaneous

As more cases of sebaceous adenitis are recognised it becomes increasingly unlikely that this poorly understood disease is caused by a single aetiologic mechanism and the proposition that it is purely a genodermatosis is no longer tenable. Treatment is frequently unrewarding but some improvement has been seen with essential fatty acid supplementation and isotretinoin. At certain stages, epidermotrophic lymphomas may produce diffuse hair loss but progression of the disease usually removes any potential confusion with the endocrinopathies. Primary acanthosis nigricans has been described in the dachshund and causes lichenification, hyperpigmentation and alopecia in the axillae and inguinal regions (Chapter 9). This must be distinguished from post-inflammatory hyperpigmentation which often occurs in the same regions. "Post-clipping alopecia" is confined almost exclusively to the sled-dog breeds but all the endocrinopathies or concurrent cytotoxic drug therapy may produce similar signs. Hair regrowth in clipped areas may take six to twelve months and may initially be darker that the original coat. Telogen defluxation is an uncommon syndrome characterised by widespread hair loss following an episode of severe metabolic stress, the most common being pregnancy, pseudopregnancy and pyrexia. Premature cessation of hair growth results in synchronisation of follicular cycles and simultaneous shedding. Provided the triggering stress factors are removed, regrowth will occur without treatment. The major differential is anagen defluxation when anagen arrest occurs in response to catastrophic disease or cytotoxic therapy. Occasionally, mature Yorkshire terriers and Silky terriers will lose the long soft hairs that are a prominent feature of their coats leaving a short but otherwise adequate pelage. The short hair syndrome may be related to a shortened hair cycle and no effective treatment is available.

ENDOCRINE ALOPECIA

Once an endocrine aetiology is considered likely, the clinician should as a priority attempt to eliminate hypothyroidism and hyperadrenocorticism from the list of differential diagnoses. These disorders are relatively common and diagnosis and treatment are both practical and effective. Furthermore, through their involvement of other body systems, the quality of life may be reduced and potentially life threatening problems may arise.

Hypothyroidism

A number of historical and clinical features may alert the clinician to the possibility of hypothyroidism (Plate 23). The problem is common in medium sized to large breeds including doberman pinschers, boxers, great Danes, Irish setters and old English sheepdogs. Affected animals are usually at least middle aged and there is no sex predisposition. The principle clinical signs, diagnostic tests and therapy are summarised in Table 3.

Total circulating thyroxine (T4) levels may be depressed by a wide variety of diseases or drugs making single basal estimations an unreliable guide to thyroid function. Although protocols vary, there is no doubt that dynamic function tests are the method of choice for diagnosing hypothyroidism. If T4 supplementation has been initiated on empirical grounds, it should be withdrawn 4-6 weeks prior to testing. The thyroid stimulating hormone (TSH) response test is the test of choice but TSH is expensive and difficult to obtain. The thyrotrophin releasing hormone (TRH) test is more difficult to interpret and produces more equivocal results but is still preferable to basal estimations alone. If neither TSH nor TRH are available, basal T4 levels must be interpreted in conjunction with other parameters and it may be advisable to seek specialist advice or consult an appropriate text.

T4 supplementation is the treatment of choice. T4 is peripherally converted to the active form, T3 and as conversion defects have not been demonstrated, there is no advantage in T3 supplementation. Crude desiccated thyroid extracts are not an acceptable substitute for T4. Improvements in activity and behaviour may be seen within a few days of starting therapy. Hair regrowth should be appreciable in 6-8 weeks but a full response may take 6 months. Significant weight loss may occur during the initial stages of therapy and it is advisable to weigh dogs regularly and adjust the T4 dose appropriately. Blood samples should be taken 6-12 weeks after treatment is initiated and at intervals throughout the dog's life to confirm that circulating T4 concentrations are in the euthyroid range 4-6 hours after treatment.

Hyperadrenocorticism

Hyperadrenocorticism (HAC)(Plates 24 and 25) is a common canine endocrinopathy and pituitary adenomas (Cushing's syndrome) account for 85-90% of spontaneously occurring cases; the remaining 10-15% are due to adrenocortical neoplasms secreting excessive amounts of cortisol. The administration of exogenous glucocorticoids unfortunately remains the most common cause of hyperglucocorticism (see Chapter 27). The dermatological manifestations are often the least serious features of this

Table 3
Clinical signs, diagnostic tests and treatment of hypothyroidism

Clinical signs
> Lethargy, exercise intolerance, mental dullness, weight gain
> Reproductive failure, irregular oestrus/anoestrus, testicular atrophy, gynecomastia
> Heat-seeking behaviour, cool skin, low body temperature
> Bilaterally symmetrical alopecia, hyperpigmentation, myxoedema
> Comedones, seborrhoea, hyperkeratotic plaques (esp. pinnae)
> Dry, brittle, dull pelage, occasionally hypertrichosis
> Mild non-regenerative anaemia, raised serum cholesterol and creatinine phosphokinase
> Recurrent pyoderma
> Keratoconjunctivitis sicca, corneal lipidosis, uveitis, retinopathy
> Bradycardia, first degree heart block, arrythmias
> Neurological abnormalities, myopathy, myalgia

Diagnostic tests
TSH response test
> Basal T4 measured. 0.1 IU/kg. of TSH administered i/v and T4 measured 6 hours later.
> Post TSH T4 should reach 1.5 x basal T4 and a minimum level of 35 nmol/l.

TRH response test
> Basal T4 measured. 0.02 mg/kg TRH given i/v and T4 measured 4 hourslater. Post
> TRH T4 should reach 1.2 x basal T4 and a minimum level of 30 nmol/l

Treatment
T4 supplementation at 10-20 µg/kg bid. After 12 weeks check T4 concentration within
> euthyroid range 4-6 hours post-treatment.

disease and untreated animals are at risk of developing a number of life-threatening problems. A wide variety of clinical signs may be seen and alopecic animals may not present with all or any of the other signs. Onset of clinical disease is usually insidious and slowly progressive. Several breeds are recognised to be at risk; these include dachshunds, poodles and boxers. Spontaneously occurring HAC is a disease of middle-aged to older dogs whilst iatrogenic cases may occur at any age. The clinical signs, diagnosis and treatment of HAC are summarised in Table 4. Diffuse truncal alopecia is also occasionally seen in diabetes mellitus. This may be due to the secondary adrenocortical hyperplasia that frequently accompanies HAC as a response to metabolic stress or may be due to other, currently unknown factors.

In addition to the diagnostic tests in Table 4, a number of other protocols have been suggested. The combined dexamethasone suppression and adrenocorticotrophic hormone (ACTH) stimulation test has few additional advantages and can produce results that are more difficult to interpret. Endogenous ACTH assays are not commercially available in Great Britain. Urinary cortisol/creatinine ratios are a sensitive method of detecting HAC. However, urinary cortisol excretion is elevated in polyuria/polydipsia secondary to non-adrenal disease and the method is not specific enough for HAC to be reliable.

The prognosis for HAC is variable. Most dogs will respond well to o'p DDD but a small number will not tolerate therapy or become resistant. Glucocorticoid supplementation is usually not necessary. The aim of therapy should be to produce a pituitary-adrenal axis unresponsive to ACTH stimulation. If a significant response persists, even if it is within normal limits, it is likely that the state of hyperadrenocorticism also persists. ACTH stimulation tests may be performed to confirm successful therapy and monitor adrenal function. Iatrogenic hyperglucocorticism requires that administration of exogenous glucocorticoids be discontinued. A gradual reduction will be necessary to avoid precipitating an adrenocortical insufficiency crisis. ACTH stimulation tests can again be used to confirm this diagnosis and monitor recovery of the pituitary-adrenal axis. A full account of the management of HAC is beyond the scope of this chapter and reference should be made to an appropriate text.

Clinical signs.
Polyuria/polydipsia (in excess of 100 ml/kg/day).
Polyphagia and weight gain.
Pot belly, muscle wasting, hepatomegaly, lethargy.
Neurological signs.
Thin fragile skin, telangectasia, comedones, prominent superficial blood vessels.
Symmetrical alopecia, dry brittle hair, change in coat colour.
Anoestrus or irregular oestrus. Testicular atrophy.
Behavioural changes, neurological signs.
Recurrent pyoderma, calcinosis cutis,
Eosinopaenia, mature neutrophilia, lymphopaenia.
Elevated serum alkaline phosphatase, alanine aminotransferase.
Hyperglycaemia, hypercholesterolaemia.

Diagnostic tests
ACTH stimulation test.
    Basal cortisol measured. 0.25 mg synthetic ACTH (Synacthen, Ciba Labs) administered i/v. Post-stimulation sample collected after 1 hour.
    Exaggerated response consistent with HAC .
    Poor or no response consistent with iatrogenic hyperglucorticoidism.

Low dose dexamethasone suppression test.
    Basal cortisol measured. 0.01 mg/kg of soluble dexamethasone administered i/v. Post suppression samples collected at 3 and 8 hours.
    Suppression at 8 hours consistent with normal response.
    Failure to suppress at 3 or 8 hours suggestive of adrenocortical neoplasia.
    Suppression at 3 hours with rebound at 8 hours suggestive of pituitary dependant HAC.

High dose dexamethasone suppression test.
    Basal cortisol measured. 0.1 mg/kg soluble dexamethasone administered i/v. Post suppression samples collected at 3 and 8 hours.
    Failure to suppress to 50% of basal concentration at 3 or 8 hours suggestive of adrenocortical neoplasia.
    Used to differentiate pituitary dependant HAC from adrenal dependant HAC

Radiography - 25% of adrenal neoplasms are calcified.

Ultrasonography - right adrenal gland often difficult to scan.

Treatment
o'p DDD (Lysodren)
    Induction therapy - 25-50 mg/kg sid for 5-10 days. Patient should be closely monitored during this period.
    Maintenance therapy - dose reduced to 25-50 mg/kg weekly in 2 or 3 divided doses.

Ketoconazole
    5 mg/kg bid Monitor success with ACTH stimulation test after 7-10 days.

Adrenalectomy
    Appropriate for unilateral adrenocortical adenomas which have not metastasised.
    Adenocarcinomas frequently metastasise prior to diagnosis

Seasonal Flank Alopecia

Symmetrical, diffuse flank alopecia may repeatedly develop in either the spring or autumn which then spontaneously resolves during the course of the year. Affected male boxers, English bulldogs, Airedale terriers and doberman pinschers start to lose hair in the autumn and alopecia persists until the following spring. In neutered bitches of several breeds including boxers and English bulldogs, hair loss starts in the spring and resolves in the autumn. Alopecic areas are usually well-circumscribed, confined to the flanks and may show mild scaling and intense hyperpigmentation. ACTH response and TSH/TRH response tests are normal. No pruritus, thickening or erythema is present. Biopsies show an atrophic pattern consistent with an endocrine aetiology. If no endocrinopathy can be demonstrated and there are compatible clinical signs and a seasonal history, a diagnosis of seasonal flank alopecia can be made.

The aetiology of this condition is unknown. It has been proposed that the antiandrogenic effects of the pineal gland hormones are responsible for suppression of testosterone production in animals with a marginal growth hormone deficiency. Pineal gland secretion is influenced by photoperiod and is at a maximum when the day length is short. Theoretically, androgen supplementation (see sex hormone imbalances) may promote hair regrowth and if given prior to the onset of shedding, may prevent hair loss. The problem is purely cosmetic and treatment is not always necessary or requested.

Sex Hormone Imbalances

Although validated assays for the major sex hormones are now commercially available, the lack of information regarding the references values of these hormones in neutered and debilitated animals continues to impede the diagnosis of sex hormone imbalances. Current understanding of the interaction between the receptors for glucocorticoids, retinoids, androgens and other steroid hormones is poor and little information relating to their numbers and distribution in the skin is available. In many of the imbalances described, serum concentrations of the major sex hormones do not consistently reflect expectations based on the proposed aetiology. Diagnosis of a sex hormone imbalance is best made on clinical and historical grounds and the elimination of differential diagnoses.

Sex hormones are produced by the gonads and the adrenal glands. Neutering does not in itself produce symmetrical alopecia despite the dramatic shift in hormonal balance it imposes. Relatively few animals develop alopecia and it would appear likely that when this does occur, it is due to an individual susceptibility, perhaps associated with inadequate adrenal sex hormone secretion or a receptor defect. Excessive adrenal secretion appears to also be a possible cause of problems.

GONADAL ORIGIN

Entire male

Unilateral atrophy or the presence of palpable masses or irregularities in one or both testes is strongly suggestive of primary testicular neoplasia but not all testicular neoplasms will be palpable, even if the testes are present in the scrotum. Bilateral testicular atrophy is more consistent with hormonal influence of non-testicular origin and particular care should be taken to eliminate hypothyroidism and HAC from consideration. If one or both testes are missing from the scrotum, care must be taken to eliminate the possibility of unilateral or bilateral cryptorchidism. If there is doubt over this issue, a human chorionic gonadotrophin (HCG) stimulation test can be performed (Table 5). The incidence of Sertoli cell tumours and seminomas increases significantly in cryptorchid testicles.

Sertoli's cell tumours (Plate 26) are the type most frequently associated with feminisation but this may occur with interstitial cell tumours and seminomas as well. One, two or all three tumour types may be present. Approximately 20% of Sertoli cell tumours metastasise; interstitial cell tumours are the least likely to do so. Seminomas and Sertoli cell tumours may produce oestrogens whereas interstitial cell tumours usually produce androgens. Pruritus has been reported as a feature of a presumed androgen hypersensitivity. Rarely, glucocorticoid-like compounds may be synthesised producing polyuria and polydipsia and adrenocortical suppression.

Table 5
Dynamic function tests for sex hormone imbalances

HCG stimulation test
Basal testosterone concentration measured. 250 IU of HCG administered i/v. Post-stimulation samples collected after 2 hours.
Normal response will show a 5-7 fold increase in serum testosterone.
Castrated dog will show little or no response.
Dog with cryptorchid testes will react in a similar fashion to normal dog.

ACTH stimulation test for adrenal sex hormones.
Basal concentrations of cortisol, oestradiol, progesterone and testosterone measured. 0.5 mg of synthetic ACTH (Synacthen, Ciba Labs) administered i/v. Post-stimulation samples collected after 1 hour.
11-deoxycortisol, 17-hydroxyprogesterone, dehydroepiandrosteronesulphate (DHEAS) and androstenedione may also be measured if assays are available.
Progesterone, 17-hydroxyprogesterone, DHEAS and androstenedione concentrations should be elevated if an adrenal sex hormone abnormality is present.

Xylazine stimulation test
Basal concentrations of GH (or somatomedin) measured. 0.1 mg/kg of xylazine administered i/v. Post-stimulation samples collected after 15 and 30 minutes.
Normal animals show a marked rise in serum GH concentrations - 10-15 fold.

Symmetrical alopecia is the most common dermatological clinical sign associated with testicular neoplasms and generally affects the perineal and genital region. Progression along the ventral trunk and neck may occur. The hair coat is dry and dull and a variable degree of hyperpigmentation may be present. Gynaecomastia, a pendulous prepuce, lactation, decreased libido and attraction of male dogs may be seen. Dogs may alter their urination posture, squatting in the female posture or fail to lift a leg. Keratinisation abnormalities, seborrhoea and a ceruminous otitis are common features. An erythematous or pigmented linear preputial dermatosis is strongly suggestive of a Sertoli cell tumour. Evidence of bone marrow suppression may be seen and prostatitis or prostatomegaly have been reported.

If testicular abnormalities can be palpated in a dog with symmetrical alopecia, bilateral castration should be advised as tumours may be present in both testes. Histopathological confirmation of testicular neoplasia should always be sought. Radiography or ultrasonography should be performed to search for metastases prior to surgery. One of serum oestradiol, progesterone or testosterone concentrations will usually, but not invariably, be elevated. This may provide supportive evidence for a diagnosis of testicular neoplasia when no abnormalities are palpable. Improvement should be seen in 3 months. Failure to improve or recurrence after an initial improvement may be evidence for the presence of functional metastases.

"Castration responsive dermatosis" is a term that has been used to describe a syndrome in young adult dogs that present with symmetrical alopecia, have no palpable testicular abnormalities and have no evidence of neoplasia on histopathological examination of the testes following castration. Pomeranians, chow chows, Alaskan malamutes, Siberian huskies, keeshonds and miniature poodles are the breeds most frequently affected. The alopecia starts in the same areas as those associated with testicular neoplasia and may progress to involve the trunk. A band of alopecia often develops around the neck. Skin hyperpigmentation and changes in coat colour are common and light or dark streaks may appear. Tufts of hair regrowth frequently occur at biopsy sites. A primary gonadal sex hormone abnormality has been proposed as the cause; many have altered basal serum concentrations of oestrogens or testosterone. In entire males, progesterone is mainly produced by the adrenals and serum concentrations are less commonly altered. A gonadotrophin releasing hormone response test may be of use in demonstrating abnormal gonadal function but this test has still to be adequately validated in the dog. The role of peripheral receptor defects in this condition has not been determined. Many affected dogs have low basal serum growth hormone (GH) concentrations and a poor GH stimulation response to xylaxine but this does not appear to be the primary defect. Castration is the only effective treatment.

A presumed androgen hypersensitivity has been described in entire dogs causing traumatic alopecia, lichenification, hyperpigmentation over the rump, ventrum, perineum and thighs. This condition is distinguished by intense glucocorticoid resistant pruritus and will not be discussed further in this chapter.

Neutered male

A small number of dogs castrated in the first year of life develop symmetrical alopecia in middle or old age. Hypoandrogenism has been proposed as a contributory factor. Normally, adrenal androgen production is thought to maintain basal androgen concentrations following castration. The late appearance of alopecia may reflect changes in adrenal androgen production or changes in peripheral androgen conversion or receptors. The alopecia affects the perineum and genital areas and may progress to the ventral neck and chest and occasionally, flanks. The coat is dry and brittle and secondary keratinisation changes may be seen. Gynaecomastia is absent.

The treatment of choice is oral methyltestosterone supplementation. An initial dose of 1 mg/kg (total dose not exceeding 30 mg) is given every 48 hours for 1-3 months until hair regrowth is seen and then reduced to twice weekly. Some dogs which do not respond to oral methyltestosterone will respond to intramuscular 2 mg/kg methyltestosterone, the total dose again not exceeding 30 mg. Exogenous testosterones are hepatotoxic and hepatic biochemistry should be monitored monthly during induction and every 4-6 months during maintenance.

Entire female

Elevations of serum oestradiol, progesterone or testosterone concentrations may be seen in bitches with ovarian cysts or functional ovarian neoplasia. Rarely, the cause is iatrogenic due to excessive administration of oestrogens or progestagens. The clinical syndrome has been called "ovarian imbalance type 1" for many years and consists of symmetrical alopecia affecting the perineal and perivulval regions. The flanks and ventral trunk and neck may become involved. Hyperpigmentation may be seen and may be localised to the flanks. Keratinisation disturbances, lichenification and a ceruminous otitis are common. Gynaecomastia and vulvar enlargement may be seen when oestrogen or progesterone is produced in excess but not when testosterone is the excess hormone. Frequently, an association with oestrus, pregnancy or pseudopregnancy may be noted and the oestrus cycle may be abnormal. Nymphomania may be reported.

Diagnosis is based on history, compatible clinical signs and demonstration of persistently elevated serum oestrodiol, progesterone or testosterone concentrations. Ovariohysterectomy is the treatment of choice and improvement should be seen in 3-6 months. If an elevated progesterone concentration alone is found, a functioning persistent corpora luteum may be responsible. If this is sustained for 3-4 months and involution does not occur, ovariohysterectomy should be performed. Topical therapy may be required if significant seborrhoea is present.

Pruritus associated with a presumed hormonal hypersensitivity may be an early clinical sign and may precede other dermatological manifestations. The pruritus develops prior to the onset of oestrus and regresses spontaneously.

Neutered female

Oestradiol, progesterone and testosterone are produced by the ovaries at different stages of the oestrus cycle. A deficiency of one or all of these may arise following ovariohysterectomy if adequate basal concentrations are not maintained by the adrenal glands. The primary defect may lie in the adrenal gland, in peripheral conversion of the hormones or in skin receptor numbers or function. The clinical syndrome that arises has been referred to as "ovarian imbalance type 2" and is characterised by symmetrical alopecia of the perivulvar and perineal region. Progression to the ventral trunk and neck and occasionally the pinnae may occur. Hyperpigmentation does not generally develop. Flank alopecia has also been reported and may fluctuate in severity during different times of the year.

Oestrogen replacement is the usual treatment. The recommended treatment regime is 0.1-1.0 mg oral diethylstilboestrol given daily for 3-4 weeks followed by a similar dose 1-2 times weekly as maintenance. Exogenous oestrogens may cause serious bone marrow suppression and a full haematology profile and platelet count should be performed every 2 weeks during the initial stages of treatment. These checks also be made every 3-6 months during maintenance. Testosterone may occasionally be effective if there is a poor response to oestrogen replacement. The dose regime is identical to that described under hypoandrogenism. The dermatological manifestations are mild and there is no serious systemic disease. In view of the potential problems with therapy, it may not always be necessary nor in the animal's best interest to initiate treatment.

ADRENAL ORIGIN

The role of adrenal sex hormones has been overlooked for many years but investigations into the aetiology of other endocrine alopecias has focused attention on the adrenal gland. In common with many other endocrine alopecias, symmetrical hair loss develops over the tail, caudal thighs, ventral abdomen, cervical area and lateral trunk. Hyperpigmentation usually develops in the alopecic areas, the coat becomes dry and brittle and may darken or lighten in colour. Irregular streaking of coat colouration may develop. Keratinisation defects and secondary infections are rare. The majority of confirmed cases have occurred in samoyeds, keeshonds, chow chows, pomeranians and their crosses.

Diagnosis is based on compatible history, clinical signs and the ruling out of other endocrinopathies, particularly "castration responsive dermatosis" and sex hormone imbalances of gonadal origin. Entire animals with elevated serum hormone concentrations should be neutered. Following neutering, elevated basal serum sex hormone concentrations persist or an exaggerated sex hormone response to ACTH stimulation can be demonstrated (Table 5).

Therapy with o'p DDD may be undertaken and has proved successful in the management of this problem. This may be due to the adrenal cytotoxic effect but o'p DDD also modifies peripheral metabolism of steroids and reduces the availability of androgen precursors and therefore the effect of peripheral androgens on the hair follicle. The relative importance of these mechanisms is unknown. An induction dose of 15-25 mg/kg is given for 5 days and control can be maintained with a similar dose every 1-2 weeks. Owners should be advised of the potential risks of o'p DDD therapy in the dog.

"GROWTH HORMONE RESPONSIVE DERMATOSIS"

It has become increasingly difficult to diagnose "GH responsive dermatosis" with any certainty. Validated assays for GH have never been commercially available in Great Britain and there has always been considerable doubt about the accuracy of the of pathogenesis that the term implies. The response to GH supplementation is variable and improvement in some individuals may be seen following castration. This must cast further doubt on the true role of GH in these dogs, despite demonstration of a poor GH response to xylazine or clonidine stimulation. It is possible that the GH abnormalities are secondary to other endocrine disturbances. The history, clinical signs and breed incidence are identical to those seen in "castration responsive dermatosis", where a sex hormone aetiology is suspected, and in adrenal sex hormone abnormalities.

It is essential to rule out these two conditions if a diagnosis of primary GH deficiency is be made. In addition, hypothyroidism, hyperadrenocorticism and gonadal sex hormone imbalance should be eliminated. An ACTH response test should be performed and serum concentrations of cortisol and the sex hormones should be measured (Table 5). If no abnormality is demonstrated, a xylazine response test (Table 5) should be performed to confirm a low GH response. No commercial GH assays are available in Great Britain but serum somatomedin concentrations closely follow GH concentrations and can be measured as an alternative.

If no other endocrinopathy can be demonstrated, GH stimulation test results are low and there is a compatible history and clinical presentation, a GH deficiency can be suspected. GH supplements are extremely expensive at present and the cost of treatment is likely to be prohibitive. In addition, GH is diabetogenic and blood glucose concentrations should be measured prior to and during therapy. The recommended dose is 0.15 IU/kg injected subcutaneously twice weekly for 6 weeks. A good response should be seen within 3 months but therapy may have to be repeated at intervals.

Response to GH does not confirm a primary GH defect; the actions of GH are so broad that a non-specific response may be induced. It is likely that the term "GH responsive dermatosis" will fall into disuse as the pathogenesis of this group of fascinating endocrine alopecias is unravelled.

SUMMARY

The root cause of most cases of non-pruritic symmetrical alopecia in the dog can be determined if a systematic diagnostic process is followed. The clinical similarity of many of the endocrinopathies is often confusing and the lack of validated assays and dynamic function tests has until recently seriously hampered the definitive diagnosis of these conditions. There has been some improvement both in the range of assays available and in our knowledge of the physiology of the endocrine systems affecting the skin. However, the complex interaction between these systems and the hair follicle is still poorly very understood. The names for many of the conditions described in this chapter will almost certainly change as current knowledge is expanded and integrated.

FURTHER READING

GRIFFIN, C.E. KWOCHKA, K.W. and MACDONALD, J.E. (1993) In: *Current Veterinary Dermatology - The Science and Art of Therapy*. Mosby Year Book, St. Louis.

MILLER, W.H. (1989) Sex hormone-related dermatoses in dogs. In: *Current Veterinary Therapy 10* (Ed. R.W.Kirk) W.B. Saunders, Philadelphia.

HERRTAGE, M.E. (1990) The adrenal glands. In: *Manual of Small Animal Endocrinology* (Ed. M. Hutchison) British Small Animal Veterinary Association, Cheltenham.

GRANT, D.I. (1990) Differential diagnosis of alopecia. In: *Manual of Small Animal Endocrinology* (Ed. M. Hutchison) British Small Animal Veterinary Association, Cheltenham.

THODAY, K.L. (1990) The thyroid gland. In: *Manual of Small Animal Endocrinology* (Ed. M. Hutchison) p25 British Small Animal Veterinary Association, Cheltenham.

MEDLEAU, L. (1989) Sex hormone associated endocrine alopecias in dogs. *Journal of American Animal Hospital Association* **25**:689.

ROSSER, E.J. (1987) Growth hormone-responsive dermatosis vs. castration responsive dermatosis. Derm Dialogue Autumn 1987.

ROSSER, E.J. (1989) Castration responsive dermatosis in the dog In: *Advances in Veterinary Dermatology Volume 1* (Eds. C. von Tscharner and R.E.W. Halliwell) Baillière Tindall, London.

SCHMEITZEL, L.P. (1990) Sex hormone related and growth hormone related alopecias. *Veterinary Clinics of North America* **20**:1579.

SCHMEITZEL, L.P., Lothrop, C.D. (1990) Hormonal abnormalities in Pomeranians with normal coat and in Pomeranians with growth hormone-responsive dermatosis. *Journal of the American Veterinary Medical Association* **197**:1333.

SCOTT, D.W. (1989) The biology of hair growth and it's disturbances. In: *Advances in Veterinary Dermatology Volume 1* (Eds. C. von Tscharner and Halliwell, R.E.W.) Baillière Tindall, London.

SCOTT, D.W. (1990) Seasonal flank alopecia in ovariohysterectomised dogs. *Cornell Veterinarian* **80**:187.

SYMMETRICAL ALOPECIA IN THE CAT

Julie I Henfrey —————————————

INTRODUCTION

Feline symmetrical alopecia (FSA) can be defined as total or partial absence of hair in a symmetric pattern in areas where hair is normally present. It is a very common presenting sign in cats and has a myriad of underlying causes. Successful treatment hinges on an accurate diagnosis which in turn relies on an accurate and detailed clinical history with a careful physical examination, followed by the rational use of laboratory tests. This chapter will discuss the differential diagnosis of FSA from a problem oriented view. The diseases causing FSA are listed in Table 1.

Table 1
Causes of feline symmetrical alopecia

PATHOLOGICAL PROCESS	DISEASE CONDITION	
Failure of hair coat production	Alopecia universalis Hereditary hypotrichosis Pili torti	
Excess shedding of hair	Folliculitis –	dermatophytosis demodicosis bacteria
	Metabolic/nutritional disorders	
	Endocrinopathy –	hyperadrenocorticism diabetes mellitus thyroid disease "endocrine alopecia"
	Miscellaneous –	telogen defluxion alopecia areata alopecia mucinosa drugs
Pruritus and self-trauma	Allergy –	fleas food atopy
	Drug eruption Psychogenic alopecia	

APPROACH TO THE CASE

A logical and meticulous approach to the history and physical examination is essential in the approach to the cat with FSA. This subject is covered in Chapter 2 and will not be repeated here, but some aspects are of particular importance and warrant highlighting in this chapter.

Clinical History

In the diagnosis of the FSA case it is crucial to establish whether the alopecia is associated with failure of hair production, excessive hair shedding or self-trauma and resulting alopecia.

At the initial consultation it should be ascertained whether the affected areas have ever had hair present, or whether the cat has been affected since a kitten. This will help to determine if one of the congenital diseases is present in which failure of production of hair occurs. The second group of conditions which may cause FSA are those which are characterised by excessive or premature shedding of the hair coat which has previously been considered normal. It is difficult to determine from the history alone that excessive shedding of the hair coat is occurring. It is important to exclude the possibility that the cat is pulling or licking the hair out. Cats may lick or pull hair out from extensive areas of the body in a perfectly symmetric pattern whilst causing little or no damage to the underlying skin and can do this completely unobserved by the owner. Pruritus and resulting licking and pulling at the hair coat is the commonest cause of feline symmetric alopecia. Determining the presence or absence of pruritus is critical in the diagnosis of the FSA case, and is not always as easy as it might appear. Most cats with pruritic FSA are not observed to be scratching, but careful questioning of the owner may reveal a pattern of excessive grooming.

PHYSICAL EXAMINATION

A full physical examination of the affected cat is mandatory. Signs of intercurrent disease may help to narrow the list of possible differential diagnoses. Most importantly, close examination of the hair coat will help differentiate between a cat which is suffering from an excessive shedding of its hair coat and one which is removing the hair coat as a result of self-trauma. Diagnostic hints which may help to determine that the hair is being shed include the observation that any remaining hairs are in telogen (the resting phase of hair development) and are easily epilated. Microscopical examination of such hairs shows a club root with no root sheaths and a keratinised sac, ie. a telogen hair. Cats which are chewing or licking the hair out will have hairs which are not easily epilated, and microscopical examination of remaining hairs from the affected areas will reveal that the tips are irregular and barbered by the cat. In addition, there may be a history of recurrent vomiting of fur balls, and faecal examination may reveal large amounts of hair. Placing an Elizabethan collar on the pruritic cat for a period of several weeks to demonstrate re-growth of hair once the self-trauma ceases will give conclusive proof that the hairs are being removed, but this is likely to be an uncomfortable experience for the cat.

ESTABLISHING THE DIAGNOSIS

Once the patient can be categorised as to the pathogenesis of the alopecia, it is much easier to establish a definitive diagnosis.

Failure of Hair Coat Production

Definitive diagnosis of all the hereditary diseases causing a failure of hair production is by biopsy. These diseases are not common, but have all been recorded in the United Kingdom.

Alopecia Universalis (Sphinx cat, Canadian hairless cat)
Alopecia universalis is a rare, congenital, hereditary disease in which affected animals show a complete absence of hair except for the whiskers and occasionally a few secondary hairs on the face, tip of the tail, scrotum and dorsum. Affected cats are reluctant to groom, and the skin may develop marked seborrhoea oleosa with large deposits of lipid material in the nail folds. Weekly bathing in anti-seborrhoeic shampoos help to control the seborrhoea, but regular manual removal

of lipids from the nail folds is mandatory in the management of affected cats. This congenital disorder has been selectively bred for, giving the Sphinx or Canadian Hairless cat.

Hereditary hypotrichosis

There are several reports of hereditary hypotrichosis in the literature. The condition, with an autosomal mode of inheritance, has been reported in Siamese cats. At birth the kittens have a thin hair coat over the entire body which is lost within two weeks. Some re-growth may be noted by eight to ten weeks of age, but by the time the cat reaches the age of six months severe hypotrichosis is present and is permanent. The condition has also been reported in a Mexican breed of cat, and also in the Devon rex (Thoday, 1981). The author has seen a Devon rex cat with hereditary hypotrichosis which suffered a generalised actinic dermatitis every summer and which eventually developed multiple squamous cell carcinomata over much of the body surface. There is no treatment for hereditary hypotrichosis, but owners of affected cats should be encouraged to use a sun block cream on their animal in the summer.

Pili torti

This rare condition has been reported in the United Kingdom (Geary and Baker 1986). It is a condition in which there is rotation of the hair along the axis of secondary hair shafts leading to diffuse thinning of the hair coat by ten days of age with rapidly developing generalised alopecia, pedal dermatitis and paronychia. All the affected kittens died or were destroyed *in extremis* within two months of birth.

Excess Shedding of Hair

The group of conditions which cause excessive shedding of the hair coat are collectively the second most common cause of FSA in cats in the United Kingdom. The selective use of laboratory tests based on features of the history and physical examination will yield a diagnosis in many cases. Excessive shedding of hair may be caused by folliculitis, metabolic and nutritional disorders, endocrinopathies and a miscellaneous group of conditions.

Folliculitis

Symmetric hair loss may be seen associated with damage to the hair and/or hair follicle with subsequent shedding of hairs. Although papules or pustules of follicular origin (ie. with a hair growing from the centre of the lesion) and epidermal collarettes may be seen in affected cats, it is not unusual for folliculitis in cats to be manifest by alopecia alone.

Dermatophytosis may have a myriad of clinical signs ranging from a virtually asymptomatic carrier state, widespread diffuse alopecia with fractured hairs to a severe inflammatory dermatosis. Symmetric alopecia affecting the groin, perineum and medial aspects of the hindlimbs has been recorded. In the UK 94% of isolates are *Microsporum canis*, of which around 60 per cent will fluoresce under a Wood's lamp. *Trichophyton mentagrophytes* may also be isolated (6% of cases), and tends to produce more severe inflammatory lesions than does *M.canis*. Occasionally other dermatophytes may be isolated.

Diagnosis is by microscopical examination of skin scrapings and hair pluckings to detect spores on infected hairs, followed by fungal culture (Chapter 3). Once the diagnosis is confirmed the affected cat should be clipped out and treated with griseofulvin at a dose of 50 - 100 mg/kg once daily with an oily meal. This dose is much higher than is recommended in the data sheets, but is thought to be more appropriate (Scott, 1980). Toxicity reactions are uncommon, and if they do occur are thought to be idiosyncratic and not dose related (Kunkle and Meyer, 1987). Treatment should be continued until the lesions resolve and fungal cultures are negative.

Demodicosis is an uncommon disease of cats that is becoming recognised increasingly frequently. There do not appear to be any age, breed or sex predilections, but most cases so far reported have been associated with an underlying immunosuppressive disorder such as diabetes mellitus (White *et al*, 1987), feline immunodeficiency virus (Chalmers *et al*, 1989), feline leukaemia virus or chronic long acting glucocorticoid use (Chesney, 1989). Two mites are involved, *Demodex cati* and an as yet unnamed short, broad *Demodex* sp. Clinical signs of feline demodicosis include alopecia of the head, ears and neck, and in some cases generalised alopecia which may be symmetric. There may be variable degrees of erythema, scaling or secondary pyoderma. Diagnosis is by microscopical examination of skin scrapings. Once the diagnosis is confirmed a careful search should be made for any possible immunosuppressive disorder. Treatment is much more simple than for canine demodicosis and success has been achieved with 0.025-0.05% amitraz, 0.75% rotenone, lime sulphur dips and 1% selenium sulphide (Chesney, 1989).

Bacterial folliculitis is uncommon in cats and pyoderma is not always visible grossly. Clinical signs are variable but may include miliary dermatitis, crusts, erosions, draining tracts or, in some cases, alopecia with or without epidermal collarettes (White, 1991). Diagnosis is by biopsy; a neutrophilic folliculitis in the absence of ectoparasites or dermatophytes on skin scrapings or fungal culture is very suggestive of a bacterial aetiology. Bacterial culture should be helpful, with *Staphylococcus aureus* the most common isolate. Haematology and serology are unhelpful. Therapy involves prolonged treatment with antibacterial agents such as one of the cephalosporins for two weeks after the last lesion has resolved. Some cats may require antibacterial therapy for an indefinite period (White, 1991).

Metabolic and nutritional disorders

Hair formation requires up to 30 per cent of the daily protein intake of adult cats. Consequently, diseases such as chronic hepatic disease, end-stage renal disease and malabsorption syndromes are particularly associated with diffuse hair loss mainly affecting the trunk. If a thorough history is taken it should indicate an underlying systemic disease and diagnostic techniques should be aimed at determining the underlying abnormality. If the systemic disease can be controlled, the hair will regrow.

Naturally-occurring Vitamin A deficiency has been reported to cause alopecia in cats, but again the history and general physical examination should reveal the anorexia, weight loss, muscle wasting, conjunctivitis, keratitis, testicular atrophy in males and anoestrous in females which are also associated with chronic hypovitaminosis A. Treatment is by intramuscular injection of 12,500 - 25,000 IU. vitamin A (Scott, 1980).

Endocrine disease

Hyperadrenocorticism is rare in cats but several cases have been described. Most affected cats are female with a mean age of 10 years. Most manifest polydipsia, polyuria, polyphagia, diabetes mellitus and lethargy with a pendulous abdomen and thin skin which is easily torn. Medial curling of the ear tips may be observed. Bilaterally symmetric alopecia affecting the trunk, neck and proximal limbs is present in 50% of cases. Diagnosis is confirmed by a dexamethasone suppression test. Management with o,p'-DDD (mitotane) or metyrapone is reported to be of no benefit although ketoconazole at a dose of 12 mg/kg *per os* bid may be helpful (Scott, 1980).

Diabetes mellitus has been reported to cause symmetric alopecia of the groin, perineum, hindlimbs and lateral abdomen (Thoday, 1986). In view of the high incidence of diabetes mellitus in cats with hyperadrenocorticism, all cats with diabetes mellitus and symmetric alopecia should be evaluated for hyperadrenocorticism.

Thyroid disease. Naturally occurring, acquired hypothyroidism has never been diagnosed in cats in the UK. Experimental thyroid ablation using radioiodine did not cause symmetric alopecia except of the pinnae (Thoday, 1986). Kittens with congenital hypothyroidism may exhibit a generalised thinning of the hair coat with only a few primary hairs scattered throughout the coat. Prognosis is good with thyroxine supplementation.

Feline hyperthyroidism is a condition which may cause changes in all body systems including the skin. Symmetric hair loss has not been reported, although patchy alopecia due to over-grooming may be seen.

"Feline endocrine alopecia" (FEA) is a descriptive term which has been used to describe the bilaterally symmetric alopecic lesions seen in the groin, ventrum, medial hindlimbs, perineum and forelegs from elbow to carpus of some cats. It is now accepted that the clinical appearance described is not invariably associated with an endocrine disease. In the last few years the term

FEA has been changed to idiopathic FSA as an endocrine aetiology has not been proven.

The condition is seen in neutered or entire animals of any age or breed, and the response to sex hormone therapy, particularly megoestrol acetate, has been cited as evidence of a sex hormone aetiology. However, megoestrol acetate is known to have mood-modifying actions as well as an antipruritic effect in cats and these cases may well have psychogenic alopecia or a hypersensitivity reaction. All the conditions mentioned in this chapter should be excluded before a diagnosis of idiopathic FSA is made. One test is particularly useful: Thoday (1986) showed that a circulating eosinophil count of >1.5 x 10^9/l has a 92% predictive value in excluding FSA as a diagnosis. Cases with eosinophilia should be carefully evaluated for hypersensitivity disorders.

If all other diagnoses are eliminated then a tentative diagnosis of idiopathic FSA or FEA may be made. In these cases there is evidence that some of these cats may respond to liothyronine sodium (T3, Tertroxin, Pitman-Moore). It is suggested that an initial dose of 20 µg per cat is used, gradually increasing to a maximum of 50 µg per cat per day. Such cases should be carefully monitored for thyrotoxicosis (Thoday, 1986). It should be noted that thyroid hormones may stimulate hair growth in non-thyroidal diseases. It is this author's opinion that the description FEA or idiopathic FSA as a diagnosis reflects our ignorance of the skin diseases of the cat and with increasing knowledge, much more specific diagnoses will be achieved.

Miscellaneous causes of excess hair shedding.

There are a variety of other causes of symmetric alopecia in cats which are caused by shedding of the hair rather than the cat licking or pulling it out. Preauricular partial alopecia is an example of one such condition in which some cats lose hair from the temporal region in a symmetric pattern. No treatment of this physiological condition is warranted or effective.

Perhaps the commonest condition in this miscellaneous group is telogen defluxion (telogen defluvium, telogen effluvium). This condition is initiated by stress such as gestation, lactation, surgery and number of other diseases, and is characterised by a shortening of the anagen phase of the hair cycle leading to large numbers of hairs entering the telogen phase at once with resultant shedding of the hair coat. The alopecia is usually generalised and transient. Skin biopsies are helpful in the diagnosis as all the hair follicles are in telogen. No specific therapy is required, except reassurance of the anxious owner. The ventral midline alopecia sometimes associated with oestrous is probably a manifestation of telogen defluxion.

Two very rare conditions which may cause symmetric alopecia are alopecia areata and alopecia mucinosa. Alopecia areata is characterised by focal or multifocal areas of alopecia which may be symmetric. The underlying skin appears normal. There are no apparent breed, age or sex predispositions. Definitive diagnosis is based on a history of insidious onset of alopecia, with skin biopsy revealing lymphoplasmacytic folliculitis. Topical and systemic glucocorticoids have been advocated for this condition in humans, dogs and cats (Nelson and Spielvogal, 1985; Muller et al, 1989) but there is little evidence they are beneficial and some cases will recover spontaneously. Alopecia mucinosa has been recognised in two cats with alopecia of the head, ears and neck (Scott, 1987). Biopsy results were typical of alopecia mucinosa, and both cats went on to develop mycosis fungoides.

Some drugs, especially those used for chemotherapy, may cause excess hair shedding.

Pruritus and Self-trauma

Pruritus and resulting licking and pulling at the hair coat is the commonest cause of feline symmetric alopecia. Although some of the diseases covered already in this chapter may involve a degree of pruritus (dermatophytosis, demodicosis, bacterial folliculitis and some of the systemic illnesses) the main problem in these conditions is that of excessive hair coat shedding due to damage to the hair or follicle in some way. The rest of the disorders covered are those in which the primary problem is pruritus and/or self-trauma to healthy hair and follicles.

Hypersensitivity disorders

Flea bite hypersensitivity is the commonest cause of skin disease in cats in the United Kingdom. It is a reasonable working principle that ALL feline dermatoses are caused by fleas until a flea eradication programme proves otherwise! The commonest presenting sign of flea bite hypersensitivity is miliary dermatitis (Chapter 16) but almost as common is bilaterally symmetric alopecia affecting the groin, ventrum, perineum, medial hindlimbs, lateral abdomen and, commonly, the medial aspect of the front limbs from elbow to carpus. Little or no damage may be detected on the underlying skin. It seems incredible that cats can induce such symmetrical lesions, but repeated trials with Elizabethan collars prove that they can. Any age, breed or sex of cat may be affected but it is uncommon to see extensive lesions in cats under eight months of age. The immunological basis of flea bite hypersensitivity involves Type I (immediate) and Type 4 (delayed) hypersensitivity, and possibly cutaneous basophil reactions as well.

All cases of FSA should be treated with a suitable antiparasitic spray such as a combination of dichlorvos and fenitrothion (Nuvan Top, Ciba Geigy) every ten days for six weeks, with all in-contact pets also being treated. Environmental control of the intermediate and adult stages of the flea is mandatory, using products such as methoprene and permethrin (Acclaim Plus, Sanofi) or dichlorvos/lodofenphos (Nuvan Staykill, Ciba Geigy).

Food hypersensitivity or food intolerance is relatively more common in the cat than the dog. In a recent study (White, 1989), 64% of all cases were alopecic with only three cats having papules and two with eosinophilic plaques. Pruritus was located principally in the head and neck region in 42% of cases. There were no age, breed or sex predilections, and in no case could owners relate the clinical signs to a recent change in diet. Definitive diagnosis involves feeding the cats a hypoallergenic diet for five to six weeks. Hypoallergenic diet composition should be tailored to the individual cat to provide a protein source the animal does not eat regularly (one of shark, rabbit or chicken is usually suitable) with a carbohydrate source (potatoes or rice). Consideration should be given to keeping the cat indoors during the trial period to avoid scavenging. If the alopecia improves, provocation with the original diet should lead to a relapse, confirming the diagnosis. The best solution for maintenance is to put the cat onto a commercial hypoallergenic diet. However, some animals with dietary hypersensitivity will manifest pruritus on these diets, therefore a balanced home made diet may be the only solution.

Atopic disease is becoming increasingly commonly recognised in cats. Clinical signs may include facial pruritus, miliary dermatitis, indolent ulcers or eosinphilic plaques and, of course, symmetric alopecia in the absence of other signs. Intradermal testing may reveal the allergen(s) responsible. Avoidance of the allergen, hyposensitisation, glucocorticoids, essential fatty acid supplements and antihistamines can all be used in therapy.

Drug eruptions may mimic any dermatosis and should be considered as a possible differential diagnosis in any animal with skin disease which is on drug therapy, especially if it fails to respond to apparently appropriate treatment. Withdrawal of the offending drug leads to resolution of the signs.

Psychogenic alopecia is a condition linked to stress and characterised by hair licking and pulling. Breeds such as the siamese and burmese are most commonly affected. Whilst some painful or irritating condition (eg. otitis) may precipitate the condition, the degree of self trauma is out of proportion to the initiating factor. Several cases have been seen associated with a new cat being introduced into the household, a new baby arriving, or a change of environment. The condition is diagnosed on history and physical examination and by ruling out all other possible diagnoses. Treatment with oral diazepam (Valium, Roche) at a dose of 1-2 mg bid may be effective. Occasionally, oral phenobarbitone at a dose of 2-6 mg/kg bid may be required. If possible, remove the inciting cause and gradually decrease the drug dosages.

INITIAL MANAGEMENT

The management of FSA is entirely dependant on making an accurate diagnosis. Until a diagnosis is achieved therapeutic attempts are likely to be unrewarding with a subsequent loss of confidence by the owner. In the author's experience good communication with the owner is essential from the time of first presentation, with a clear statement that FSA is a syndrome with many underlying causes for which there is no universal panacea. Once a specific diagnosis is made specific therapy is indicated and an accurate prognosis can be given.

REFERENCES

CHALMERS, S., SCHICK, R.O. and JEFFERS, J. (1989). Demodicosis in two cats seropositive for feline immunodeficiency virus. *Journal American Veterinary Medical Association,* **194**, 256.

CHESNEY, C.J. (1989). Demodicosis in the cat. *Journal of Small Animal Practice,* **30**, 689.

GEARY, M.R. and BAKER, K.P. (1986). The occurrence of pili torti in a litter of kittens in England. *Journal of Small Animal Practice,* **27**, 85.

KUNKLE, G.A. and MEYER, D.J. (1987). Toxicity of high doses of griseofulvin in cats. *Journal American Veterinary Medical Association,* **191**, 322.

MULLER, G.H., KIRK, R.W. and SCOTT, D.W. (1989). *Small Animal Dermatology,* Fourth Edition, W. B. Saunders, Philadelphia.

NELSON, D.A. and SPIELVOGAL, R.L. (1985). Alopecia areata. *International Journal of Dermatology,* **24**, 26.

SCOTT, D.W. (1980). Feline dermatology 1900-1978: a monograph. *Journal of American Animal Hospital Association,* **16**, 331.

SCOTT, D.W. (1987). Feline dermatology 1983-1985. *Journal of American Animal Hospital Association,* **23**, 255.

THODAY, K.L. (1981). Skin diseases of the cat. *In Practice,* **3**, 22.

THODAY, K.L. (1986). Differential diagnosis of symmetric alopecia in the cat. *Current Veterinary Therapy* IX, (Ed. R.W. Kirk) W.B. Saunders, Philadelphia.

WHITE, S.D., CARPENTER, J.L., MOORE, F.M. and OGILVIE, G. (1987). Generalised demodicosis associated with diabetes mellitus in two cats. *Journal American Veterinary Medical Association,* **191**, 448.

WHITE, S.D. (1989). Food hypersensitivity in cats: 14 cases (1982-1987). *Journal American Veterinary Medical Association,* **194**, 692.

WHITE, S.D. (1991). Pyoderma in five cats. *Journal of American Animal Hospital Association,* **27**, 141.

CHAPTER FOURTEEN

FACIAL DERMATOSES

Ross Bond ─────────────────────────────

INTRODUCTION

The face is a frequent site of skin disease in the dog and cat (Plates 40-45). The aim of this chapter is to outline an approach to the diagnosis of the skin diseases which are confined to, or predominately involve, the face or which may first affect the face prior to becoming more generalised. The principal skin diseases of this region are listed in Tables 1 to 3; this is not exhaustive as virtually any skin disease may affect the face. More detailed information on the conditions discussed below can be found in the standard textbooks.

Table 1
Hypersensitivity diseases and autoimmune/immune mediated
dermatoses which may affect the face

Disease	Usual lesion type	Incidence and main diagnostic features
Atopy	Erythema, lesions of self-trauma, often secondary pyoderma	Common. Rule-out other pruritic dermatoses, intradermal tests
Contact dermatitis*	Erythema, macules, papules, rarely erosions	Uncommon. Contact restriction, patch testing (rarely)
Dietary hypersensitivity	Erythema, lesions of self-trauma, often secondary pyoderma	Uncommon. Response to elimination diet, relapse on challenge
Drug eruption	Varies widely. May mimic almost any skin disease	Uncommon. History of drug exposure, resolution on drug withdrawal. Biopsy
Discoid lupus erythematosus	Nasal hyperkeratosis, erosions, depigmentation	Rare. Lesions often confined to face. Biopsy, ANA negative
Eosinophilic granuloma complex	Ulcer, plaque or nodule	Common in cats, rare in dogs. Biopsy
Eosinophilic furunculosis of the face (dogs)	Papules, pustules	Rare. Eosinophils predominant on cytology. Biopsy
Pemphigus erythematosus/foliaceus	Crusts, collarettes, erosions, vesicles, pustules	Rare. Rule-outs. Biopsy
Systemic lupus erythematosus	Erosions, scaling, ulceration, crusts	Rare. Other systems affected, biopsy, ANA positive
Vogt-Koyanagi-Harada-like syndrome	Depigmentation, erosion, crusting	Rare. Biopsy. Also uveitis

*Contact dermatitis may also result from irritant reactions.
ANA, antinuclear antibody.

Table 2
Facial dermatoses caused by micro-organisms and parasites

Disease	Usual lesion type	Incidence and main diagnostic features
Bacterial folliculitis/furunculosis	Papules, pustules, collarettes, furuncles	Common. Cytology. Culture. Biopsy. Response to treatment
Demodicosis	Scale/crust, alopecia, comedones, hyperpigmentation	Common. Skin scrapings
Dermatophytosis	Scale, alopecia, erythema, crusts	Common. Culture. Biopsy. Scrapings. Wood's light
Feline poxvirus infection	Papules with central ulcer and crust ("pock")	Rare. Cellulitis may preceed papules. Serology. Biopsy. VI, EM
Leishmaniasis	Diffuse dry scaling, periocular alopecia	Rare (imported dogs only in U.K). Serology. Biopsy. Bone marrow and lymph node aspirates
Malassezia dermatitis	Erythema, scaling, alopecia	Unclear (underdiagnosed?). Cytology. Culture. Response to treatment
Scabies	Crust, scale, fine erythematous papules	Common. Skin scrapings. Response to treatment. History of contagion

VI, virus isolation. EM, electron microscopy

Table 3
Miscellaneous facial dermatoses

Disease	Usual lesion type	Incidence and main diagnostic features
Canine acne	Papules, furuncles, comedones	Common. Rule-out demodicosis
Dermatomyositis	Alopecia, crusts, vesicles, scarring	Rare (UK). Breed and age, rule-outs, biopsy
Facial/lip fold dermatitis	Erythema	Common. Clinical signs diagnostic
Juvenile cellulitis	Vesicles, pustules, swelling	Uncommon. Age of onset, enlarged submandibular nodes
Nasal hyperkeratosis	Hyperkeratosis	Uncommon. Confined to nasal planum, non-inflammatory
Necrolytic migratory erythema	Crusts, erosions, fissures	Rare. Biopsy, evidence of hepatic disease or diabetes mellitus
Neoplasia	Varies with type	Uncommon. Biopsy
Vitiligo	Depigmentation	Rare. Non-inflammatory, non-pruritic, biopsy
Zinc-responsive dermatosis	Crusting	Rare. Response to treatment

The aim of the clinician should be to establish a definitive diagnosis so that specific therapy may be instituted, which in turn increases the likelihood of successful management. However, the diagnosis and treatment of facial dermatoses can be challenging as differential diagnoses are often numerous and may include some diseases which are rarely encountered.

APPROACH TO THE CASE

In common with dermatoses of other regions of the body, many facial disorders of differing causes may appear clinically similar. A logical and methodical approach involving a full history and clinical examination followed by appropriate laboratory tests is often necessary if an accurate diagnosis is to be obtained.

HISTORY

Signalment

A breed predilection exists for a number of diseases which involve the face (Table 4), and this may be of value when listing the principle differential diagnoses. The age of onset of the condition may be useful as some disorders tend to develop within a particular age range (Table 4). For example, demodicosis is most commonly seen in dogs of less than 15 months of age (Henfrey, 1990), whereas metabolic and neoplastic diseases usually affect animals in the later years. The gender of the patient is seldom helpful in the diagnosis of facial dermatoses.

Table 4
Facial dermatoses with breed and age predilections.

Disease	Breed predilection*	Usual age of onset#	References
Atopy	English setter, terriers, retrievers, boxer, GSD	1-3 years	Nesbitt et al (1984)
Canine acne	Boxer, bulldog, great Dane, doberman	3-12 months	Muller et al (1989)
Demodicosis	Doberman, bull terriers, OES	<15 months	Henfrey (1990)
Dermatomyositis	Rough collie, shetland sheepdog	3-6 months	Kunkle et al (1985)
Dermatophytosis	Jack Russell terrier¶	-	Wright (1989)
Discoid lupus erythematosus	GSD, rough collie, shetland sheepdog, siberian husky	-	Scott et al (1983b)
Facial fold dermatitis	Brachycephalic breeds, Shar-Pei	-	Ihrke (1983), Muller (1990)
Juvenile cellulitis	Retriever, dachshund	1-4 months	Kunkle (1985)
Lip fold dermatitis	Spaniels, setters	-	Ihrke (1983)
Pemphigus foliaceus	Bearded collie, akita, Newfoundland, schipperke	-	Ihrke et al (1985)
Systemic lupus erythematosus	Rough collie, shetland sheepdog	-	Scott et al (1983a)
Vitiligo	Siamese	-	Muller et al (1989)
Vogt-Koyanagi-Harada-like syndrome	Akita, samoyed, Siberian husky	-	Vercelli and Taraglio (1990)
Zinc responsive dermatosis	Siberian husky, Alaskan malemute	-	Kunkle (1980)

* Breed predilections may vary according to regional gene pool
\# Clinical signs may first develop at other ages in some cases; (-) denotes wide age of onset
¶ Predisposed to *Trichophyton* sp and *M. persicolor*.
GSD, German Shepherd dog; OES, Old English Sheepdog

General medical history

A general medical history should be obtained to determine whether there are any abnormalities of other organ systems, which may be related or unrelated to the skin disease (Table 5). This is of particular importance when systemic lupus erythematosus, canine familial dermatomyositis, canine necrolytic migratory erythema (also known as the "hepatocutaneous" syndrome, superficial necrolytic dermatitis, metabolic epidermal necrosis), leishmaniasis, Vogt-Koyanagi-Harada-like syndrome and adverse drug reactions are suspected.

Table 5
Table 5
Facial dermatoses with associated systemic disease

Disease	Possible associated abnormalities
Adult onset demodicosis	Immunosuppression eg. hyperadrenocorticism, neoplasia
Dermatomyositis	Muscle atrophy and weakness, sometimes dysphagia
Leishmaniasis	Weight loss, anaemia, diarrhoea, ocular, hepatic or renal disease
Necrolytic migratory erythema	Hepatic disease or pancreatic tumour ± diabetes mellitus
Systemic lupus erythematosus	Polyarthritis, anaemia, thrombocytopaenia, glomerulonephritis, pyrexia
Vogt-Koyanagi-Harada-like syndrome	Uveitis

Family history/contagion

A familial history may be a feature of inherited diseases such as atopy, juvenile-onset generalised demodicosis and dermatomyositis. In-contact animals or humans may be affected by contagious diseases such as ectoparasitic infestations, dermatophytosis and feline poxvirus infection.

Management

A complete list of all dietary components is needed if food sensitivity is suspected, so that an appropriate elimination diet can be formulated. Although nutritional dermatoses are uncommon in dogs and cats fed with commercially-prepared diets (Chapter 28), zinc responsive dermatosis may occur in dogs fed on cereal or soya based diets (Thoday, 1989).

The indoor and outdoor environment of the patient should be determined. Food bowls, chews or toys may cause contact dermatitis of the muzzle area. Animals in a rural environment with access to wild animals (rodents, hedgehogs, foxes) may be at risk from contagious diseases such as dermatophytosis, cowpox and scabies. In the UK, sporadic cases of leishmaniasis are seen only in dogs imported from Mediterranean countries.

Dermatological history

The duration of skin disease should be determined. This may vary from hours, in the case of an acute eruptive process such as eosinophilic furunculosis (Gross, 1992), to years with allergic skin diseases. The initial location and nature of skin lesions and their progression or spread should be recorded. Observant owners may describe transient primary lesions such as vesicles and pustules which are no longer present at the time of examination.

Pruritus may be the main complaint in many facial dermatoses. Pruritus may be severe in atopy, food hypersensitivity and scabies but absent in nutritional dermatoses and vitiligo. The severe muzzle pruritus shown by some dogs with *Malassezia* dermatitis can be so intense that they may be misdiagnosed as having neurological disease (Mason, 1992). Variable degrees of pruritus may be present in other inflammatory facial dermatoses, such as infectious and immune mediated conditions.

The owner may report seasonal variations in the occurrence or severity of diseases of more than twelve months duration. Atopic patients with pollen sensitivities may have clinical signs confined to the spring or summer months, and immune mediated dermatoses such as lupus erythematosus and the pemphigus complex may be exacerbated by exposure to sunlight. In cats, lesions of the eosinophilic granuloma complex associated with flea hypersensitivity or atopy may recur on a seasonal basis.

A knowledge of the response to previous therapy may be helpful. Response to antibacterial agents may be observed in animals with superficial or deep pyoderma; however, most cases recur and must be evaluated for an underlying cause. Atopy may respond well to anti-inflammatory doses of glucocorticoids, whereas dietary sensitivities and the immune mediated dermatoses such as pemphigus and lupus erythematosus are often poorly responsive. Demodicosis, dermatophytosis and feline poxvirus infection may be exacerbated by glucocorticoid therapy. Recent treatment may have influenced the appearance of the lesions and interfere with diagnostic tests such as bacterial culture and intradermal allergy tests.

PHYSICAL EXAMINATION

Skin disease of the facial region may be directly or indirectly associated with abnormalities of other body systems (Table 5) and a full physical examination should accompany the dermatological examination to ensure that important findings elsewhere are not overlooked.

The entire skin surface should be examined and the nature and extent of any primary and secondary lesions recorded. Identification of the lesion type is of fundamental importance in formulating the differential list. A symmetrical distribution usually indicates a systemically mediated disease. A summary of the most common lesion type for each condition is given in Tables 1 to 3.

Involvement of the nasal planum is most useful in narrowing the list of differential diagnoses (Table 6). For example, follicular diseases such as superficial and deep bacterial infections and demodicosis do not affect this region, due to the absence of hair follicles. Although fungal hyphae may invade the keratinized layers of the nasal planum in rare cases, this area is usually spared in dermatophyte infections of the face.

Erythema with or without other lesions

Atopic dogs frequently present with pruritus and erythema of the muzzle and periorbital areas, although non-lesional pruritus may occur in the early stages of the disease. The ears, interdigital skin and ventrum are also frequently affected and, with chronicity, may become alopecic, lichenified and hyperpigmented. Contact dermatitis caused by a food bowl or toy will lead to pruritus and erythema of the muzzle area only. Facial pruritus is a relatively common manifestation of dietary sensitivity in cats; self-trauma may lead to marked alopecia, excoriations and crusting. The commensal yeast *Malassezia pachydermatis* has emerged as an occasional cause of facial and more generalised dermatitis in dogs, which may mimic or complicate atopy and dietary sensitivity (Mason, 1992).

Papular lesions

Papules may dominate the clinical picture in dogs with nasal pyoderma, eosinophilic furunculosis, and canine acne. In nasal pyoderma and eosinophilic furunculosis, lesions may develop rapidly

Table 6
Facial dermatoses which may affect the nasal planum

Frequently involved	Sometimes involved
Discoid/systemic lupus erythematosus	Contact dermatitis
Pemphigus foliaceus/erythematosus	Dermatophytosis
Vitiligo	Drug eruption
Vogt-Koyanagi-Harada-like syndrome	Leishmaniasis
Nasal hyperkeratosis	Zinc responsive dermatosis
	Neoplasia

and coalesce to involve large areas of the bridge of the nose, whereas the lesions of canine acne are accompanied by comedones and furuncles and are often chronic, asymptomatic and confined to the chin.

Feline poxvirus (cowpox) infection is a sporadic disease of cats believed to originate from contact with infected wild rodents (Bennett *et al,* 1990). Typically, an initial bite wound usually found on the head, neck or limb develops into an abscess or area of cellulitis, and after 10-20 days numerous secondary lesions develop. These consist of widely distributed, circular, erythematous, large papules which ulcerate and crust; occasional vesicles may also be seen.

Vesicular and pustular lesions

Vesicles and pustules are transient, fluid filled lesions of considerable diagnostic value. Vesicles may be seen in the pemphigus group of diseases, occasionally in systemic lupus erythematosus and drug eruptions and rarely in dermatomyositis and contact dermatitis. Vesicles may evolve into pustules as inflammatory cells accumulate in the epidermis. As these lesions readily rupture, epidermal collarettes and focal crusts usually predominate and careful or repeated inspections may be needed to locate the intact primary lesion. A hair protruding from a pustular lesion is indicative of folliculitis; follicular pustules usually indicate bacterial infection, demodicosis or dermatophytosis.

Juvenile cellulitis (juvenile pyoderma, puppy strangles) is an acute, vesicopustular disease of puppies between one and four months of age, the cause of which is unknown (Kunkle, 1985; Muller *et al,* 1989). Cases may first present with swelling of the lips and eyelids, and there may be a purulent blepharitis and ulcerative otitis. Systemic signs (pyrexia, anorexia) may occur, and submandibular and a more generalised lymphadenopathy is frequently present; affected nodes may rupture and drain. One or more pups in the litter may be affected.

Scaling and crusting dermatoses

Leishmaniasis is a severe, often fatal, systemic disease caused by protozoan parasites of the genus *Leishmania* which are endemic in Mediterranean countries (Ferrer, 1992). In the United Kingdom, the disease occurs only in imported dogs. Skin lesions are common and are most often characterised by symmetrical, non-pruritic, dry scaling which begin on the head and extend to affect wide areas of the body surface. Less commonly, nodules, papules and ulcers may develop (Ferrer *et al,* 1988). Systemic signs are variable and may include weight loss, lymphadenopathy, ocular lesions, diarrhoea, renal failure, hepatic failure, epistaxis and anaemia (Ferrer, 1992). Some dogs with systemic lupus erythematosus may also present with symmetrical scaling of the face accompanied by systemic disease (Scott *et al,* 1983a).

Diffuse scaling of the face and other regions may be seen in dogs with dermatophytosis due to *Microsporum canis* and *M. persicolor* (Wright, 1989; Bond *et al,* 1992). In contrast, *Trichophyton mentagrophytes* and *T. erinacei* often induce severe inflammatory lesions of the face or limbs characterised by a well demarcated, peripherally-expanding area of alopecia, crusting and erythema which initially becomes smooth and shiny during the healing process (Wright, 1989).

Dogs and cats with scabies often present with intensely pruritic lesions of the head and pinnae, either alone or in addition to other sites. Skin lesions usually consist of marked scaling and crusting, erythematous papules and excoriations, sometimes accompanied by peripheral lymphadenopathy. *Sarcoptes scabiei var canis,* the sarcoptid mite of the dog, may occasionally infest immunosuppressed cats. The sarcoptid mite of cats, *Notoedres cati,* is rarely encountered in the UK.

Zinc responsive dermatosis are characterised by symmetrical, often non-pruritic, yellowish crusts which affect the face, pinnae, scrotum and limbs (Kunkle, 1980; Thoday, 1989). Hyperkeratosis of the foot pads and nasal planum has also been reported (Kunkle, 1980). Rarely, deficiencies or imbalances of other nutrients may result in scaling or crusting dermatoses.

Periocular and perioral crusting with fissures and ulceration is a frequent feature of dogs with necrolytic migratory erythema (the "hepatocutaneous syndrome"), a rare dermatosis associated with underlying hepatic disease or a glucagon producing pancreatic neoplasm, with or without concurrent diabetes mellitus (Walton *et al*, 1986; Gross *et al*, 1990; Miller, 1992). Facial lesions may be preceded by severe footpad hyperkeratosis and skin lesions elsewhere, accompanied by systemic signs of anorexia, weight loss and polyuria.

Canine familial dermatomyositis is a rare, possibly inherited disease which almost exclusively affects rough collies, Shetland sheepdogs and their crosses and usually begins between 3-6 months of age (Kunkle *et al*, 1985). Skin lesions often consist of facial crusts and alopecia, which evolve from pustules or vesicles. Lesions may also affect pressure points and the tips of the tail and ears, and there may be evidence of concurrent muscle disease (Table 5). One or more pups within the litter may be affected, and there may be considerable variation in the severity of clinical signs.

Depigmentation

Depigmentation (Chapter 9) is a feature of some of the less common facial dermatoses. Vitiligo is characterised by non-inflammatory macular areas of depigmentation, often affecting the nasal planum, lips, footpads and elsewhere in a symmetrical pattern. The cutaneous features of vitiligo may be indistinguishable from those of the Vogt-Koyanagi-Harada-like syndrome, a rare disorder also believed to be associated with an immune mediated assault on melanin containing-tissues (Kern *et al*, 1985). In the latter disease however, uveitis may occur prior to or simultaneously with the skin disease, and cutaneous erosions and crusting are sometimes seen (Kern *et al*, 1985; Vercelli and Taraglio, 1990). Nasal depigmentation accompanied by erosions, crusting, alopecia and erythema may also occur in systemic or discoid lupus erythematosus or pemphigus foliaceus/erythematosus. Depigmentation of the nasal planum has also been reported in a dog with epitheliotropic lymphoma (DeBoer *et al*, 1990).

ESTABLISHING THE DIAGNOSIS

A careful consideration of the history and clinical signs should allow the clinician to list the differential diagnoses to be considered and, in some cases, the diagnosis will be straightforward (for example, facial fold dermatitis). However, a number of laboratory tests will usually be required. Simple laboratory techniques such as the microscopical examination of skin scrapings and cytological preparations should be performed routinely, although a wider range of tests may be necessary depending on the nature and severity of the disease. The diagnostic tests discussed below are described in more detail in Chapter 3.

Skin scrapings are essential in virtually every dermatology case. Several scrapings should be taken, and adequate time set aside for careful microscopical examination. Fungal hyphae and arthroconidia may be observed in scrapings from animals with dermatophytosis, although direct examination was positive in only 41% of cases in one study (Wright, 1989).

Cytological techniques such as impression smears are rapid and inexpensive methods of obtaining useful information which may support a clinical diagnosis and allow institution of specific therapy early in the course of the disease. Pustules can be opened with a fine needle and the contents smeared onto a glass slide and stained. Neutrophils with intracellular cocci (or less commonly rods) indicate bacterial infection. Although culture may confirm the identity of bacteria seen on cytology, antimicrobial agents can often be selected empirically and culture and sensitivity testing may only be necessary in severe or poorly responsive cases (Ihrke, 1983). Large numbers of acantholytic keratinocytes, accompanied by healthy neutrophils and sometimes eosinophils, *in the absence of bacteria*, may support a diagnosis of pemphigus and is an indication for confirmatory biopsy. As the name suggests, eosinophils may be found in large numbers in eosinophilic furunculosis.

Tape strippings are useful for recovering *Malassezia* organisms from the skin surface. Clear adhesive tape is pressed onto the skin surface following gentle clipping, removed and stained with a suitable agent such as Diff Quik. The tape is then stuck to a glass slide and examined under the oil immersion lens for the presence of the characteristic peanut-shaped yeast. If the organism is detected, a therapeutic trial may be indicated to determine the significance of the yeast (Mason, 1992).

If a diagnosis is not established by the above measures then further investigations must be considered. Fungal culture is the most reliable method for the diagnosis of dermatophytosis and should be routinely performed in every unexplained case of facial dermatitis. Identification of the pathogen may be useful in establishing the source of infection; for example, most canine cases of dermatophytosis due to *Microsporum canis* result from contact with infected cats and wild rodents are the usual source of *Trichophyton mentagrophytes* (Wright, 1989).

Skin biopsy may play a pivotal role in the diagnosis of a number of skin diseases of the face. Biopsy is necessary for the definitive diagnosis of most autoimmune and immune mediated diseases, neoplasia and dermatomyositis and should be performed whenever these conditions are suspected. However, careful lesion selection is important if useful information is to be gained; in general, intact primary lesions should be sampled. Nasal planum involvement is an indication for biopsy as histopathological examination is often necessary to differentiate the diseases of this area (Table 6). Distinctive histopathological features may also be observed in necrolytic migratory erythema, leishmaniasis, feline poxvirus infection, demodicosis, dermatophytosis and deep bacterial and fungal infections. However, diagnostic pathology may only be found following the examination of several sections and the use of special stains and may be absent in some cases. Biopsy is less helpful when hypersensitivity disorders and *Malassezia* dermatitis are suspected as, although the histological pattern may support these diagnoses, other methods are necessary for confirmation. The reader is referred to Chapters 4, 16 and 31 for a discussion of the diagnostic approach to allergic skin disease.

Routine haematological and biochemical profiles and urinalyses should be obtained from animals suspected of having systemic diseases. Serological tests are available for the diagnosis of leishmaniasis (Ferrer, 1992) and feline poxvirus infection (Bennett et al, 1990). A positive antinuclear antibody (ANA) titre, in addition to other criteria, is required for the definitive diagnosis of systemic lupus erythematosus (Halliwell and Gorman, 1989). Dogs and cats with pemphigus erythematosus may also be ANA positive (Scott *et al*, 1987).

While awaiting results of laboratory tests, care should be taken to ensure that any empirical therapy (such as glucocorticoids) will not exacerbate the disease or interfere with further investigations. However, therapeutic trials can be of considerable diagnostic value when a number of conditions are suspected. Mites may be difficult to find in some cases of canine scabies and trial therapy is justified if there is a high index of suspicion for this disease. All in-contact dogs and the environment should be treated (Chapter 29). Zinc responsive dermatosis may be confirmed by response to oral zinc sulphate (Zincomed, Medo Pharmaceuticals Limited, 10 mg/kg sid with food) while leaving the original diet unchanged (Thoday, 1989). Dietary alterations may be sufficient for sustained control, although some huskies and malamutes require lifelong supplementation.

Mason (1992) suggests a two week course of oral ketoconazole (10 mg/kg bid, with food) as trial therapy for dogs suspected of having *Malassezia* dermatitis. This product is not licensed for veterinary use. Vomiting and malaise are occasionally seen. Alternatively, selenium sulphide or tar and sulphur shampoos, applied two to three times per week, or miconazole cream, twice daily, may be used. Predisposing factors such as underlying hypersensitivity disorders should be addressed where identified.

INITIAL MANAGEMENT

A definitive diagnosis allows the clinician to provide the client with a prognosis and to consider specific therapeutic options. Although appropriate treatment will result in resolution of many infectious and ectoparasitic diseases, certain facial dermatoses such as hypersensitivities and immune mediated disorders may require lifelong therapy. If a diagnosis is not established and the condition persists, the clinician should then check the history, re-examine the patient and re-evaluate the laboratory data in case some important findings have been overlooked. Alternatively, the case may be referred to a veterinary dermatologist. A detailed discussion of therapy of the various facial dermatoses is beyond the scope of this chapter; the reader is directed to other chapters in Part Three of this manual and to the standard texts.

REFERENCES

BENNETT, M., GASKELL, C.J., BAXBY, D., GASKELL, R.M., KELLY, D.F. and NAIDOO, J. (1990) Feline cowpox virus infection. *Journal of Small Animal Practice.* **31**, 167.

BOND, R., MIDDLETON, D.J., SCARFF, D.H. and LAMPORT, A.I. (1992) Chronic dermatophytosis due to *Microsporum persicolor* infection in three dogs. *Journal of Small Animal Practice.* **33**, 571.

DeBOER, D.J., TURREL, J.M. and MOORE, P.F. (1990) Mycosis fungoides in a dog: demonstration of T-cell specificity and response to radiotherapy. *Journal of the American Hospital Association.* **26**, 566.

FERRER, L. (1992) Leishmaniasis. *Current Veterinary Therapy XI.* (Eds. R. W. Kirk and J.D. Bonagura.) W.B. Saunders, Philadelphia.

FERRER, L., RABANAL, R., FONDEVILA, D., RAMOS, J.A. and DOMINGO, M. (1988) Skin lesions in canine leishmaniasis. *Journal of Small Animal Practice.* **29**, 381.

GROSS, T.L. (1992) A proposed arthropod etiology for canine eosinophilic furunculosis of the face. In: *Advances in Veterinary Dermatology, Volume 2* (Eds. P.J. Ihrke, I.S. Mason and S.D. White), in press. Pergamon, Oxford.

GROSS, T.L., O'BRIEN, T.D., DAVIES, A.P. and LONG, R.E. (1990) Glucagon-producing endocrine tumors in two dogs with superficial necrolytic dermatitis. *Journal of the American Veterinary Medical Association.* **197**, 1619.

HALLIWELL, R.E.W. and GORMAN, N.T. (1989) *Veterinary Clinical Immunology.* W. B. Saunders, Philadelphia.

HENFREY, J.I. (1990) Canine demodicosis. *In Practice* **12**, 187.

IHRKE, P.J. (1983) The management of canine pyodermas. *Current Veterinary Therapy VIII* Ed. R. W. Kirk. W.B. Saunders, Philadelphia.

IHRKE, P.J., STANNARD, A.A., ARDANS, A.A. and GRIFFIN, C.E. (1985) Pemphigus foliaceus in dogs: a review of 37 cases. *Journal of the American Veterinary Medical Association.* **186**, 59.

KERN, T.J., WALTON, D.W., RIIS, R.C., MANNING, T.O., LARATTA, L.J. and DZIEZYC, J. (1985) Uveitis associated with poliosis and vitiligo in six dogs. *Journal of the American Veterinary Medical Association.* **187**, 408.

KUNKLE, G.A. (1980) Zinc-responsive dermatoses in dogs. *Current Veterinary Therapy VII* (Ed. R. W. Kirk). W. B. Saunders, Philadelphia.

KUNKLE, G.A. (1985) Problem oriented approach to canine pediatric dermatology. *Compendium on Continuing Education.* **7**, 377.

KUNKLE, G.A., GROSS, T.L., FADOK, V. and WERNER, L.L. (1985) Dermatomyositis in collie dogs. *Compendium on Continuing Education.* **7**, 185.

MASON, K.V. (1992) *Malassezia* dermatitis and otitis. *Current Veterinary Therapy XI* (Eds. R. W. Kirk and J. D. Bonagura.) W.B. Saunders, Philadelphia.

MILLER, W.H. (1992) Necrolytic migratory erythema in dogs: a cutaneous marker for gastrointestinal disease. *Current Veterinary Therapy XI* (Eds. R.W. Kirk and J. D. Bonagura.) W.B. Saunders, Philadelphia.

MULLER, G.H. (1990) Skin diseases of the Chinese Shar-Pei. *Veterinary Clinics, North American Small Animal Practice.* **20**, 1655

MULLER, G.H., KIRK, R.W. and SCOTT, D.W. (1989) *Small Animal Dermatology.* 4th edition, W.B. Saunders, Philadelphia.

NESBITT, G.E., KEDAN, G.S. and CACIOLO, P. (1984) Canine atopy. Part 1. Etiology and diagnosis. *Compendium on Continuing Education.* **6**, 73.

SCOTT, D.W., WALTON, D,K., MANNING, T.O., SMITH, C.A. and LEWIS, R.M. (1983a) Canine lupus erythematosus. I. Systemic lupus erythematosus. *Journal of the American Hospital Association.* **19**, 461.

SCOTT, D.W., WALTON, D,K., MANNING, T.O., SMITH, C.A. and LEWIS, R.M. (1983b) Canine lupus erythematosus. II. Discoid lupus erythematosus. *Journal of the American Hospital Association.* **19**, 481.

SCOTT, D.W., WALTON, D.K., SLATER, M.R., SMITH, C.A. and LEWIS, R.W. (1987) Immune-mediated dermatoses in domestic animals: ten years after - part 1. *Compendium on Continuing Education.* **9**, 424.

THODAY, K.L. (1989) Diet related zinc-responsive skin disease in dogs: a dying dermatosis? *Journal of Small Animal Practice.* **30**, 213.

VERCELLI, A. and TARAGLIO, S (1990) Canine Vogt-Koyanagi-Harada-like syndrome in two Siberian Husky dogs. *Veterinary Dermatology.* **1**, 151.

WALTON, D.K., CENTER, S.A., SCOTT, D.W. and COLLINS, K. (1986) Ulcerative dermatosis associated with diabetes mellitus in the dog: a report of four cases. *Journal of the American Hospital Association.* **22**, 79.

WRIGHT, A.I. (1989) Ringworm in dogs and cats. *Journal of Small Animal Practice.* **30**, 242.

OTITIS EXTERNA

Patrick J McKeever ────────────────────

INTRODUCTION

Otitis externa is an inflammation of the epithelial lining of the external auditory canal, which is that portion of the external ear located between the pinna and the tympanic membrane.

Incidence of otitis externa in the canine has been reported to be from 4 to 16% of hospital admissions and up to 20% of the general population (Grono, 1969). Incidence in cats has been reported to be from 2 to 6.6% of hospital admissions (Baxter and Lawler, 1972). Variance of incidence between authors may be due to such factors as time of year when the surveys were taken, breed popularity in a given area, and the differences in criteria concerning diagnosis.

Diagnosis and symptomatic treatment of otitis externa based only on a superficial otic examination may resolve some cases of otitis, but often this response will only be temporary. Therefore, otitis externa has the potential to become a frustrating diagnostic and therapeutic challenge. This is due to the numerous aetiological agents that are responsible for its development. Failure to diagnose and treat the primary disease or environmental factors will result in less than satisfactory results.

ANATOMY OF THE EXTERNAL EAR

The pinna is formed from the distal flaring of the auricular cartilage and is funnel-shaped; it serves to receive air vibrations and transmit them via the ear canal to the tympanic membrane. The pinna can be controlled independently and is highly mobile (Macy and Seim, 1985). The shape of the pinna is breed specific. It is covered on both sides with skin that is tightly attached to the perichondrium. The skin that lines the inner surface of the pinna generally contains fewer hairs.

The diameter of the ear canal or external acoustic meatus formed from the auricular and annular cartilages is 5-10 mm, depending on the age, breed and size of the dog. It is approximately 2cm in length and ends proximally with the tympanic membrane or ear drum (Getty *et al*, 1956).

The tympanic membrane is thin and semitransparent; it is elliptical in outline and serves as a wall between the tympanic cavity and the external acoustic meatus. The tympanic membrane is thinnest in the centre and becomes progressively thicker peripherally, where it is attached to a fibrocartilaginous circular pad that is, in turn, fastened to a definite collar of bone in the external acoustic meatus (Getty *et al*, 1956). The manubrium of the malleus can be seen as a white fingerlike projection extending out into the tympanic membrane.

The skin that lines the deep or proximal portion of the ear canal is thinnest. It becomes thicker as it progresses to the distal or superficial part of the canal and reaches its greatest thickness on the distal third of the concave surface of the pinna (Fernando, 1966). Close to the tympanic membrane, the skin is aglandular and, in the shorthaired breeds, possesses no hair follicles. However, in longhaired dogs, very fine hairs are present (Fernando, 1966). Sebaceous glands form the superficial glandular bed in the dermis of the ear canal and are especially prominent in the more distal or superficial areas of the canal. The apocrine glands occur below the sebaceous glands in the deeper dermis. These glands open directly to the skin surface either immediately adjacent to the opening of an associated hair follicle or at some distance from it (Fraser, 1961). The number of sebaceous and apocrine glands that are present vary, depending on the breed. Longhaired and finehaired breeds, like spaniels and Irish setters, have relatively better developed and higher numbers of glands than do the shorthaired breeds (Fernando, 1966).

PATHOPHYSIOLOGY OF OTITIS EXTERNA

In the early acute stages of otitis, irritation due to the inciting or predisposing factors results in hyperplasia of both epidermis and sebaceous glands, as well as hyperkeratinisation of the infundibulum of the hair follicle. A superficial dermal infiltrate of lymphocytes, plasma cells, polymorphonuclear leukocytes and histiocytes develops (Fernando, 1967). Chronic otitis is characterised by extensive epidermal hyperplasia (5 to 6 times its normal thickness) with or without the formation of distinct rete pegs extending between the dermal papillae (Fraser, 1961). Ulceration of the epidermis is frequently observed in chronically affected ears especially if *Pseudomonas* or *Proteus* are present. Sebaceous glands are usually smaller and less active in chronic otitis and are displaced in the superficial dermis by the apocrine glands, which become hyperplastic and dilated. Changes in the apocrine glands further decrease the diameter of the ear canal. If the cystic apocrine glands rupture, they become surrounded by a dense infiltrate of histiocytes, polymorphonuclear leucocytes, mast cells, giant cells and fibroblasts. Reduction of the diameter of the ear canal is further exacerbated by fibroplasia of the dermis (Fernando, 1966). In severe, longstanding cases of chronic otitis externa, ossification of the external ear canal and associated cartilages may occur.

EXTERNAL FACTORS PREDISPOSING TO OTITIS EXTERNA

It has generally been assumed that otitis externa is a primary condition with micro-organisms and parasites being aetiological agents . However, with the exception of parasites, otitis is generally secondary to predisposing factors or other disease states. In dogs, one or more of the following may be involved (Fraser, 1961a; Fraser *et al*, 1961; Rycroft and Saben, 1977; Griffin, 1981; Woody and Fox, 1986):

1. Foreign bodies (weed awns, seeds, excess hair, and dried wax)

2. Parasites (mites, ticks, chiggers and biting flies)

3. Physiological disturbances (nutritional deficiencies and concomitant disease)

4. Trauma (iatrogenic or self induced)

5. Abnormally small or restrictive ear canals

6. Ear tumours

7. Excessive moisture in the ear (animals which swim frequently, animals with pendulous ears [which results in poor air circulation] and increased environmental humidity)

DISEASES PREDISPOSING TO OTITIS EXTERNA

Atopic Dermatitis

The disease that otitis externa is most likely to be secondary to is atopic dermatitis. Approximately 55% of the cases with this condition develop concurrent otitis and in 3% of the cases of atopic dermatitis, otitis is the only manifestation of this disease (Scott, 1981). Inflammation of the pinna, associated with atopic dermatitis, causes hyperplasia of epidermis, dermis and the sebaceous and apocrine glands (Fraser, 1965; Rycroft and Saben, 1977). The increased secretions and decreased ventilation resulting from a narrowing of the ear canal create an ideal environment for the proliferation of bacteria and yeast. Otitis secondary to atopic dermatitis develops in conjunction with the pruritic skin disease. Initially, it appears as erythema and or hyperplasia with minimal exudation, but some animals may have excessive wax production by the skin of the pinna. Ear lesions respond to topical or systemic steroids or hyposensitisation (Chapter 31).

Endocrinopathies

Hypothyroidism, male feminizing syndrome, Sertoli cell tumour, and ovarian imbalances are often associated with a chronic otitis externa (Griffin, 1981; Macy and Seim 1985). Of these, hypothyroidism is the most frequently encountered. The exact pathogenesis leading to the development of endocrine-related otitis is unknown. Most likely, it involves changes in glandular activity and keratinisation because most animals with otitis externa due to endocrinopathies have seborrhoea as well. In two reported cases of hypothyroidism, otitis was the only clinical sign noted (Griffin, 1981).

Immune Mediated Diseases

Diseases of the pemphigus complex as well as systemic or discoid lupus erythematosus may cause vesicular, pustular, ulcerative, or crusting lesions of the pinna and ear canal (Griffin, 1981; Rycroft and Saben, 1977; Macy and Seim, 1985). Of the diseases that make up the pemphigus complex, pemphigus foliaceous and pemphigus erythematosus are most likely to be associated with ear lesions and otitis. Lesions almost always involve other parts of the body as well, although cases of pemphigus foliaceous involving only the ear have been reported (Griffin, 1981). The clinical signs of systemic lupus are variable, but when ear lesions are observed, they are associated with one or more of the following:

1. Concomitant skin lesions

2. Polyarthritis

3. Fever

4. Proteinuria

5. Anemia

6. Thrombocytopenia

Drug eruptions that result in ear lesions are uncommon but can occur as the result of either topical or systemic medications. Lesions are confined to the ears if the reaction is to a topical otic preparation, but in the case of a systemic drug, lesions may also be found in the skin of other areas of the body and mucocutaneous junctions. The diagnosis is dependent upon confirming an appropriate history of recent drug use and response to drug withdrawal (Macy and Seim, 1985).

Foreign bodies

Foreign bodies such as plant material, dirt, sand and dried medications are frequently responsible for otitis externa (Rycroft and Saben, 1977; Wilson, 1985). In some locales grass awns are the most common cause of foreign body otitis. Most cases are acute and unilateral, but many dogs in areas with a high density of grass awns will have chronic bilateral disease. Penetration of the tympanic membrane by grass awns may occur.

Otodectes

Otodectes cynotis (ear mites) are large, white freemoving psoroptid mites that live on the surface of the epithelial lining of the ear canal, or in rare instances, on the skin surface. These mites are highly transmissible, and studies have shown that they lack specificity among carnivore host species (Muller *et al*, 1989). Ear mites are responsible for approximately 10% of the cases of otitis in dogs and 50% in cats (Rose, 1976; Griffin, 1981; August, 1988). The incidence may actually be higher than this because otitis can be produced by only 2-3 mites, which would be difficult to demonstrate (Griffin, 1981). In addition, the mites will often leave the ear canal if severe inflammation and a purulent bacterial or yeast infection develops (August, 1988). The life cycle is completed in 3 weeks (Muller *et al*, 1989). The egg is laid with a cement that attaches it to a substrate and after 4 days it hatches into a six legged larva. Within 3 to 10 days this larva develops into an eight legged protonymph. After 3 to 5 days, the protonymph molts into the deutonymph. After an additional 3 to 5 days the deutonymph becomes attached, end to end, with an adult male. If a male adult is produced from the deutonymph, the attachment has no significance. However, if a female is produced, she is, and must be, fertilised at the moment of ecdysis or she will not be able to produce eggs (Muller *et al*, 1989).

Mites feed on lymph and whole blood thereby exposing the host to mite antigens. Therefore animals may become sensitised to the mites with the production of IgE reaginic antibodies (Powell *et al*, 1980). Immediate wheal and flare responses to mite antigens are found in 87% of random source cats. This response is unrelated to infestation with mites (Weisbroth *et al*, 1974). It has been proposed that almost all cats are exposed to small numbers of mites early in life. Some cats develop immune responses that can create an aural environment sufficiently hostile to prevent mite colonisation and clinical disease. Other cats may have defective or lesser immune responses that allow the mites to colonise and produce clinical disease (Powell *et al*, 1980).

Tumours

Tumours of the ear should be considered in any chronic case of otitis externa that does not respond to appropriate therapy. Ear tumours can develop either from the skin or its adnexal structures. Squamous cell carcinomata, histiocytomata, sebaceous gland adenomata and adenocarcinomata, basal cell carcinomata, mast cell tumours, chondromata, chondrosarcomata, trichoepitheliomata, apocrine gland adenocarcinomata, fibromata, fibrosarcomata and papillomata have all been reported (Rycroft and Saben, 1977; Rose, 1978; Griffin, 1981; Macy and Seim, 1985). In general, ear tumours in the dog are more common but less malignant than those observed in the cat (Van der Gaag, 1986).

Squamous cell carcinomata are more common in cats than dogs and are frequently found on the pinnal margins of white-haired cats.

Inflammatory polyps are unique but common ear tumours of cats. The stroma of this tumour consists of either myxomatous or dense fibrous connective tissue. Inflammatory cells and dilated capillaries are found throughout the connective tissue. The stroma is covered by either ciliated or nonciliated columnar epithelium or by stratified squamous, nonkeratinizing epithelium. Inflammatory polyps have been diagnosed in cats, ranging in age from 3 months to 5 years of age; approximately 45% of these cases are found in cats less than 2 years of age. No sex or breed predisposition has been noted. If extensive they may occupy the external ear canal, middle ear, eustachian tube, and nasopharynx (Harvey and Goldschmidt, 1978).

Bacteria and Yeast Associated With Otitis

The presence of bacteria and yeast in the ear canal does not necessarily mean that these organisms are playing a causal role in the development of the otitis. This is because many normal dogs have low numbers of commensal and potentially pathogenic bacteria and yeast present in the ear canal (Dickson and Love, 1983). These organisms can quickly colonize the ear canal if its lining or microclimate becomes altered (August, 1988). Their growth then exacerbates and perpetuates the inflammatory response within the ear (August, 1988). Although these bacteria and yeast may not be the principle aetiological agents, there is a high probability that they are involved in the subsequent disease process.

Staphylococcus. In one study, coagulase-positive *Staphylococcus* spp. were isolated from 9.6% of animals with normal or clean ears, 14% of dogs with waxy ears, and 22% of dogs with otitis externa (Sharma and Rhoads, 1975). Other studies show that *Staphylococcus* spp. are present in about 20% of normal ears and 40% of ears with otitis externa (Dickson and Love, 1983).

Ears populated with *Staphylococcus* spp. generally have exudates that are light brown or yellow in colour. Exudates produced due to copopulation of *Streptococcus* spp. tend to be light in colour, while exudates due to copopulation of *Malassezia* will be brown to dark-brown (Pugh *et al*, 1974; Rycroft and Saben, 1977; August, 1986).

134

Streptococcus. When data are averaged from several studies, it is found that *Streptococcus* spp. can be isolated from approximately 16% of normal ears and 10% of ears with otitis externa (Sharma and Rhoads, 1975; Dickenson and Love, 1983). This may indicate that otitic ears are less favourable for the growth of *Streptococcus* spp. in some cases than the environment of the normal ear. If present, the exudate associated with *Streptococcus* spp. tends to be light yellow to light brown in colour.

Pseudomonas. *Pseudomonas aurogenosa* is isolated from normal ears in only 0.4% of the dogs studied (Woody and Fox, 1986). In contrast, *Pseudomonas* is isolated in 20% of otitic ears (August, 1988). It is isolated frequently from chronic recurrent cases of otitis and those cases in which there has been long-term treatment with topical antibacterial drugs (August, 1988). Otitic ears populated with *Pseudomonas* are generally quite painful and have copious amounts of pale or light yellow-colored secretions (Fraser *et al*, 1961). Extensive ulceration of the ear canal epithelium is also commonly associated with this organism.

Proteus. *Proteus* spp. have not been cultured from normal ears and are present in only 11% of otitic ears (Fraser, 1965). Like *Pseudomonas*, they often often found in cases of chronic ulcerated otitis with light yellow secretions (August, 1988).

Malassezia. *Malassezia pachydermatis* (formerly called *Pityrosporum pachydermatis*) is an oval or peanut-shaped budding, Gram-positive, nonmycelial yeast. It has been isolated frequently from both normal and otitic ears. This has created controversy as to the role it plays in perpetuating otitis. There is no general agreement between various studies as to its incidence either in normal (15 to 49%) or in otitic (2 to 80%) ears. If data are averaged, the incidence in normal and otitic ears would be 17 and 24% respectively. The author concurs with others who have found the incidence of *Malassezia* in otitic ear canals to be about 50% (Baxter and Lawler, 1972). The frequency of *Malassezia canis* in relation to the amount of wax within the ear canal has been investigated, and it was concluded that the organism is most easily demonstrated in ears with excess wax (Baxter and Lawler, 1972).

One investigator suggested that *Malassezia* is a nonpathogenic, normal commensal because its incidence was the same for both normal and otitic ears (Baxter and Lawler, 1972). Another study showed that *Malassezia* may be pathogenic because clinical cures for otitis were obtained in cases where *Malassezia* was isolated in monoculture, and topical nystatin was the only treatment (Gedek *et al*, 1979). It was concluded that although *Malasezzia* is usually a commensal, it may become pathogenic and contribute to or produce lesions in the ear if the microclimate is favourable. Ears with high populations of *Malassezia* will have large amounts of chocolate-brown waxy discharge.

APPROACH TO THE CASE

A complete history with an emphasis on dermatology and a complete physical examination are the initial steps required to obtain information necessary for the development of a differential diagnosis of primary diseases and predisposing environmental factors (Chapter 2).

The history will often provide as many clues to the cause as any other diagnostic procedure. However, due to time restraints of a busy practice schedule, the history is often dealt with in a superficial manner. This problem can be overcome by having a history form that the client fills out either at home or in the waiting room. This form can then be scanned by the attending clinician to obtain the pertinent historical information. Only clarifying questions or questions specific to the ears will have to be asked of the client. Once the dog has been evaluated as a whole the focus can be directed to the ears.

Environment can be important as animals that are frequently in fields are more apt to have foreign bodies, such as grass awns, causing problems. Animals who swim frequently are predisposed to otitis due to maceration caused by the continual presence of water in the ear.

Chronicity and whether the otitis is unilateral or bilateral is also important. Acute, unilateral otitis is frequently associated with foreign bodies, especially grass awns. A unilateral otitis of gradual onset is more suggestive of a neoplastic process. Bilateral otitis is frequently associated with either parasites or as a problem secondary to some other disease. Also, it is important to obtain information pertaining to any previously used medications and the animal's response to them. Finally, according to the differential diagnosis developed, appropriate diagnostic plans can be formed for any primary disease.

PHYSICAL EXAMINATION

As with a general physical examination for other body systems, the examination of the ears should be done in a systematic fashion and the findings recorded. To ensure this and to minimize the time necessary for the recording of findings, it is very helpful to have an ear examination form.

Equipment

The standard otoscope is the preferred piece of equipment for the routine examination of the vertical and horizontal ear canals and the tympanic membrane. A halogen light source is desirable as it is bright enough to reach to the depths of the long canine ear canal. An operating head (Operating Otoscope: WelchAllyn) is suggested by the author because it allows for observation while removing foreign materials from the ear or aspirating the ear with suction. Cones for the veterinary otoscope are needed in a variety of lengths, diameters, and shapes to accommodate the various sizes and shapes of canine and feline ears. Because the lumina of the ear canals are often narrowed by hyperplastic tissue, the author routinely uses a cone that is 4mm in diameter and 5.5 cm in length (Veterinary Speculum:WelchAllyn). Cones designed for human ears are unsatisfactory for use in the majority of canine ears as they are too short for adequate viewing of the horizontal ear canal and the tympanic membrane.

Restraint

Physical restraint may suffice for examination of even tempered dogs with minimal problems and for cursory examination of most other animals. However, to perform a complete and through examination of the horizontal canal and tympanic membrane, almost all animals will require chemical restraint. This will also allow for cleaning of the ear at the same time; this is often necessary so that the horizontal canal and tympanic membrane can be visualised. In dogs, ketamine (1.4 to 2.2 mg/kg) in combination with diazepam (0.045 mg/kg) and acepromazine (0.023 mg/kg) mixed in the same syringe and given i/v has been used satisfactorily by the author for both the examination and cleaning of ears. The higher dose of ketamine (2.2 mg/kg) is preferred and provides ample restraint for about 20 minutes.

Examination of ear canal and tympanic membrane

To properly visualise the ear canal with an otoscope the pinna should be pulled up and out from the head so that the canal is straight. While looking into the otoscope, its cone is slowly inserted to the depth necessary for examination of the horizontal canal and tympanic membrane.

The normal ear canal may contain small amounts of pale yellow or yellow-brown wax. Some breeds of dogs such as the poodle, schnauzer and terriers (Airedale, wirehair and fox) normally have hair growing in the canals and this may have to be removed with alligator forceps before complete examination can be made.

The normal tympanic membrane is translucent, glistening, pearlgray in colour and slightly concave. Cloudiness, opacity, colour change or bulging are signs that generally indicate pathological changes in the middle ear. Rupture of the tympanic membrane may appear as a small tear in its surface, or it may be so complete that it is difficult to determine where the horizontal canal ends and the middle ear begins.

ESTABLISHING THE DIAGNOSIS

Primary disease

From the differential diagnoses, appropriate diagnostic and laboratory procedures can be performed to rule out the various primary diseases that are potentially responsible for or predispose an animal to otitis.

Cytology

Cytological evaluations of otic exudate provide immediate diagnostic information about the inflammatory response as well as types of micro-organisms and ectoparasites present within the ear canal. Smears stained with either a modified Wright's stain (Diff Quick) or Gram's stain and should be examined carefully for numbers and morphology of bacteria, yeast, leucocytes and neoplastic cells. Generally, the presence of cocci on smears indicates that either *Staphylococcus* spp. or *Streptococcus* spp. are present; rods usually indicate either *Pseudomonas* spp. or *Proteus* spp. Yeast are almost always *Malassezia* spp. but *Candida* spp. are also a possibility. In addition to stained smears, debris from the ear canal can be mixed with mineral oil and examined for ectoparasites and their eggs or larvae.

Cultures

Although cytology will provide clues as to which bacteria are present, culture and sensitivity tests are still very appropriate because a greater proportion of bacteria are becoming resistant to the routine antibacterials used for the treatment of otitis (Blue and Wooley, 1977). If Gram-negative rods, which have a high probability of being *Pseudomonas* spp., are present on the smears, a culture and sensitivity is mandatory as *Pseudomonas* spp. are often resistant to the majority of antibacterials.

Biopsy

In order to diagnose a tumour or confirm proliferative tissue in the ear canal, a small pinch biopsy may be obtained by passing endoscopic biopsy forceps through the otoscope cone.

INITIAL MANAGEMENT

Successful treatment of otitis externa is based on four fundamental principals:

1. Diagnosis and treatment or correction of any primary disease or environmental factors that are predisposing to the otitis.

2. Accurate identification of specific bacteria, yeast, parasites or foreign bodies within the ears.

3. Thorough cleaning of all debris, exudate and wax from the pinna, vertical and horizontal ear canals.

4. Complete client education concerning the aetiology of otitis, the anatomy of the ear, as well as instruction in the proper techniques of cleaning the ears at home and applying appropriate medications.

Ear Cleaning

All hair, wax, debris, exudate, and foreign material must be removed from the horizontal and vertical ear canals so that: a complete examination of the ear canal and tympanic membrane can be made; topical medication can penetrate to the affected tissues; there is no debris left to serve as a focus for reinfection, and bacterial toxins, degenerating cells and free fatty acids do not serve as a stimulus for further inflammation.

The use of a bulb syringe or a dental water-propulsion device (Water Pik:Teledyne) to flush the ears has been advocated (Neer, 1982; August, 1986). Other equipment necessary for cleaning the ears include a bulb syringe, mosquito and alligator forceps for plucking hair and removing foreign objects from the ears.

Technique

With the animal sedated and in lateral recumbency, the upper ear is filled with a solution containing dioctyl sodium sulfosuccinate, carbamide peroxide and tetracaine (Clear$_x$ Ear Cleansing Solution, DVM [USA]). In the UK, a lactic acid, salicylic acid in docusate sodium and propylene glycol is available as an ear cleaning fluid (Epi-Otic, Virbac). The canal is then massaged for 2 minutes. If the pinna has exudate or wax on its surface, the cleaning solution should be applied to it also. The pinna can then be folded on itself and massaged for 1 minute to loosen the debris. The carbamide peroxide has a foaming action that helps to break down larger clumps of debris and float it to the opening of the canal. After massaging the canal, excess cleaning solution and any exudate and debris that has floated to the surface should be wiped away with a cotton ball. The ear canal is then flushed twice with warm water using a bulb syringe. Next, debris, exudate, and any water that is still present are removed by suction using the bulb syringe. The ear is then examined to verify that it is completely clean. If not the process should be repeated. This procedure should then be followed for the other ear if it needs cleaning. Once this technique has been mastered by either a technician or veterinarian, it should be possible for both ears to be completely cleaned in less than 20 minutes.

If the tympanic membrane is ruptured a cleaning solution of either propylene glycol, malic acid, benzoic acid, salicylic acid (Oticlens, Beecham [USA]; Dermisol Multicleanse Solution, SmithKline Beecham; Epi-Otic; Virbac; Oterna Ear and Wound Cleanser, Pitman Moore [UK]) or diluted povidine-iodine solution (1 part to three parts water) can be used for the cleaning of both the external and middle ear (Wilson, 1985). The cleaning technique is the same as just previously described. A short-term head tilt or transient ataxia has been observed in about 1% of the cases when the middle ear is flushed (Neer, 1982). The owners of animals with a ruptured tympanic membrane should be warned that some animals may swallow or cough when liquid solutions are instilled in their ears. This is due to the solution flowing through the ruptured tympanum, to the middle ear and down the eustachian tube into the pharynx. Although a ruptured tympanum increases the likelihood of middle ear infection, it is not a serious problem in a clean ear and will heal in 5 to 10 days (Neer, 1982; August, 1988).

Surgical intervention may be necessary if the tissues lining the ear canal are so hyperplastic that the canal cannot be completely cleaned.

Although useful for cleaning the folds of the antihelix, the longstanding practice of using cotton swabs (Qtips or cotton buds) to clean the ear canal should be abandoned. Even if done carefully, this technique invariably packs exudate and debris further down the canal next to the tympanum. If the tympanic membrane is diseased, pressure of the debris may cause it to rupture. If this occurs or if the tympanum is already ruptured, the debris can be pushed by the swab into the middle ear where it may contribute to the development of otitis media. The physical presence of the swab in the canal also tends to traumatise and often ulcerate the epithelium lining the canal.

Treatment

Initial treatment should be based on stained smears of the ear exudate. If cocci are present, formulations containing neomycin, gentamicin or chloramphenicol would be appropriate. If rods are present, gentamicin or polymyxin B would be the antibacterials of choice . The aminoglycosides (neomycin, polymyxin and gentamicin) should not be used for treatment of otitis if the tympanic membrane is ruptured because of their ototoxicity. If yeast are found, topicals such as miconazole or clotrimazole should to used. Once culture and sensitivity findings are known, treatment can be changed, if necessary, to more appropriate antibacterial or antifungal agents. If at any point, response to therapy is not as good as would be expected, another culture and sensitivity should be performed. Another approach to treatment is the use of 2 to 5% solutions of acetic acid to lower the pH within the ear canal. This treatment is especially beneficial for the treatment of infections with *Pseudomonas* spp. when the organism becomes resistant to antibacterials. Inflammation, sometimes severe, is an occasional side effect of otic treatment with acetic acid. It is more likely to occur when a 5% solution is used.

Silver sulfadiazine and ticarcillin are two additional antibacterials used frequently by the author for the treatment of *Pseudomonas* spp. A 1% solution of silver sulfadiazine is made by adding 1 g of silver sulfadiazine powder to 100 ml of water and shaking well. Depending on the size of the ear canal 4-12 drops are instilled twice daily. Ticarcillin is an injectable antibacterial that is supplied lyophilised. Sterile water is added to the bottle to reconstitute the drug. Six ml of this is then added to 120 ml of a solution containing propylene glycol, malic, benzoic, and salicylic acid (see above), and this is used to both clean and treat the ears twice daily. The remaining ticarcillin can be frozen for use at a later date. The author has used both of these to treat animals with ruptured tympanic membranes and no adverse effects have been noted.

Topical glucocorticoids will benefit most cases of otitis by reducing the inflammation in the tissues of the ear canal resulting in less pruritus, swelling, exudation, and tissue proliferation. Flucinolone acetonid in 60% dimethylsulfoxide (Synotic; Syntex Animal Health [USA]) is especially beneficial as the dimethylsulfoxide serves as a vehicle to allow the flucinolone to penetrate into the tissues. Its use will often result in the reduction of the hyperplastic tissue response associated with chronic otitis externa. Owners are instructed to fill the affected ear canal with the solution and massage the canal for 30 to 60 seconds 2 to 3 times daily. Its use has also been beneficial to decrease wax build up in the ear which often results in a concomitant *Malassezia* infection. No equivalent licenced product is available in the UK. Even if an infected ear is completely cleaned and treated with appropriate medications, it may still continue to produce small amounts of exudate or wax. To prevent this from accumulating and interfering with treatment, it has to be removed by inhome cleaning. Ear cleaners can be dispensed and the client is instructed to clean the ears by filling the canal with the cleanser, massaging the ear canal for 1 to 2 minutes and then wiping the cleansing solution and debris from the outer ear and pinna with a cotton ball. The interval between cleanings will vary from 3 to 7 days depending on the state of the ears and rate of accumulation of wax or exudate.

When *Otodectes cynotis* infestation is diagnosed, the author recommends that the ears should first be cleaned of excess wax and then treated for 20 days with a mixture containing 1 ml of rotenone (Canex Solution; Pitman Moore [USA]) and 10 ml of a solution containing procaine penicillin, neomycin sulfate, polymyxin B, and glucocorticoids (Forte Topical; Upjohn [USA]). In the UK a number of ear treatments combining acaricidal agents, antibiotics and glucocorticoids are available. Again treatment for 20 days is advised. Alternatively, two doses of ivermectin, 300 ug/kg can be given subcutaneously two weeks apart (Paradis, 1989). However, this drug is not licenced for use in dogs and cats in the UK. All contact animals, both dogs and cats, should be treated because asymptomatic carriers may often be sources for reinfection.

CLIENT EDUCATION

No matter how through the veterinarian has been in diagnosis, cleaning and dispensing medications, the efforts will be in vain unless the owner properly cleans and treats the ears at home. To help assure client compliance the veterinarian or an experienced veterinary technician should carefully explain the cleaning and treatment instructions, demonstrate how cleaning and treatment are supposed to be performed and then watch as the owner repeats the process.

All instructions pertaining to the cleaning or treatment of the ears should be typed or clearly printed for the owner. To save time, these instructions can be printed on a form designed for handing out to the client: the clinician has only to write in the names, amounts and frequency of medications to be used.

Finally, re-examinations should be scheduled at appropriate intervals so that progress can be monitored and any problems with cleaning or treatment can be addressed.

REFERENCES

AUGUST, J.R. (1986). Evaluations of the patient with otitis externa. *Dermatology Reports* **5**; 1.

AUGUST, J.R. (1988). Otitis externa in the dog and cat, Part II: *Pathogenesis of the disease*. Western Veterinary Conference. Las Vegas, 162.

BAXTER, M. & LAWLER, D.C. (1972). The incidence of otitis externa of dogs and cats in New Zealand. *New Zealand Veterinary Journal* **20** ; 29.

BLUE, J.L. & WOOLEY, R.E. (1977). Antibacterial sensitivity patterns of bacteria isolated from dogs with otitis externa. *Journal of The American Veterinary Medical Association* **171**; 362.

DICKSON, D.B. & LOVE, D.N. (1983). Bacteriology of the horizontal ear canal of dogs. *Journal of Small Animal Practice* **24**; 413.

FERNANDO, S.D.A. (1966). A histological and histochemical study of the glands of the external auditory canal of the dog. *Research in Veterinary Science* **7**; 116.

FERNANDO, S.D.A. (1967). Certain histopathologic features of the external auditory meatus of the cat and dog with otitis externa. *American Journal of Veterinary Research* **28**; 278.

FRASER, G. (1961). The histopathology of the external auditory meatus of the dog. *Journal of Comparative Pathology* **71**; 55.

FRASER, G. (1961a). Factors predisposing to canine external otitis. *Veterinary Record* **73**; 253.

FRASER, G., WITHERS, A.R., & SPREULL, J.S.A. (1961). Otitis externa in the dog. *Journal of Small Animal Practice* **2**; 32.

FRASER, G. (1965). Aetiology of otitis externa in the dog. *Journal of Small Animal Practice* **6**; 445.

GEDEK, B. BRUTZEL, K., GERLACH, R., NETZER, F., ROCKEN, H., UNGER, H. & SYMOENS, J. (1979). The role of *Pityrosporum pachydermatitis* in otitis externa of dogs: Evaluation of a treatment with Miconazole. *Veterinary Record* **104**; 138.

GETTY, R., FOUST, H.L., PRESTLEY, E.T., & MILLER, M.E. (1956). Macroscopic anatomy of the ear of the dog. *American Journal of Veterinary Research* **17**; 364.

GRIFFIN, C.E. (1981). Otitis externa. *Compendium on Continuing Education and the Practicing Veterinarian* **3**; 741.

GRONO, L.R. (1969). Observations on the incidence of otitis externa in the dog. *Australian Veterinary Journal* **45**; 417.

HARVEY, C.E. & GOLDSCHMIDT, M.H. (1978). Inflammatory polypoid growths in the ear canal of cats. *Journal of Small Animal Practice* **19** ; 669.

MACY D.W. & SEIM, H.B. (1985). Medical and surgical aspects of the ear. Scientific Proceedings *American Animal Hospital Association*.

MULLER, G.H., KIRK, R.W. & SCOTT, D.W. (1989). Cutaneous parasitology. In: *Small Animal Dermatology 4th Edn.* W.B. Saunders, Philadelphia.

NEER, M.T. (1982). Otitis media. *Compendium on Continuing Education and the Practicing Veterinarian* **4**; 410.

PARADIS, M. (1989). Ivermectin in small animal dermatology. In: *Current Veterinary Therapy X: Small Animal Practice.* (Ed. R.W. Kirk) W.B. Saunders, Philadelphia.

POWELL, M.B., WEISBROTH, S.H., ROTH, L.& WILHELMSEN, C. (1980). Reaginic hypersensitivity in *Otodectes cynotis* infestation of cats and mode of mite feeding. *American Journal of Veterinary Research* **41**; 877.

PUGH, K.E., EVANS, I.M., HENDY, P.G. (1974) Otitis externa in the dog and cat: An evaluation of a new treatment. *Journal of Small Animal Practice* **15**; 387.

ROSE, W.P. (1976). Otitis Externa: Otoacariasis. *Veterinary Medicine and Small Animal Clinician* **71**; 1280.

ROSE, W.R. (1978). Small animal clinical otology: Tumors. *Veterinary Medicine and Small Animal Clinician* **73**; 427.

RYCROFT, A.K. & SABEN, H.S. (1977). A clinical study of otitis externa in the dog. *Canadian Veterinary Journal* **18**; 64.

SCOTT, D.W. (1981). Observations on canine atopy. *Journal of the American Animal Hospital Association* **17**; 91.

SHARMA, V.D. & RHOADS, H.E. (1975). The occurrence and microbiology of otitis externa in the dog. *Journal of Small Animal Practice* **16**; 241.

VAN DER GAAG, I. (1986). The pathology of the external ear canal in dogs and cats. *Veterinary Quarterly* **8**; 307.

WEISBROTH, S.A., POWELL, B., ROTH, L.& SHER, S. (1974). Immunopathology of naturally occurring otodectic otoacariasis in the domestic cat. *Journal of The American Veterinary Medical Association* **165**; 1088.

WILSON, J.F. (1985). A practitioner's approach to complete ear care. *Dermatology Reports* **4**; 1.

WOODY, B.J. & FOX, S.M. (1986). Otitis externa: Seeing past the signs to discover the underlying cause. *Veterinary Mediciane and Small Animal Clinician* **87**; 616.

MILIARY DERMATITIS IN THE CAT

Richard G Harvey

INTRODUCTION

A papulocrustous "miliary" dermatitis is a common presenting sign and represents about 25% of the feline dermatological case load in practice (Scott, 1980). The condition is recognised to be the common cutaneous manifestation of a number of allergic and infectious diseases (Table 1) although flea allergy dermatitis is by far the most common cause, accounting for some 80% of cases (Muller *et al*, 1989 and Grant, 1991). The approach to the condition should take this into account and every effort should be made to assess and treat a flea infestation before considering other aetiologies. In a number of instances however, it may not be possible to establish an definite cause and in these cases symptomatic therapy may be required. Symptomatic treatment may also be indicated in cases of severe flea allergy where total control of the parasite may not be possible, for instance in households with many cats or where cats have free access to other non-treated cats.

APPROACH TO THE CASE

A detailed history of the cat should be ascertained, in particular the details of any medications that have been given or are currently being administered, the diet being offered and the details of the other animals in the house, their species and age. These findings may suggest whether dietary idiosyncrasy, drug eruption or the infectious dermatoses should be considered in the differential diagnosis.

The presence of other cats is a much greater risk factor for exposure to fleas than is the presence of a dog in the house. Young, elderly and infirm cats carry higher flea burdens than healthy adults, perhaps due to poor grooming skills in juvenile cats, and, in the case of elderly or infirm cats, less frequent and less effective grooming. The lifestyle of the cat should be enquired into as the degree of control over the cat's movement in and out of doors will allow evaluation of the probability of exposure to fleas. Are there any fleas on the cat in question or on other animals in the house? Do other animals in the house have evidence of skin disease? Has the owner or other member of the household been bitten by fleas? Cat fleas can bite humans and the lesions are often on the lower leg where they appear as pruritic papules. What is the level of flea control? The application of a flea collar and the occasional spray with a topical ectoparasiticide does not constitute effective flea control.

The details of the lesions and the their history may be helpful in arriving at a diagnosis. For instance, are the lesions seasonal and do they respond to therapy? If so, to what? A study of the clinical records will often reveal patterns to the disease that the owner cannot recall. Thus a cat with lesions confined to the summer months would not be an obvious candidate for dietary intolerance whereas flea allergy dermatitis, atopy and trombiculidiasis would be considered.

PHYSICAL EXAMINATION

Having established the natural history of the disease and obtained details of the cat's management,

Table 1

The differential diagnosis of feline miliary dermatitis

---

1. Hypersensitivities

Flea allergy dermatitis
Atopy
Dietary intolerance
Drug eruption
Endoparasite hypersensitivity

2. Infectious dermatoses

i. Ectoparasite infestations
Felicola subrostratus
Cheyletiella spp. particularly *Ch.blakei*
Otodectes cynotis
Notoedres cati
Trombicula autumnalis
Lynxacarus radovsky

ii. Other infectious conditions.
Bacterial folliculitis
Dermatophytosis

3. Nutritional aetiologies

Biotin deficiency
Essential fatty acid deficiency

4. Disorders of unknown pathogenesis

Feline hypereosinophilia

5. Idiopathic feline miliary dermatitis

---

attention should turn to the examination of the animal. A general clinical examination should be made and any evidence for the presence of systemic disease assessed. Superficial lymphadenopathy has been reported to occur in cases of flea allergy dermatitis as well as in cases of systemic disease. The external ear canals should be examined for the presence of *Otodectes cynotis*, since ectopic infections (those in which the parasite colonises areas of the body surface other than those normally infected) can result in a papulocrustous reaction.

The characteristic lesion of miliary dermatitis is a crusted papule that is often more easily felt than seen. In some cases lesions are more aptly described as focal points of crusting and no obvious underlying papule can be found. Many cases have crusted lesions under normal coats with no associated pruritus being apparent. In other animals the coat may be greasy to the touch. Some cats display evidence of self trauma with patchy, often stubbled alopecia and, on occasion, severe excoriations. These may particularly be found on the head and neck, areas of the body which are easy for the cat to scratch. Severe self trauma is less common in the dorsal lumbo-sacral region.

The distribution and nature of the cutaneous lesions may suggest the nature of the underlying disease. Crusted lesions need not always be confined to the dorsal lumbosacral region, as in some cases of flea allergy dermatitis, for example. They may be found in a generalised pattern or confined to a localised area such as the head and neck and in these instances *Otodectes cynotis*, atopy or dietary intolerance should be considered in addition to flea allergy dermatitis.
During the clinical examination the clinician may observe the presence of fleas or note the presence of flea faeces. Flea faeces often fall onto the examination table during the clinical examination and suspicious particles can be collected with damp cotton wool and examined for

the presence of blood (Chapter 3). Although a careful search for fleas may reveal evidence of infection it is frequently difficult to demonstrate the presence of fleas on cats with flea allergy dermatitis. It is often more fruitful to examine the apparently uninfected and asymptomatic cat from the household, if there is one.

The minimum procedures required for a new case would be to take a history and complete a physical examination, examine skin scrapings and hair shafts for the presence of ectoparasites. Other tests that might be indicated are examination under Wood's light and the fungal culture of fluorescent hairs and scale, the imposition of a restricted diet and intradermal skin testing to screen for dietary intolerance and atopy, faecal flotation and haematology and biochemistry to assess hepatic and renal function or detect abnormalities such as eosinophilia. The detailed procedures for many of these tests are discussed in Chapter 3.

ESTABLISHING THE DIAGNOSIS

The differential diagnosis of feline miliary dermatitis is summarised in Table 1 and a number of the possible diagnoses can be ruled out on the basis of a careful history and physical examination. For example, biotin deficiency and essential fatty acid deficiency are highly unlikely to occur in cats fed commercially balanced cat food. Relative deficiency of essential fatty acids, perhaps due to metabolic disease, might be suspected if evidence of hepatic and renal disease is noted during the taking of the history or the conducting of the physical examination.

Infectious Dermatoses

Ectoparasites may be demonstrated by inspection of the hair and coat and by the microscopical examination of skin scrapings. These procedures should reveal evidence of pediculosis, cheyletiellosis, otodectic mange, trombiculidiasis and infestation with *Lynxacarus radovsky*, the cat fur mite. The presence of pediculosis may be inferred by the observation of characteristic ova on the hair shafts, confirmation being made by examining hair pluckings under the microscope. Examination is facilitated by affixing the hair shafts or plucked hairs to transparent adhesive tape such as Sellotape and then laying the tape sticky side down onto a glass slide.

Lynxacarus radovsky might present similarly and may be differentiated by microscopical examination and the identification of adult fur mites rather than eggs on the hair shafts. In addition, the mite has a restricted geographical distribution; it appears to be confined to the Southern United States, Hawaii and Australia. Examination of the hair shafts under the low power objective of a microscope may also reveal the presence of the eggs of *Cheyletiella* spp. and these are differentiated from those of the louse *Felicola subrostratus* by being smaller and only attached to the hair shaft at the lower pole, rather than along the entire length of the egg as is the case for *Felicola subrostratus*.

Skin scrapings should be taken with both liquid paraffin and 10% potassium hydroxide (KOH) as moistening agents. Examination of the liquid paraffin preparation under a microscope will allow demonstration of *Cheyletiella blakei* (the commonest member of the genus that is be found on the cat), *Otodectes cynotis* and *Neotrombicula autumnalis*. The use of 10% KOH is advisable if dermatophytosis is suspected.

The use of a nit comb and the examination of combings are a useful method of demonstrating fleas and flea faeces on the cat and, as mentioned above, these parasites or their faeces may also drop onto the consulting table during the course of the examination.

The provisional diagnosis of flea allergy dermatitis in the cat is based on two findings;

i. The presence of compatible clinical signs

ii. The demonstration of fleas or flea faeces on the individual or its close contacts

In the case of the dog it is also useful to record a positive reaction to the intradermal injection of aqueous flea allergen but the reliability of available preparations in the cat is open to question. Other findings that would support a diagnosis of flea allergy dermatitis are the presence of zoonotic lesions on the members of the household, the presence of *Dipylidium caninum* infection, the lack of adequate flea control, contact with other animals in the household and regular contact with other cats in the neighbourhood.

Dermatophytosis may be suspected after examination of the KOH preparation which may be facilitated by adding Quink ink to the potassium hydroxide (Chapter 3). If any suspicion exists that the cat may have dermatophytosis then samples of crust and hair should be incubated on Sabouraud's medium or submitted to a laboratory for culture.

The other infectious cause of crusting lesions is bacterial folliculitis which is regarded as being rare in the cat. Suspicion may be aroused by the observation that the crusting papule is only a transient lesion, there being a progression from macules and papules, through crusting papules to lesions which are resolving. The condition is so unusual that culture and sensitivity and biopsy are indicated to allow definitive diagnosis.

INITIAL MANAGEMENT

If a definitive diagnosis can be made on the first consultation then specific therapy can be provided and its effect ascertained at future examinations. Failure to establish a clear aetiology for the lesions should prompt the suspicion of a hypersensitivity, in particular flea allergy dermatitis. Because it be extremely difficult to demonstrate fleas on cats with flea allergy dermatitis it should be the first consideration in the absence of a definitive diagnosis to the contrary. Details of flea treatment are covered in Chapter 29 but a summary is presented in Table 2.

The animal should be re-examined after three weeks and if there is any sign of improvement then flea control should be continued for a further three weeks. If there is no improvement at this stage consideration of other hypersensitivities is warranted; dietary intolerance and atopy being the major differential diagnoses.

Dietary intolerance may occur in any cat of any age. Although it is uncommon, the lack of response to flea control and the absence of an alternative diagnosis should prompt its consideration. It is important to emphasise that a commercial diet should not be used when screening an animal for dietary intolerance. A diet comprising a single source of protein such as chicken, fish, turkey or rabbit should be chosen, based on a knowledge that it does not constitute a regular part of the cat's diet. Milk should be withdrawn and only fresh water allowed. Access to feeding bowls in neighbouring houses and hunting should be controlled if at all possible. This diet should be fed for a minimum of three weeks.

Resolution of the clinical signs is suggestive of a dietary intolerance and the original diet should be re-instituted. Relapse should follow if dietary intolerance is indeed the cause. If this occurs then the restricted diet is again fed until improvement occurs and then individual dietary components are fed in sequence to document the causative substance. A typical list might contain milk, cheese, egg, brown bread, beef, fish, dried cat food and commercial canned food.

Having established which items cause relapse then it usually proves possible to find a suitable commercial diet which the animal can tolerate. Care should be taken not to precipitate metabolic crises such as hepatic lipidosis that may occur if the cat steadfastly refuses the unusual foodstuffs. It is important to try to identify a commercially balanced diet for the long term management of cats since their metabolic idiosyncrasies make them prone to nutritional deficiencies (particularly of essential fatty acids and taurine) if they are fed unbalanced diets for prolonged periods.

Atopy is not uncommon in the cat and is second in frequency to flea allergy dermatitis as a cause of miliary dermatitis. There is no breed predisposition but there is an age predisposition with the majority of cases beginning to exhibit clinical signs before two years of age. In addition to the presence of crusted papules over the dorsal lumbosacral area there may be self trauma to the head, neck and interscapular region. This tendency for self trauma in addition to crusted papules may be of diagnostic value in that it is not common in cats with flea allergy dermatitis alone. Lack of response to flea control, the absence of other ectoparasites, failure to improve after the imposition of a restricted diet and the failure to demonstrate dermatophytosis will suggest the possibility of atopy. The diagnosis is confirmed on the basis of a positive response to the intradermal injection of aqueous allergen extracts.

Table 2

A summary of flea control for the domestic house

1. Vacuum clean the entire property
2. Dispose of the contents of the collecting bag
3. Apply methoprene, as directed
4. Do not vacuum clean for 7 days
5. Repeat steps 1-3 after this period
   and
6. Apply a suitable topical aerosol product or a sytemically absorbed product, according to the manufacturer's recommendation, to all of the animals

Hypersensitivity to endoparasites has been recorded on rare occasions and miliary dermatitis may be one of the manifestations. The diagnosis is based on the failure to identify an alternative aetiology, the presence of ova in the faeces and the resolution of clinical signs after antiparasitic therapy. The signs will recur if re-infestation takes place.

Drug eruption is not commonly reported but may occur more frequently than this suggests since many cases escape diagnosis (Mason, 1990). Any animal may exhibit a systemic or cutaneous reaction to any drug and the signs are unpredictable but may include crusting papules and pruritus. The condition should be suspected in any case where medications or supplements are being or have been administered. This should be established during the initial taking of the history and if it is suspected that a drug eruption is occurring the administration of the agents should be suspended. Resolution of the clinical signs, and failure to establish an alternative diagnosis suggests drug eruption and the animal's medical records should be suitably flagged to record this. Re-exposure is dangerous and may result in a systemic and potentially fatal recurrence.

Feline hypereosinophilic syndrome is a very rare systemic disease in which there is an autonomous production and liberation of mature eosinophils into the circulation and an eosinophilic infiltration into various organs. Typically these are the abdominal organs but on two occasions crusting papules have been recorded. Diagnosis is by demonstrating a persistent, circulating, mature eosinophilia and by an inability to demonstrate an underlying aetiology, since the condition is idiopathic.

Idiopathic and refractory miliary dermatitis may be encountered occasionally. This is particularly true of flea allergy dermatitis where it may prove particularly difficult to provide complete control. Even a greatly reduced challenge may still be more than sufficient to cause clinical signs. Similarly with atopy it may prove impossible to remove the allergen from the cat's environment and immunotherapy may not be successful in inducing remission. In these cases symptomatic control is indicated and essential fatty acids, antihistamines, glucocorticoids have all been shown to be effective.

FURTHER READING

GRANT, D.I. (1991). *Skin Diseases in the Dog and Cat* 2nd Edn, Blackwell Scientific Publications, Oxford.

HARVEY, R.G., (1991). Management of feline miliary dermatitis by supplementing the diet with essential fatty acids. *Veterinary Record,* **128**, 326.

MASON, K.V. (1990). Cutaneous drug eruptions. *Veterinary Clinics of North America*, **20**, 1633.

MULLER, G.H., KIRK, R.W. and SCOTT, D.W. (1989). *Small Animal Dermatology* 4th Edn, W.B. Saunders, Philadelphia.

SCOTT, D.W. (1980). Feline Dermatology 1900-1978: monograph. *Journal of the American Animal Hospital Association* **16, 331.**

CHAPTER SEVENTEEN

PODODERMATITIS

Stephen D White ──────────────────────

INTRODUCTION

Pedal dermatoses (pododermatoses) are frequently encountered diseases in small animal practice (Anderson, 1980; Scott, 1980) (Plates 46-51). The clinician must remember that there are many causes for disease involving the feet and that determining the aetiology of the dermatosis is the best way of achieving a rational therapeutic plan.

HISTORY AND PHYSICAL EXAMINATION

A thorough history and physical examination are vital in the diagnosis of a pododermatitis. Details extracted from the history may suggest possible causes of the pododermatitis (Table 1).

Table 1
Pododermatitis: Important aspects of medical history

The Environment:	
Rough or unsanitary housing	trauma, *Pelodera*
Hunting dogs	trauma, contact irritants
Incontact dogs	hookworms
The History of the Lesions:	
Seasonal	inhalant allergy, contact allergy contact dermatitis
Responsive to antibiotics	pyoderma
Responsive to glucocorticoids	allergy, irritants, sterile pyogranuloma, autoimmune
Lesions Affecting Other Sites:	
Axilla, face	inhalant allergy, food allergy
Dependant / ventral areas	contact irritant or allergen, hookworms, *Pelodera*
Mucocutaneous junctions	auto immune disease, superficial necrolytic dermatosis, zinc responsive dermatitis, thallium poisoning, leishmaniasis, demodicosis
Otitis externa	atopy (inhalent allergen) atopy, *Malassezia pachydermatitis*
Diet	generic dog food dermatosis, dietary hypersensitivity

Physical examination should include a thorough search for lesions elsewhere on the body, palpation of lymph nodes and determination of how many feet are involved. Laboratory tests should include skin scrapings, fungal culture and a stained smear of any exudate or pustule contents. Dependent upon history and physical examination, other tests might include faecal examination, biopsy (for histopathology, bacterial and fungal culture and possibly for immunopathology), instituting a hypoallergenic diet, intradermal testing for inhalant allergies or endocrine tests. The author generally approaches skin scrape negative cases in the dog by classifying them as either with or without nodules (or fistulas, thickening, purulence, etc). Those without these lesions tend to be pruritic and allergic in nature. Those with these lesions should be biopsied for histopathology and bacterial or fungal cultures. The presence of thick crusts and/or vesicles are also indications for biopsy. In the cat, pedal dermatosis is relatively rare and the author biopsies all cases.

Successful therapy of pedal dermatoses is dependent upon pursuing a definite diagnosis. In the author's practice, most cases of pododermatitis in the dog are associated with allergies, pyoderma, demodicosis or pemphigus, roughly in that order.

ESTABLISHING THE DIAGNOSIS AND INITIAL MANAGEMENT

INFECTIOUS DISEASE

Pyoderma

Pyoderma will frequently involve the feet in dogs and this may be the only body area involved (Plates 50 and 51). Nodules with or without fistulous tracts may be present. So called interdigital "cysts" are actually interdigital pyoderma and histological examination reveals purulent material covered by friable, alopecic erythematous skin (White and Ihrke, 1987). *Staphylococcus intermedius* is the usual pathogen. Diagnoses is by biopsy and culture. Therapy involves long term (six weeks or more) antibiotics, based on culture and sensitivity. Suggested antibiotics are discussed in Chapter 25). If several species of bacteria with differing sensitivities are isolated an antibiotic should be chosen that is effective against the staphylococcal species. In recurrent cases a defect in the immune system may be suspected and testing for hypothyroidism and hyperadrenocorticism is indicated (Chapter 3). If these tests reveal no abnormalities, immunostimulants such as autogenous vaccines or bacterins may be used (Kirk, 1983). Some cases will need life long antibiotics. In these rare cases, and **only** in these cases, a gradual reduction in frequency of administration of the antibiotic may be attempted once clinical remission is achieved. Owners should be aware that recurrence of the disease or the emergence of resistant strains is a possibility. However, in some cases with financial restraints, gradual reduction of drug frequency may be the only alternative to euthanasia.

Bacterial infections caused by mycobacteria (White, 1986), *Nocardia* sp, (Attleberger, 1983), or *Actinomyces* sp (Attleberger, 1983; Brennan and Ihrke, 1983) may affect the feet. While such infections are uncommon, actinomycosis may be associated with grass awn foreign bodies (Brennan and Ihrke, 1983) (see below under environmental disease). Diagnosis is based on histopathology and culture, with antibiotic therapy chosen on the basis of sensitivity testing. Surgical removal of the affected toes/foot may be indicated in severe cases. Diagnosis and therapy of the mycobacteria may be difficult.

Dermatophytes

Dermatophytes may affect the feet in dogs and cats (Lewis *et al*, 1991) (Plate 48). Lesions are variable, with alopecia, erythema, scaling or even inflammatory plaques (termed "kerions") as possible manifestations. The triad of alopecia, scale and nail abnormalities is especially suggestive of dermatophytosis. Diagnosis is by demonstration of the fungi on culture media. Therapy is both systemic (griseofulvin 50-110 mg/kg, q 24 h) and topical (captan 50% wettable powder, two tablespoons in one gallon of water, applied one to two times weekly as a dip (Not available in the UK). Therapy should be continued for two weeks past clinical cure. Any in-contact animals should also be dipped; any other pets having lesions should also be given griseofulvin. Captan may cause a rash in some people; protective gloves are advised. In rare cases of griseofulvin resistant dermatophytes, ketoconazole (a benzimidazole derivative) may be used. Dosage is 5 to 30 mg/kg every 12 to 24 hours (Foil, 1986).

Malassezia dermatitis may affect the feet, and mimic an allergic dermatitis. Diagnosis is achieved by superficial skin scraping the affected area, smearing the debris onto a microscope slide, heat-fixing then staining with a cytological stain followed by microscopical examination with immersion oil. Therapy with various topicals (chlorhexidine, selenium sulfite) and/or (ideally) ketoconazole 5mg/kg BID, per os is recommended.

Intermediate mycoses (sporotrichosis, mycetoma) and **deep** (systemic) **mycoses** (blastomycosis, cryptococcosis) may also cause pedal dermatoses. Lesions may be nodules and/or draining tracts and are resistant to antibiotic therapy. Diagnosis is by histopathology and culture. Therapy varies, with sodium iodide, potassium iodide, ketoconazole, or amphotericin B recommended for sporotrichosis (Attleberger, 1988) and amphotericin B, 5-fluorocytosine and/or ketoconazole used against the deep mycoses (Legendre *et al*, 1984).

Parasitic

Parasitic causes of pedal dermatoses include *Demodex canis*, *Pelodera strongyloides*, and hookworms (*Ancylostoma* and *Uncinaria sp*).

Demodectic pododermatitis in dogs, usually presents with lesions similar to bacterial pododermatitis as secondary bacterial infection is frequently a complicating factor (White and Stannard, 1983) (Plate 46). Older dogs with demodicosis and deep pyoderma limited to the feet should be evaluated for hyperadrenocorticism (White *et al*, 1989).

Occasionally, erythema and alopecia may be the only signs of pedal demodicosis. In chronic cases, skin scrapings may not be able to penetrate the fibrous or granulomatous tissue surrounding the mites and microscopy of the roots of plucked hair or biopsy must be used as a diagnostic tool. Therapy consists of antibiotics based on culture and sensitivity for the pyoderma and a solution of amitraz (Derasect Demodectic Mange Wash, 0.05%; SmithKline Beecham, U.K.: Mitoban, 0.025%; Upjohn, U.S.A.) for the *Demodex* (Kwochka, 1986). In severe demodectic pododermatitis, the author prefers to apply the amitraz to the **entire body surface of the clipped** dog once weekly, with application of an amitraz lotion (1.0 ml of concentrate in 25 ml of mineral oil) twice weekly to the feet. Female dogs should be spayed, both to prevent future affliction of future generations as well as to prevent the exacerbation of the disease that often occurs with oestrus (Kwochka, 1986). Vitamin E (200 IU five times daily) may also be helpful (Figueiredo, 1993, in press). Extensive involvement of the feet usually denotes a poorer chance of cure.

Pelodera and **hookworm** infestations usually occur in dogs maintained in an unclean environment, often containing vegetation (especially straw) (Scott, 1980) (Plate 47). Dogs with *Pelodera* dermatitis have intense pruritus, with an erythematous papular eruption involving those areas of the body in contact with the ground, including the feet. Diagnosis is by skin scraping or demonstration of the organisms on histopathology. Therapy consists of destroying bedding, spraying the environment with an insecticide such as malathion and treating the patient with a parasiticidal dip at least twice on a weekly basis. Hookworm pododermatitis is usually mildly pruritic with alopecia and erythema evident on the paws as well as other parts of the body in contact with the ground. Diagnosis is based on clinical signs, environment and positive faecal tests for hookworms. Rarely is the organism demonstrated on histopathology. Therapy is appropriate anthelmintic treatment as well as cleaning the premises and frequent removal of faeces.

Leishmaniasis, caused by the protozoal organisms *Leishmania donovani* and *L. tropica* has been reported in the dog. Lesions affecting the feet include erosions, ulcerations, erythema, scale, and toenail hypertrophy (Ferrer *et al*, 1988). Diagnosis may be made by demonstration of the organism in histopathological specimens, aspirates of lymph nodes or joints, culture of the organism from body tissues, and/or serum titers (Mancianti and Meciani, 1988). Therapy is parenteral antimony compounds (Glucantime: Rhodia, Madrid; Pentostam: Wellcome, UK) (Ferrer, 1992). This disease is potentially zoonotic, the prognosis is poor and recurrence is frequent.

Anatrichosomiasis has been reported as causing necrosis, sloughing and ulceration of the foot pads on all four feet of a cat (Lange *et al*, 1980). Histopathology showed numerous worms and eggs within migrating tracts in the epidermis.

ALLERGIC DISEASE

Any allergic condition can cause a pedal dermatitis. The feet are usually erythematous and alopecic, secondary to pruritus. "Fox-red" salivary staining may be present. Inhalant allergy (atopy) and food allergy are the most common allergic causes of pedal dermatitis in the author's experience. Both these conditions may involve only the feet.

Inhalant allergies

Inhalant allergies may be seasonal or year round and are diagnosed by intradermal skin testing (Willemse, 1987) (Plate 49). The most appropriate therapy is usually hyposensitisation injections but, if these fail or if the owner refuses this therapy, antipruritic drugs may be necessary. While prednisone or prednisolone (1 mg/kg once daily, then tapered to the lowest effective alternate day day dosage) is usually effective, occasionally antihistamines will give relief from clinical signs. The author has the most success with diphenhydramine (2.2 mg/kg tid), hydroxyzine hydrochloride (2.2 mg/kg tid), chlorpheniramine (0.2 to 0.8 mg/kg bid to tid), or clemastine (1.34 mg tablet; dogs < 10 kg: 0.5 tab bid; 10-25 kg: 1 tab bid; >25 kg: 1.5 tab bid) (See Chapter 31). Chlorpheniramine (1-2 mg/cat, bid) may control pruritus in atopic cats.

Recently, products containing essential fatty acids (EFA) (DermCaps: DVM; EfaVet: Efamol Vet; EfaCaps: Allerderm) have been used as nonsteroidal antipruritics (Lloyd and Thomsett, 1989; Miller *et al*, 1989). These drugs apparently interfere with the production and metabolisation of arachidonic acid and other "pro-inflammatory" substances. In the author's experience, approximately 25% of dogs with inhalant allergies show clinical improvement with antihistamine and/or EFA supplementation.

Food allergy

Food allergy in cats and dogs may be diagnosed by being fed a "hypoallergenic" or limited allergen diet (White, 1992). This will vary somewhat depending on which foods were fed previously and the local availability of alternative diets but, basically, one protein and one starch source that the animal has not been fed in the past are used. The author prefers lamb (or tofu) and (non-minute) rice for dogs and lamb baby food for cats. The pet is kept on this diet with all other food excluded for 4-6 weeks. Clinical signs should abate within that time. Owners may then elect to challenge the animal with a new food stuff each week to determine the offending food(s). Alternatively, the diet may be changed to some of the prescription diets available through veterinarians such as d/d or c/d (Hills Pet Products), or Selected Protein Diet (Waltham). However, the author has **not** found these prepared diets to be effective for diagnosis as there are some pets which **only** tolerate a home-prepared protein and starch diet. In such cases a vitamin-mineral supplement should be added to the home-prepared diet and, in cats, 60-100 mg taurine/cat/day is also required for proper retinal function. The previous recommendation of 0.5 teaspoon of clam juice per day is NOT adequate taurine supplementation.

Contact allergy

Contact allergy is probably uncommon as a cause of pedal dermatoses. Erythema, papules, alopecia and pruritus are seen on the ventrum of the feet (though not usually on the pads) and, depending on the method of contact, on the dorsum of the foot as well. Other areas of the body may be involved, particularly if the dog is lying on the allergen. The ventral aspects of the lower jaw, tail and inguinal area are especially susceptible. The sensitisation period to contact allergens may be as long as two years, thus recent changes in the environment are not necessary to suspect this diagnosis (Kunkle, 1988). Because contact allergy is a delayed type hypersensitivity, a 48-hour patch-test is usually necessary for diagnosis (Olivry *et al*, 1990). Unfortunately, patient compliance is often a problem so that contact allergy is usually a diagnosis based on history, physical exam and exclusion of other causes of pedal dermatosis. Reduction of the clinical signs after a period of 2-3 weeks in a concrete run or stainless steel cage is also suggestive of contact allergy. However cases of atopy may also improve under such circumstances. As a last resort, corticosteroids may be given to control pruritus if the allergen cannot be determined.

AUTOIMMUNE DISEASES

These diseases may all affect the feet, especially the nail beds or the foot pads and these may be the only or the initial body sites involved (Ihrke *et al*, 1985; Scott *et al*, 1987). Crusts and ulcerations are the most common lesions but occasionally intact blisters or bulla are seen. In the **pemphigus** and **pemphigoid** group, these lesions are produced by autoantibodies directed against the epidermal intercellular cement substance (pemphigus) or the basement membrane zone (pemphigoid). In **systemic** and **discoid lupus erythematosus,** the autoantibodies are directed against nuclear or cytoplasmic proteins and the antibody-antigen complexes which result are subsequently trapped in the basement membrane zone of the skin (and/or other organs) (Muller *et al*, 1989). Despite the differing pathomechanisms, the lesions of these diseases may look identical. Diagnosis is based on history, clinical signs, haematology, urinalysis, serology and, most importantly, biopsy. For definitive diagnosis of these diseases, a portion of the biopsy sample should be placed in Michel's medium for detection of autoantibodies using direct immunofluorescence. A 10% formalin solution should be used for routine histopathology.

Note: Peroxidase-antiperoxidase [PAP] is another method of distinguishing the presence of autoantibodies (Moore et al, 1987). It uses an enzyme-linked color change, rather than a fluorescent dye as its marker. For PAP, the tissue sample does NOT need any special medium but can be placed in 10% buffered formalin. Another advantage to PAP is its higher percentage of confirmation of autoimmune diseases, perhaps as high as 95%. However, its greater sensitivity lowers its specificity; that is, other disease processes (pyoderma, scabies, etc.) will also give positive results. Therefore, just as in direct immunofluorescence, histopathological and clinical findings must be taken into account before a final diagnosis is made.

Systemic lupus may cause hematological or serological changes. It may involve other organ systems such as the hematopoietic (autoimmune hemolytic anemia, autoimmune thrombocytopenia), renal (glomerulonephropathy), musculoskeletal (arthropathy and myopathy) and others. A positive serum anti-nuclear antibody (ANA) test is usually seen in systemic lupus but not in any other autoimmune disease affecting the feet.

Histopathology of the lesions of pemphigus will reveal intraepidermal pustules or clefts containing rounded epidermal cells termed acantholytic cells (Ihrke *et al*, 1985). These pustules may occur below the stratum corneum (pemphigus foliaceus) or above the basal cell layer (pemphigus vulgaris). In bullous pemphigoid, a cleft is present within, directly above or below the basement membrane zone. Acantholytic cells are not seen (Muller *et al*, 1989). In systemic or discoid lupus, intracellular edema of the basal cell layer (termed hydropic or liquefactive degeneration) and thickening of the basement membrane zone is seen. Immunological testing of the biopsy specimens for autoantibodies will reveal an intercellular pattern in pemphigus, and a basement membrane zone pattern in bullous pemphigoid and lupus (Muller *et al*, 1989).

Generally therapy consists of high dose oral corticosteroids (prednisone or prednisolone 1 mg/kg bid) with gradual tapering down to a low dose (the author uses 0.5 mg/kg alternate days). If the disease cannot be controlled on the initial high dose or the dose cannot be lowered without recurrence of clinical signs or (even with very low doses) side effects such as polyuria and polydipsia are induced then other immune-suppressive drugs may be used. These include oral 6-mercaptopurine or azathioprine (2 to 2.5 mg/kg once daily for 2 to 4 weeks, then on alternate days indefinitely), or gold (aurothioglucose) as a **weekly** intramuscular injection (1 mg/kg until 6 to 12 weeks of therapy are complete, then decrease the frequency). The oral gold salt, auranofin (0.12 to 0.2 mg/kg bid) may be used in dogs. The author does not use azathioprine in cats due to the side effects seen in this species (Beale *et al*, 1992). Complete blood and platelet counts, serum enzyme profiles and (in gold injections) urinalysis (for evidence of glomerulonephropathy) are used to monitor these drugs.

ENDOCRINE DISEASES

Hypothyroidism and hyperadrenocorticism

Both hypothyroidism and hyperadrenocorticism may be underlying diseases of pododermatitis caused by bacterial or dermatophyte infections, and hyperadrenocorticism should be suspected in cases of pododemodicosis in older dogs (White S. D. *et al*, 1989). A thyroid stimulating hormone (TSH) stimulation test and a low-dose dexamethasone suppression test are the preferred diagnostic procedures to determine whether hypothyroidism and hyperadrenocorticism, respectively, are present (Rosychuk, 1983; White *et al*, 1989). The author's protocol for the TSH stimulation test is to determine the levothyroxine (T4) concentration before and 6 hours after IV injection of TSH (1 unit/dog). Failure of the post injection T4 value to be at least greater than 38.7 nmol/L is considered to be indicative of hypothyroidism. For the low-dose dexamethasone suppression test serum cortisol concentrations are determined before and 3 and 8 hours after IV injection of 0.01 mg dexamethasone/kg of body weight. A value > 40nmol/l at 8 hours is considered nonsuppression and indicative of hyperadrenocorticism. Determination of the type of hyperadrenocorticism (pituitary dependent vs adrenal tumor) is made by the high dose dexamethasone suppression test and plasma adrenocorticotropin (ACTH) levels.

Therapy for hypothyroidism entails T4 supplementation at 20 µg/kg bid, although a reduced dose (to approximately 50%) has been recommended in elderly patients or those with cardiac disease). Pododermatitis due to hypothyroidism may take a minimum of 6 weeks to show clinical improvement and adjunctive antibacterial therapy is usually indicated.

Therapy for adrenal tumors is surgical removal. Therapy for pituitary dependent hyperadrenocorticism in dogs weighing less than 20 kg is a daily dosage of 25 mg/kg of mitotane (Lysodren) for seven days, then 12.5 mg/kg twice weekly for 3 weeks. At this point an ACTH stimulation test is performed (cortisol levels determined before and two hours after IM injection of ACTH gel, 1 unit/ 2.2 kg). If both the pre- and post-injection cortisol concentrations are between 0.0276 mc mol/ l and 0.138 mc mol/l, the dog is maintained on its dosage and rechecked 1 month later with another ACTH stimulation test. If the cortisol values are still in the previous range, the mitotane dosage is maintained and the ACTH stimulation test repeated in 6 months. If the ACTH results indicate that under- or overdosage is occurring, the **weekly** dose is increased or decreased respectively by 50-100% and the dog rechecked with an ACTH stimulation test in one month. This process is repeated until both cortisol values are in the previous range. For dogs weighing more than 20 kg, the daily and weekly dosages are initially 15 mg/kg (White *et al*, 1989).

Superficial necrolytic dermatitis

Superficial necrolytic dermatitis (hepatocutaneous syndrome, diabetic dermatosis) is a rare condition in old dogs (Walton *et al*, 1986; Miller *et al*, 1990; Gross *et al*, 1990). The cutaneous lesions include erythema, crusting, oozing and alopecia of the face, genitals and distal extremities, as well as hyperkeratosis and ulceration of the footpads. The skin disease may precede the onset of the signs of the internal disease. Histopathological findings are diagnostic, and include superficial perivascular-to-lichenoid dermatitis, with marked diffuse parakeratotic hyperkeratosis and striking inter- and intracellular oedema limited to the upper half of the epidermis. Superficial necrolytic dermatitis resembles the glucagonoma syndrome (necrolytic migratory erythema) of humans, which is usually associated with hyperglucagonaemia and a glucagon secreting alpha-cell neoplasm of the pancreas. Hyperglucagonemia has also been documented in dogs with this syndrome, However, dogs tend to have hepatic cirrhosis/parenchymal damage more commonly than gluconomas. In dogs, therapy is unrewarding, and the prognosis is grave.

ENVIRONMENTAL DISEASES

Irritant contact dermatitis

Irritant contact dermatitis is usually seen in animals with a history of exposure to fertilizer, salts or herbicidal sprays. Ulceration, erythema, pain and/or pruritus may be severe. Diagnosis is based on history and physical examination (other in-contact parts of the body may also be involved). Treatment is to remove the offending material by lavage (when possible), avoidance of re-exposure (where practical), and corticosteroids for their anti-inflammatory effects.

Trauma

Trauma may result in secondary pyodermas and/or introduction of keratin and hair into the dermis, where these materials will function as foreign bodies. Trauma is especially common in hunting dogs housed on rough surfaces (wire, stone, wood chips, etc).

Plant awns

Plant awns of various species (foxtails, spear grass, etc) may cause lesions if lodged interdigitally (Brennan and Ihrke, 1983). These lesions may appear as ulcerations, proliferative nodules, swellings or draining tracts. Animals usually present with lameness. Diagnosis may be evident on physical examination, although exploration and/or biopsy of the draining tracts with demonstration of plant material on histopathological examination may be necessary to confirm the diagnosis. Removal of solitary plant material is the preferred therapy, however, if multiple numbers of microscopic splinters are involved, long-term oral low dose corticosteroids may relieve clinical signs, as has been reported in man (Snyder and Schwartz, 1983). Eventually the corticosteroids may be discontinued.

Thallium

Thallium is a rodenticide which often (but not always) produces cutaneous and oral lesions when ingested as a chronic toxin (Zook et al, 1968). (Acute thallium poisoning generally kills the animal within four to five days with little time for cutaneous lesions to develop.) In chronic thallium poisoning, the animal may be ill for three to six weeks before death. Pedal lesions consist of alopecia, erythema, crusts and eventual ulceration of the interdigital areas. Lesions are also located on the axillae, ears, genitalia and mucocutaneous junctions. The lesions are usually not pruritic. Histopathology of these lesions is rather classic, consisting of marked parakeratosis with intraepidermal microabscesses. Antemortem diagnosis is most easily made by determination of urine thallium. **Any** thallium found is diagnostic for thallium toxicosis. (Gabriel's test with rhodamine B may give false positives in cats [Muller et al, 1989]). Therapeutic recommendations consist of supportive therapy (especially fluids) and the administration of Prussian blue (100 mg/kg orally tid). Thallium toxicosis has a grave prognosis, as the animal frequently dies of multiple organ failure.

HYPERKERATOTIC, NODULAR AND PIGMENTARY DISEASES

Zinc responsive dermatosis consists of two syndromes (Kunkle, 1980). Syndrome I has been identified in Siberian huskies, Alaskan malamutes and occasionally other breeds and is typified by crusting and scaling of the mucocutaneous junctions, elbows and foot pads. These dogs are thought to have a genetic defect in zinc absorption from the intestines. Therefore, this disease can occur in dogs fed normal, balanced diets. Diagnosis is based on breed, physical examination and histopathology, which shows marked follicular and epidermal parakeratotic hyperkeratosis. Therapy is the addition of zinc supplement to the diet indefinitely. Zinc sulphate or zinc methionine may be used. Clinical signs usually are greatly improved within four to six weeks. Syndrome II occurs in rapidly growing puppies that are often fed poor-quality dog food or over-supplemented (especially with calcium) diets. These dogs are thought to have a relative zinc deficiency, possibly caused by a combination of low zinc intake and calcium or phytate (plant protein) binding to the zinc rendering it unavaiable for absorption from the gut. Clinical signs are generalized crusting plaques with extensive crusting and fissuring of the foot pads. Diagnosis is by history, clinical signs and histopathology (which resembles that of Syndrome I). Response to zinc therapy is dramatical, though changing to a balanced diet may be all that is necessary. Supplementation with zinc is usually not needed after maturity.

Generic dog food dermatosis has been reported in dogs being fed such foods (Sousa et al, 1988). Clinical signs and histology are similar to dogs with zinc-responsive dermatosis. Some dogs develop pyrexia, lymphadenopathy and pitting oedema of dependent areas. All signs regress after changing to a national brand dog food meeting the National Research Council's (USA) minimum nutritional requirements.

Digital hyperkeratosis occurs spontaneously in some adult dogs. The keratin may be verrucous, grooved, ridged or feathered. The pads of large breed dogs may become fissured and painful. There may be a predisposition in Kerry blue and Irish terriers. Diagnosis is based on histopathology and ruling out such diseases as lupus, pemphigus, zinc-responsive dermatitis and "hard-pad" distemper. Canine ichthyosis may also cause such lesions but this is a congenital disease which involves large areas of the body. Therapy is palliative and involves trimming away non-viable keratotic tissue, the use of wet dressings followed by the application of a thin layer of petroleum jelly and/or a glucocorticoid-antibiotic ointment.

Sterile pyogranulomas involving the feet have been seen in several breeds, especially the English bulldog, great Dane, boxer and dachshund (Scott, 1980). Clinical signs are nodular lesions usually without draining tracts. Diagnosis is based both on histopathology, which shows a pyogranulomatous, nodular to diffuse dermatitis which tends to track the appendages, and on culture, which is negative for bacteria and fungal organisms. Prednisone or prednisolone at a dosage of 1 mg/kg bid are usually effective to induce lesion regression. Some dogs may be tapered off corticosteroids entirely, while others will need to be on a long-term, alternate day, low-dose regimen. An apparent variant of this syndrome is seen primarily in German shepherd dogs and consists of draining tracts usually occurring immediately proximal to the metacarpal or metatarsal pads (Kunkle *et al*, in press). Histopathology usually shows a pyogranulomatous dermatitis, and bacterial cultures are negative. Therapy is similar to that for sterile pyogranulomas of other breeds.

A generalised **nodular dermatofibrosis syndrome** has been reported in German shepherds (Lium and Moe, 1985). These dogs usually have concurrent renal cyst adenocarcinomas. Nodular growths may affect the feet as well as other areas of the body. Histopathology reveals dense collagenous dermal fibrosis. Corticosteroid therapy is equivocal in its success. The author has also seen this syndrome in mix breed dogs.

Neoplasia is an uncommon cause of pedal dermatoses. The lesions are usually nodules, with or without ulceration or pruritus. While usually only one foot is involved squamous cell carcinomas occurring spontaneously on several feet has been reported in dogs (Madewell *et al*, 1982). Rarely, cats with primary lung tumours will have metastases to both front paws (Gauguere *et al*, 1992). Diagnosis is by biopsy, with therapy (surgical excision, digit or limb amputation, radiotherapy or chemotherapy) dependent upon the type of tumour (Chapter 7).

Plasma cell pododermatitis is a rare idiopathic cause of foot pad swelling and ulceration in cats (Gauguere *et al*, 1992). The initial condition is a soft nonpainful swelling of the foot pads, which may progress to ulceration and granulation tissue. Ulceration may lead to pain and lameness. Usually the metacarpal or metatarsal pads are involved but the digital pads may also be affected. Diagnosis is by biopsy, which reveals a diffuse dermatitis with a massive plasma cell infiltration. The best mode of therapy is still undetermined. Glucocorticoids have not been particularly beneficial. Some cases will regress spontaneously. Chrysotherapy in a regimen similar to that of the treatment of autoimmune disease, or surgical removal of affected tissues, have both been reported to be effective.

Table 2
Drugs for use in the treatment of acral lick dermatitis

DRUG	DOSE	SUCCESS RATE
amitriptyline	2 mg/kg bid	30%
naltrexone*	2 mg/kg s-bid	63%
clomipramine*	1-3 mg/kg/day	66%
fluoxetine*	1 mg/kg sid	20%
hydrocodone/homatropine	5 mg/20 kg tid	66%

* These drugs are moderately to greatly expensive
_ These rates are based on the author's (and others') experience

Vitiligo (idiopathic loss of pigment) may affect the foot pads or nails. Important differential diagnoses are the autoimmune diseases. No therapy is proven effective in veterinary medicine, nor is any needed, since this is a benign disease without systemic signs.

PSYCHOGENIC/NEUROLOGIC DERMATOSES

Rarely, a pedal dermatosis will apparently be self-induced. This is usually a nervous dog with a nervous owner. Poodles, German shepherd dogs and small terriers have been reported to be the breeds most commonly affected (Scott, 1980).

Acral lick dermatitis (lick granuloma) is a common dermatitis in dogs that frequently is frustrating for both the owner and the veterinarian. The clinical appearance of acral lick dermatitis (ALD) is that of a thickened, moderately well-circumscribed alopecic and occasionally ulcerated area, typically in a large breed dog on the dorsal aspect of one of the front legs. The dog seemingly "causes" the lesion by excessive licking and chewing at the area involved. Occasionally there is an organic cause to this disease (underlying neoplasm, osteomyelitis, or deep pyoderma). However, the vast majority of these cases must be termed idiopathic. Traditionally, these have been linked to behavioral problems, such as boredom, introduction of a new person or pet into the household, confinement in a cage or kennel (Muller *et al*, 1989). Therapies have been primarily palliative and have generally included various anti-inflammatory drugs such as glucocorticoids and DMSO (Scott and Walton, 1984).

Recently, two new theories have been put forward on ALD. One compares acral lick dermatitis with various self-mutilative syndromes in people in which the mutilation releases endorphins which establish a positive feedback system for the aberrant behaviour. Oral and parenteral administration of endorphin antagonists has been shown to cease or decrease licking behavior in some but not all dogs with ALD (White, 1990; Brignac, 1992). The other theory involves sensory nerve dysfunction. In 10 dogs with ALD, sensory dysfunction (sensory axonal polyneuropathy) was documented in all cases (Van Ness, 1986).

The author's current diagnostic approach to ALD includes a radiograph of the affected area (to rule out osteomyelitis or bone neoplasm) and a biopsy (to rule out folliculitis/furunculosis, which should be amenable to antibiotic therapy). If these tests are negative or normal, the drugs in Table 2 may be used.

Acral mutilation syndrome is an unusual sensory neuropathy reported in German shorthaired and English pointers (Cummings *et al*, 1981). There are histopathologic changes (fiber degeneration, decrease in nerve cell bodies and fibre density) noted in the spinal cord, spinal roots, ganglia and peripheral nerves. The syndrome occurs in affected pups at three to five months of age. The dogs bite and lick their paws and there is total loss of temperature and pain sensation to the toes (and sometimes to the proximal legs and trunk). There may be auto-amputation of the toes. Therapy using restraining devices or sedation is not effective and euthanasia is usually requested by the owners. Parents of affected pups should not be used as breeders.

REFERENCES

ANDERSON, R.K. (1980). Canine pododermatitis. *Compendium on Continuing Education and the Practicing Veterinarian*, **2**: 361

ATTLEBERGER, M.H. (1983). Actinomycosis, nocardiosis, and dermatophilosis. In: *Current Veterinary Therapy VIII*. (Ed. R. W. Kirk), W.B. Saunders, Philadelphia

ATTLEBERGER, M.H. (1988). Subcutaneous mycoses. In: *Manual of Small Animal Infectious Diseases*, (Ed. Greene), Churchill Livingstone, New York

BEALE, K.M., ALTMON, D. and CLEMMONS, R.R. (1992). Systemic toxicosis associated with azathioprine administration in domestic cats. *American Journal of Veterinary Research*, **53**: 1236

BRENNAN, K.E. and IHRKE, P.J. (1983). Grass awn migration in dogs and cats: a retrospective study of 182 cases. *Journal of the American Veterinary Medical Association*, **182**: 1201

BRIGNAC, M.M. (1992). Hydrocodone treatment of acral lick dermatitis. *Proceedings of the Second World Congress of Veterinary*, 2 (Eds. K.W. Kwochka and S. D. White), p. 50.

CUMMINGS, J.F., deLAHUNTA, A. and WINN, S.S. (1981). Acral mutilation and nociceptive loss in English pointer dogs. *Acta Neuropathology* (Berl) **53**: 119

FERRER, L., RABANAL, R. and FONDEVILA, D. (1988). Skin lesions in canine leishmaniasis. *Journal of Small Animal Practice*, **29**: 381

FERRER, L. (1992). Leishmaniasis. In: *Current Veterinary Therapy XI*, (Eds. R.W. Kirk and J.D. Bonagura), W.B. Saunders, Philadelphia

FIGUEIREDO, C. Clinical evaluation of the effect of vitamin E in the treatment of generalized canine demodicosis. In. *Advances in Veterinary Dermatology*, Vol 2 (Eds. P.J. Ihrke, I.S. Mason and S.D. White), in press. Pergamon Press, Oxford

FOIL, C.S. (1986). Antifungal agents in dermatology. In: *Current Veterinary Therapy IX.*, (Ed. R. W. Kirk), pp. 560. W.B. Saunders, Philadelphia

GAUGUERE, E., HUBERT, B., and DELABRE, C. (1992). Feline pododermatitis. *Veterinary Dermatology*, **3**: 1

GROSS, T.L., O'BRIEN, T.D. and DAVIS, A.P. (1990). Glucagon-producing pancreatic endocrine tumors in two dogs with superficial necrolytic dermatitis. *Journal of the American Veterinary Medical Association*, **197**: 619

IHRKE, P.J., STANNARD, A.A. and ARDANS, A.A. (1985). Pemphigus foliaceus of the foot pads in three dogs. *Journal of the American Veterinary Medical Association*, **186**: 67

KIRK, R.W. (1983). Systemic therapy of skin disorders. In: *Current Veterinary Therapy VIII*, (Ed. R. W. Kirk), W.B. Saunders, Philadelphia

KUNKLE, G.A. (1980). Zinc-responsive dermatoses in dogs. In: *Current Veterinary Therapy VII*, (Ed. R. W. Kirk). W.B. Saunders, Philadelphia

KUNKLE, G.A. (1988). Contact dermatitis. *Veterinary Clinics of North America*, **18**: 1061

KUNKLE, G.A., WHITE, S.D. and CALDERWOOD-MAYS. Focal metatarsal fistulas in the German Shepherd dog. *Journal of the American Veterinary Medical Association*, in press.

KWOCHKA, K.W. (1986). Canine demodicosis. In: *Current Veterinary Therapy IX.* (Ed. R. W. Kirk), W.B. Saunders, Philadelphia

LANGE, A.L., VERSTER, A. and VANAMSTEL, S.R. (1980). *Anatrichosoma sp* infestation in the foot pads of a cat. *Journal of the South African Veterinary Association*, **51**: 227

LEGENDRE, A.M., SELCER, B.A. and EDWARDS, D.F. (1984). Treatment of canine blastomycosis with amphotericin B and ketoconazole. *Journal of the American Veterinary Medical Association*, **184**: 1249

LEWIS, D.T., FOIL, C.S. and HOSGOOD, G. (1991). Epidemiology and clinical features of dermatophytosis in dogs and cats at Louisiana State University (1981-1990). *Veterinary Dermatology*, **2**: 53

LIUM, B. and MOE, L. (1985). Hereditary multifocal renal cystadenocarcinomas and nodular dermatofibrosis in the German shepherd dog: macroscopic and histopathologic changes. *Veterinary Pathology*, **22**: 447

LLOYD, D.H. and THOMSETT, L.R. (1989). Essential fatty acid supplementation in the treatment of canine atopy; a preliminary study. *Veterinary Dermatology*, **1:** 41

MADEWELL, B.R., POOL, R.R. and THEILEN, G.H. (1982). Multiple subungual squamous cell carcinomas in five dogs. *Journal of the American Veterinary Medical Association*, **180**: 731

MANCIANTI, F.and MECIANI, N. (1988). Specific serodiagnosis of canine leishmaniasis by indirect immunofluorescence, indirect hemagglutination, and counterimmunoelectrophoresis. *American Journal of Veterinary Research*, **49**: 1409

MILLER, W.H. JR., GRIFFIN, C.E. and SCOTT, D.W. (1989). Clinical trial of DVM DermCaps in the treatment of allergic disease in dogs; a nonblinded study. *Journal of the American Animal Hospital Association*, **25**: 163

MILLER, W.H. JR., SCOTT, D.W. and BUERGER, R.G. (1990). Necrolytic migratory erythema in dogs; a hepatocutaneous syndrome. *Journal of the American Animal Hospital Association*, **26**: 575

MOORE, F.M., WHITE, S.D. and CARPENTER, J.L. (1987). Localization of immunoglobulins and complement by the peroxidase antiperoxidase method in autoimmune and nonautoimmune canine dermatopathies. *Veterinary Immunology and Immunopathology,* **14**: 1

MULLER, G.H., KIRK, R.W and SCOTT, D.W. (1989). *Small Animal Dermatology,* 4th Edn. W.B. Saunders, Philadelphia

OLIVRY, T., PRELAUD, P. and HERIPRET, D. (1990). Allergic contact dermatitis in the dog: Principles and diagnosis. *Veterinary Clinics of North America,* 1443

ROSYCHUK, R. (1983). Management of hypothyroidism. In: *Current Veterinary Therapy VIII* (Ed. R. W. Kirk), pp. 869. W.B. Saunders, Philadelphia

SCOTT, D.W. (1980). Canine pododermatitis. In: *Current Veterinary Therapy VII* (Ed. R. W. Kirk), W.B. Saunders, Philadelphia

SCOTT, D.W., and WALTON, D.K. (1984). Clinical evaluation of a topical treatment for canine acral lick dermatitis. *Journal of the American Animal Hospital Association,* **20**: 565

SCOTT, D.W., WALTON, D.K. and SLATER, M.R. (1987). Immune-mediated dermatoses in domestic animals: ten years after - part I. *Compendium on Continuing Education and the Practicing Veterinarian,* **9**: 424

SNYDER, R.A. and SCHWARTZ, R.A. (1983). Cactus bristle implantation *Archives of Dermatology,* **119**: 152

SOUSA, C.A., STANNARD, A.A. and IHRKE, P.J. (1988). Dermatosis associated with feeding generic dog food: 13 cases (1981 to 1982). *Journal of the American Veterinary Medical Association,* **219**: 676

VAN NESS J.J. (1986). Electrophysiological evaluation of sensory nerve dysfunction in 10 dogs with lick dermatitis. *Journal of American Hospital Association* **22**: 197

WALTON, D.K., CENTER, S.A. and SCOTT, D.W. (1986) Ulcerative dermatosis associated with diabetes mellitus in the dog: a report of four cases. *Journal of the American Animal Hospital Association,* **22**: 79

WHITE, S.D., STANNARD, A.A. (1983). Canine demodicosis. In: *Current Veterinary Therapy VIII,* (ED. R. W. Kirk), W.B. Saunders Company, Philadelphia

WHITE, S.D. (1986). Cutaneous mycobacteriosis. In: *Current Veterinary Therapy IX,* (Ed. R. W. Kirk), W.B. Saunders Company, Philadelphia

WHITE, S.D., IHRKE, P.J. (1987). Pyoderma. In: . *Contemporary Issues in Small Animal Practice: Dermatology,* (ED. G. H. Nesbitt). Churchill Livingstone, New York

WHITE, S.D., CERAGIOLI, K.L., STEWART, L.J., *et al.* (1989). Cutaneous markers of canine hyperadrenocorticism. *Compendium on Continuing Education and the Practicing Veterinarian,* **11**: 446

WHITE, S.D. (1990). Naltrexone for treatment of acral lick dermatitis in dogs. *Journal of the American Veterinary Medical Association,* **196**: 1073

WHITE, S.D. (1992). Food Hypersensitivity. In: *Current Veterinary Therapy XI,* (Eds. R. W. Kirk and J. D. Bonagura), pp. 513. W.B. Saunders, Philadelphia

WILLEMSE, T.A. (1987). Atopic dermatitis. In: *Contemporary Issues in Small Animal Practice: Dermatology,* (Ed. G. H. Nesbitt), pp. 57. Churchill Livingstone, New York

ZOOK, P.C., HOLZWORTH, J. and THORNTON, G.W. (1968). Thallium poisoning in cats. *Journal of the American Veterinary Medical Association,* **153**: 285

DISORDERS OF THE NAILS AND NAILBED

Richard G Harvey ————————————————————

INTRODUCTION

Diseases of the nail alone are rarely encountered in practice but they may be extremely frustrating to manage when they do occur. Disorders which affect the distal digit and nail fold are more common and will often have an effect on the nail, being associated with accumulations of odourous lipid, infection of the nail bed, abnormal nail growth and even shedding of the nail.

Nail is produced from a specialised continuation of the digital epidermis, the nail matrix, at a rate of about 1.9 mm per week in young beagles (Muller, *et al.*1989). Nail growth resembles that of the stratum corneum, being a product of basal cell division, although the nail undergoes a process of keratinisation more akin to that of the hair than that of the epidermis. Keratin fibrils are laid down in maturing keratinocytes and these impart both strength and rigidity to the nail. In contrast to the cornified epidermis, the nail possesses relatively little of the intercellular lipid that contributes greatly to both the epidermal permeability barrier and cell to cell adhesion in the stratum corneum. This relative lack of an effective barrier to water loss makes the nails potentially at risk from the effects of dehydration which is surprising for such a hard tissue. The constant production of nail tissue and its highly specialised structure and function may also make it a sensitive indicator of nutritional status.

Chronic inflammation of the skin of the distal digit may cause inflammation of the adjacent nail bed (paronychia) and this may result in abnormal nail growth. Such inflammation may result from many causes (for example: physical agents, infectious conditions, hypersensitivity or autoimmune diseases [Table 1]) and will often be accompanied by a degree of secondary bacterial infection. The pathological significance of any bacteriological results obtained from affected nails should therefore be treated with caution, particularly if several nails are affected. However knowledge of the antibacterial sensitivity of any bacteria present is of value in the management of secondary infection.

Nail disorders may take a number of forms, such as the production of abnormally soft nail (onychomalacia) or very brittle nail (onychorrhexis). Other cases may be characterised by cracking and splitting of the horizontal layers of distal nail (onychoschizia), analogous to split ends of the hair shaft. Abnormal growth of the nail may be due to infection with dermatophytes (onychomycosis) or as a consequence of the chronic irritation accompanying longstanding paronychia. The resultant nail growth may result in thickened abnormal nails (onychogryposis) or even sloughing of the entire nail (onychomadesis). The investigation of nail bed disorders and paronychia should also include consideration of systemic disorders such as defects in keratinisation, feline leukaemia virus infection, the immunosuppressive effects of endocrine disorders and of debilitating internal disease.

APPROACH TO THE CASE

There is no reported age or sex incidence but animals whose nails are subject to repeated trauma such as racing greyhounds, working dogs and the larger breeds may be predisposed. The management

Table 1

Causes of nail disorders and paronychia

1. Environmental agents

Acute trauma
Prolonged immersion
Exposure to very hot water
Prolonged exposure to a dry environment
Exposure to caustic agents
Overzealous clipping

2. Infectious agents

i. Viruses

Cowpox
Feline herpesvirus and calicivirus
Feline leukaemia virus
Feline immunosuppressive virus

ii. Bacteria

Typically secondary to any primary cause of nailbed or pedal inflammation or to systemic diseases and immunosuppression.

iii. Fungi

Dermatophytes
Candida spp.

iv. Protozoa

Leishmania spp.

v. Helminths

Ancylostoma spp., *Uncinaria stenocephala*

vi. Arthropods

Demodex canis

3. Hypersensitivities

Atopy
Dietary hypersensitivity and intolerance
Contact hypersensitivity
Drug eruption

4. Immune mediated disorders

Pemphigus complex, particularly foliaceus
Bullous pemphigoid
Discoid lupus erythematosus
Systemic lupus erythematosus

5. Systemic diseases

Endocrine disorders particularly canine hypothyroidism, feline hyperthyroidism, acromegaly and diabetes mellitus
Superficial necrolytic dermatitis (hepato-cutaneous syndrome) any serious internal disease that potentially compromises either nutrition or immunity

of the animal should be considered and details of housing, cleaning routines and exercise patterns should be obtained as chemical irritants and prolonged wetting may cause paronychia. Scalding may result in onychomadesis of several nails.

Although no association between nail dystrophies and nutrition has been reported in small animals, dietary causes should not be ruled out and an evaluation of the diet should be made early in the course of the investigation. If there are doubts about the quality of the diet a commercially balanced diet should be fed as this is a much easier task than attempting to correct an unbalanced home prepared diet .

It is important to establish whether there is evidence of internal disease such as hepatic or renal dysfunction or endocrinopathy, particularly hypothyroidism. It is possible that an acute, severe systemic illness may result in a period of compromised metabolism in the nail matrix and if this leads to the production of poor quality nail it may subsequently splinter or fracture. However, the slow turnover of nail tissue will result in a lag period of weeks or months before the damage becomes apparent.

In addition to collating this detailed history, the owner should be informed that the current status of our knowledge of nail disorders of the dog and cat is poor and that in many instances an identifiable aetiology is not recognised. In consequence, treatment tends to be supportive and non-specific, although this should not preclude a thorough investigation. Furthermore, even with identification and the successful treatment of a specific condition or effective symptomatic therapy the owner should be cautioned that a period of several months should be allowed for normal nail growth to re-establish.

PHYSICAL EXAMINATION

A full clinical examination should be carried out, the aim being to identify any evidence of systemic disease. The lymph nodes should be palpated. The nasal planum, the lips, pinnae and perineum should be examined for evidence of lesions such as vesicles, ulcers or crusts that may suggest the presence of autoimmune disease such as pemphigus foliaceus or discoid lupus erythematosus.

Attention should be paid to the texture of the hair as abnormalities in hair keratinisation may accompany nail dystrophies, for example onychomalacia may be seen in 'woolly-coated' cavalier King Charles spaniels. The animal may show evidence of defects in keratinisation of the skin and associated sebaceous glands such as seborrhoeic scale, follicular casts, comedones or accumulations of lipid around the nipples. Defects in keratinisation may equally well affect the nail matrix resulting in onychorrhexis. Some cats, particularly sphinx, may manifest seborrhoeic disease solely as accumulations of malodourous lipid in the nail fold.

All four feet should be examined and the pads, interdigital regions, nail folds and nails inspected for signs of inflammation, self trauma or damage. It may be necessary to sedate the animal to do this properly. The hair from the distal digits and interdigital region should be carefully clipped so that complete examination is possible. This will also facilitate collection of any samples that may be necessary.

ESTABLISHING THE DIAGNOSIS

The history and distribution of the condition may help to suggest a diagnosis; thus a history of lesions on several nails over a protracted period of time would be consistent with an underlying and probably internal disease. However many of these cases defy definitive diagnosis. Internal diseases can be identified by consideration of history, clinical findings and laboratory investigations. In contrast, external causes and recent managemental influences are more likely to be confined to one nail or to one foot.

Infectious agents may be suggested from the history (if, for example the animal originates from an area where *Leishmania* is endemic) and physical findings (frayed edges to the foot pads in association with paronychia, onychogryposis and some onychomadesis are characteristic of hookworm dermatitis). Skin scrapings should be taken and examined under a microscope for *Demodex canis*. Careful inspection under Wood's light and microscopical examination of 10% potassium hydroxide preparations may suggest dermatophytosis and fungal culture will support this. Onychomycosis may also be diagnosed by histopathological examination of nail sections.

When taking samples for microbiology or fungal culture it is important to minimise collection of environmental contaminants. Swabs of exudate may be taken once a loose nail is removed but samples of surface exudate from around the base of the nail are less useful. The nail should be swabbed with spirit and allowed to air-dry before samples of freshly expressed exudate are taken. Similar precautions should precede taking nail samples such for fungal culture.

INITIAL MANAGEMENT

Initial management will depend on the severity of the case and the differential diagnosis. If systemic disease is suspected then the definitive diagnosis should be pursued. If examination and skin scrapings are non-diagnostic then samples for fungal culture and bacteriological examination should be collected. If nails are on the point of being shed then removal under anaesthesia is indicated as this will ease the animal's discomfort as well as allowing access to deeper tissue for sampling. Pending laboratory results gentle topical cleansing with ethyl lactate, triclosan, chlorhexidine or povidone iodine may be of value. Bathing the feet in magnesium sulphate solution is also helpful.

If dermatophytosis is confirmed then specific treatment is indicated with both topical and systemic therapy (Chapter 30). Isolation of significant bacteria such as coagulase-positive staphylococci or enterobacilli should prompt treatment based on culture and sensitivity results. Any suggestion that more than one nail is infected or cases of multiple infected paronychia should prompt a reconsideration of the possibility of immunosuppression and the animal re-appraised with this in mind. Owing to the slow turnover of nail tissue, treatment with either antifungal or antibacterial agents should be continued for several weeks before being stopped. In the case of dermatophytosis then treatment is continued until negative culture is reported. Samples should be submitted for culture at three week intervals to assess progress. With regard to the duration of antibacterial therapy then three or four weeks is a reasonable first course.

If there is no dermatophytosis and there is no response to initial antibacterial therapy as outlined above then biopsy should be considered. In cases of chronic inflammation of the dital digit then there is no question that this is helpful. Where the nail alone is affected there is less certainty, primarily because of the lack of published information on the topic. Histopathological examination of the nail matrix is required if useful information is to be gained and this is not readily accessible unless the distal digit is amputated. The advantages and disadvantages should be explained to the owner. The obvious advantage is the ability to define a diagnosis such as discoid lupus erythematosus or a defect in keratinisation while the disadvantage to be weighed is the possibility of not obtaining a significant result. It would be worthwhile discussing the case with a histopathologist before taking samples.

An alternative approach when faced with a chronic or multiple-nail disorder which defies definitive diagnosis is to prescribe anti-inflammatory doses of prednisolone for a period of one to two months as a trial therapy. Response may follow and gradual reduction to alternate day therapy with eventual withdrawal as the aim. Supplementing the diet with vitamin A, zinc and biotin also may be useful, even in cases where a balanced diet is being fed. If there is no improvement to these measures then biopsy should be reconsidered.

FURTHER READING

DANIEL, C.R. (1985). The Nail. In: *Dermatologic Clinics*, **3**, 3. W.B. Saunders, Philadelphia.

MCNEIL, N.A. (1987). Nail Disease in Small Animals. In: *Veterinary Dermatology Newsletter.* **11**, 18.

MULLER, G.H., KIRK, R.W. and SCOTT, D.W. (1989) *Small Animal Dermatology 4th. Edn,* W.B. Saunders, Philadelphia.

SCOTT, D.W. (1990). Nail disorders in dogs and cats. In: *Proceedings 7th. Annual Meeting of The European Society of Veterinary Dermatology.*

Symmetrical alopecia in the dog (Chapter 12)

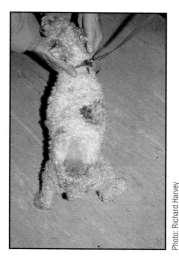

Plate 22
Flea allergic dermatitis

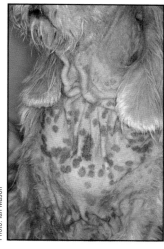

Plate 23
Hypothyroidism: alopecia and skin
thickening. Note skin folds

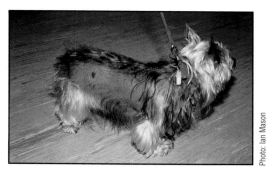

Plate 24
Hyperadrenocorticism

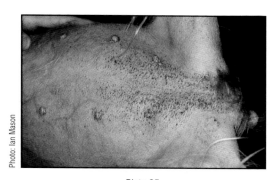

Plate 25
Hyperadrenocorticism (ventral abdomen). Note
abdominal distension, comedones, epidermal collarette,
aopecia and prominent cutaneous vasculature

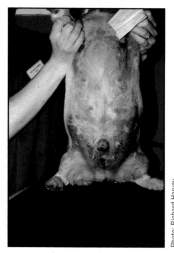

Plate 26
Sertoli cell tumour. Note alopecia
and abdominal distension

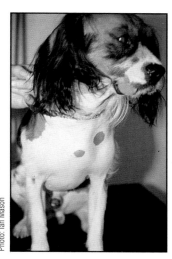

Plate 27
Congenital alopecia

Focal alopecia in dogs and cats
(Chapter 10 and 11)

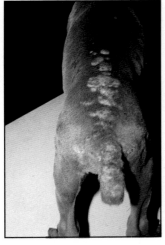

Photo: Richard Harvey

Plate 28
Superficial folliculitis in a great Dane puppy

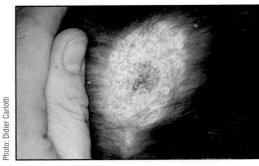

Photo: Didier Carlotti

Plate 29
Classical *Microsporum canis* infection in a European cat:
a numular, erythematous, scaly, peripherally
expanding lesion.

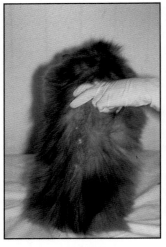

Photo: Didier Carlotti

Plate 30
Symmetrical scaly extensive alopecia due to
Microsporum canis infection in a Persian cat.

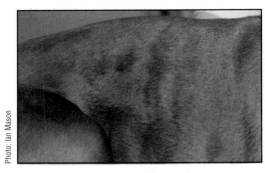

Photo: Ian Mason

Plate 31
Idiopathic flank alopecia

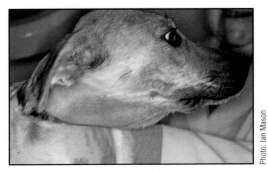

Photo: Ian Mason

Plate 32
Demodectic mange

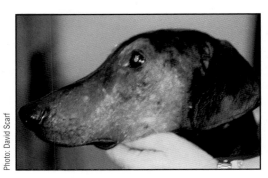

Photo: David Scarf

Plate 33
Doberman with alopecia areata; note loss of tan hair.

Cutaneous scaling disorders
(Chapter 5)

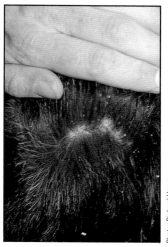

Plate 34
Cheyletiellosis in a Yorkshire terrier

Photo: Richard Harvey

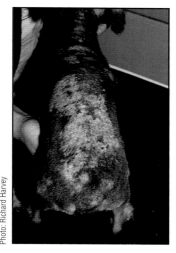

Plate 35
Demodicosis in a Norfolk terrier

Photo: Richard Harvey

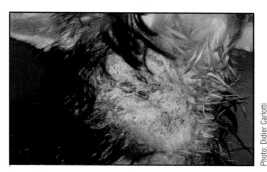

Plate 36
Microsporum canis infection in a Yorkshire terrier:
regional alopecia with erosions and crusting.

Photo: Didier Carlotti

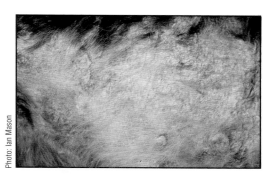

Plate 37
Epidermotropic lymphoma
(mycosis fungoides): flank of Airedale terrier

Photo: Ian Mason

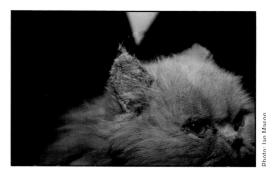

Plate 38
Pemphigus foliaceus in a Persian cat

Photo: Ian Mason

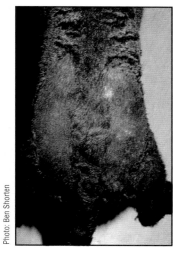

Plate 39
Sebaceous adenitis in a standard poodle

Photo: Ben Shorten

Facial dermatoses
(Chapter 14)

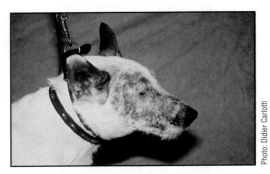

Photo: Didier Carlotti

Plate 40
Localised seborrhoeic and erythematous regional alopecia
on the face of a terrier infected with *Microsporum persicolor*

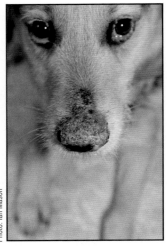

Photo: Ian Mason

Plate 41
Pemphigus foliaceus

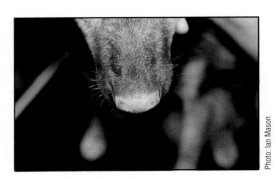

Photo: Ian Mason

Plate 42
Discoid lupus erythematosis

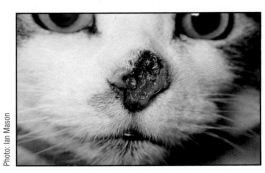

Photo: Ian Mason

Plate 43
Squamous cell carcinoma

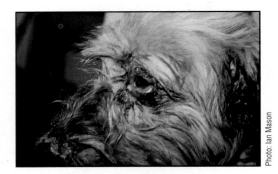

Photo: Ian Mason

Plate 44
Deep pyoderma secondary to generalised lymphoma

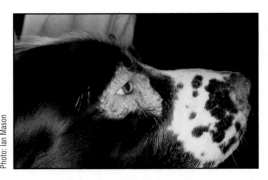

Photo: Ian Mason

Plate 45
Zinc responsive dermatosis

CHAPTER NINETEEN

DISORDERS OF THE ANAL SACS

Patrick J McKeever

INTRODUCTION

Canine anal sacs are paired cutaneous diverticula which form a reservoir and excretory duct into which apocrine and sebaceous glands empty. The secretion of these glands is believed to play a role in social recognition among dogs in the scentmarking and anointing of territory (Donovan, 1969). Expression of normal sacs occurs when the overlying external anal sphincter contracts and squeezes the sacs against stool in the anal canal (Ashdown, 1968).

Disease of the anal sacs manifested as either impaction, infection, or abscessation are a common finding in the dog. Reported incidence varies from a low of 1.3% to a high of 12.5% of admissions to veterinary hospitals (Kirk, 1939; Halnan, 1976a).

Anatomy and Normal Secretions

The anal sacs in the normal dog lie almost evenly above and below a horizontal plane through the anus, and not in a ventrolateral position (Halnan, 1978). They are located between the smooth internal muscle of the anal canal and striated muscle of the external anal sphincter (Nielson, 1953). Each sac is connected to the surface by a duct that opens into the lateral margins of the anus at the level of the mucocutaneous junction.

The lumen of the anal sac serves as a reservoir for glandular secretions from the wall, which is the true parenchyma. Numerous large coiled apocrine glands empty via tubules into the lumen and are known as the anal sac glands. Sebaceous glands are found around and empty into the anal sac duct (Anderson, 1984). The normal volume for the lumen of an anal sac of a 17 kg dog is reported as 0.25 to 0.5 ml (Halnan, 1978).

Contents of the anal sac and its duct consist of apocrine and sebaceous secretions plus desquamated cells of the stratified squamous epithelium that lines the anal sac. In the normal anal sac it is a serous to slightly viscid, clear to pale yellow or brownish liquid with a disagreeable odour (Archibald and Horney, 1974; Anderson, 1984). A crude analysis of the secretion showed it to be 87.8% water and the dried substance was 96.1% organic and 3.9% inorganic (Halnan, 1978). Normal anal sacs should not be distended as the thin consistency of their secretions allows for easy expression via the action of the external anal sphincter muscle during defaecation.

Pathogenesis

The aetiology and exact pathogenesis of anal sac disease is not the same in all animals. However, retention of secretion is probably the inciting factor in the majority of cases. Retention may occur if secretions become so thick and pasty that they will not easily flow through the anal sac ducts; if the ducts become plugged with flocculent or granular material; if the stools are soft (due to, for example, dietary factors or gastrointestinal disease so that proper expression does not occur upon defaecation) and if there is loss of tone in the external anal sphincter muscle so that proper compression of the anal sacs does not occur.

Retention of secretions leads to enlargement of the anal sacs, thinning of the epithelial lining and, finally, rupture. The resulting inflammatory response to the anal sac contents in the surrounding tissues may lead to ulceration of the overlying skin and direct drainage.

Bacterial flora of normal anal sacs resembles that of the lower intestinal tract (Anderson, 1984). *Escherichia coli*, *Proteus* spp., *Streptococcus faecolis*, *Clostridium welchii*, *Staphylococcus* spp., and *Pseudomonas* spp. are the predominant bacteria that have been cultured from infected anal sacs (Halnan, 1976a). Infection may be limited to the lumen of the anal sac, spread to the apocrine glands lining the sac wall or to the surrounding tissues (Anderson, 1984). If infection is extensive, abscess formation and resultant fistulation to the skin surface may occur.

Anal sac disease has been produced experimentally by introduction of pathogenic bacteria directly into the sac and by ligation of the anal sac duct (Halnan, 1976b).

One study showed that anal sac disease, especially anal sac infection and abscess formation, is more common in smaller breeds of dogs, with a higher incidence in the poodle and chihuahua. A lower than expected incidence was found in German shepherd dogs (Harvey, 1974). However, another study showed no relationship between anal sac disease and breed, sex, or age (Halnan, 1976a).

APPROACH TO THE CASE

Owners usually will be the first to note signs of anal sac disease. Thus historical information is of prime importance to the clinician. The classic complaint is that the animal frequently scoots, drags, or rubs its rear on the ground or carpet. Often these actions will allow the dog to evacuate the anal sacs and thus obtain relief. Other signs that may be noticed by the owner include constant licking of the anal area, tenesmus, pain associated with defaecation, tail chasing, biting or licking at the flank or lumbosacral area, discharge from the perianal area, discomfort when sitting and rubbing of the back against the underside of a chair or table. In addition, behavioural changes such as an aggressive attitude towards someone handling the caudal half of the body, a sudden startled action followed by licking or biting at the caudal half of the body and periodic staring at the anal area may be noted (Halnan, 1976a).

PHYSICAL EXAMINATION

On physical examination, the anal sacs may be found to be enlarged and the animal may evidence moderate to severe pain when they are palpated. An area of acute moist dermatitis may be noted over the diseased anal sac from an animal's constant licking. Necrotic, sometimes oedematous, skin may be noted if an abscess of the anal sac has formed but has not yet ruptured. Finally a fistula overlying the anal sac with a serosanguinous to mucopurulent discharge will be found if the anal sac abscess has spontaneously ruptured.

ESTABLISHING THE DIAGNOSIS

The presence of anal sac disease may be assessed by evaluation of history, enlargement of the sacs, presence of abnormal secretions, concomitant skin disease overlying the anal sac area, rupture of an anal sac abscess and abnormal bacterial flora. Assessment of anal sac size is subjective, but an anal sac may be considered to be enlarged when it can be easily palpated through the skin of the anal region (Anderson, 1984). Bilateral enlargement most often suggests impaction or sacculitis while unilateral enlargement may be associated with anal sac abscess or tumour.

After determining the size of the anal sacs their contents should be examined. Simultaneous expression of both sacs via outside pressure on the overlying skin should be avoided because excessive amounts of unnecessary pressure are required. The preferred method of examination and expression of the anal sac is to introduce a lubricated, gloved index finger into the anus and squeeze the anal sac between the index finger and the thumb which is placed on the skin surface overlying the anal sac. In most cases application of gentle pressure will result in expression of the anal sac contents. Massage of the anal sac with the index finger may be required for complete evacuation.

A thick, pasty, brown or greyish brown secretion is generally associated with impaction. In some cases the secretions may become inspissated and appear as a thin ribbon like material that is expressed with difficulty.

Acute infection of the anal sac wall results in secretions that are purulent, often blood streaked and foul smelling.

Chronic infections are characterized by secretions that vary from a thin watery consistency to a creamy purulent material. In these cases the wall of the anal sac often feels thick on palpation.

Microscopical examination of secretions from infected anal glands reveals numerous leucocytes and bacteria. In contrast, secretions from normal anal sacs contain cellular debris but few bacteria and leucocytes.

Presence of bacteria in cultures from animals with anal sac disease does not confirm an infectious aetiology because they are found in normal anal sacs. However, cultures are helpful for assessing the potential pathogenicity of isolated organisms and sensitivity testing may help in the selection of appropriate antibacterial therapy (see Chapter 25).

INITIAL MANAGEMENT

In cases of impaction or mild closed infection the manual expression of anal sac contents is the essential first procedure. If manual expression is successful in establishing free drainage through the anal sac ducts no other treatment may be necessary to obtain a cure. This procedure may have to be repeated several times at weekly intervals until normal secretions and normal function return. Routine expression may be necessary in some dogs as a preventative measure.

If the anal sac content is so thick that it cannot be expressed with reasonable pressure, a softening agent such as mineral oil or a lipophilic and solubilising agent such as hexamethyltetracosane (Seb-O-Sol, Butler, USA) can be instilled into the sac using a lacrimal cannula or a tom cat catheter. The anal sac is then massaged, using the same technique as for expression, until the contents have mixed with the softening or solubilising agents sufficiently to allow passage out of the duct.

After infected sacs have been manually expressed, they should be irrigated via a lacrimal cannula or tom cat catheter with a mild antiseptic solution such as 0.5% chlorhexidine. Infusion of an antibiotic corticosteroid ointment promotes resolution of the anal sacculitis by reducing the inflammatory response and decreasing bacterial numbers (Anderson, 1984). A solution of 0.01% flunocinolone acetonide with 60% dimethyl sulphoxide in a propylene glycol vehicle has also been reported as being useful for the treatment of impacted or inflamed anal sacs and is especially effective in counteracting the offensive odour of the infected anal sac secretions (Anderson, 1984).

The use of systemic antibiotics is a matter of clinical judgement, but is rarely needed in the treatment of impaction or mild infection.

Manual expression of anal sacs, irrigation and instillation of treatment solutions can be accomplished in a majority of dogs without sedation. If, however, the animal is intractable or the anal sac is painful sedation may be required. The author prefers a combination of ketamine (1.4 to 2.3 mg/kg), diazepam (0.045 mg/kg), and acepromazine (0.023 mg/kg). All of these are combined in one syringe and given intravenously. Effective sedation lasts for approximately twenty minutes.

Exact treatment of anal sac abscesses will depend on whether or not the animal is presented with external rupture of the abscess. If cellulitis is present, a warm wet compress can be applied to the affected area three to four times daily, for five to ten minutes until the abscess has developed enough that it can be drained. A needle aspirate of the swollen mass will confirm whether or not an abscess has formed to the extent that it can be lanced (see Chapter 3).

In order to thoroughly treat an abscess a suitable sedative such as that previously described should be administered. An incision is made through the skin to establish ventral drainage. After the abscess is lanced, or in animals where the abscess has ruptured externally, it should be flushed thoroughly with an antiseptic solution such as 0.5% chlorhexidine. Once the abscess is lanced and thoroughly cleaned the anal sac duct should also be flushed with the antiseptic solution to assure its patency. Cauterisation, with caustic agents such as silver nitrate or phenol should be avoided as they can cause extensive cellular necrosis and delay healing.

Systemic antibacterial therapy for ten to fourteen days is indicated in the treatment of anal sac abscesses. Ideally it should be based on culture and sensitivity results, but the author has had good success treating empirically with ampicillin or amoxicillin.

With cooperative dogs, owners can irrigate the wound daily with the antiseptic solution to cleanse the area and promote healing from within.

Anal sacculectomy may be indicated if there are recurrent episodes of severe impaction, infection, or abscessation of the anal sacs. Various surgical procedures have been advocated with no general agreement on the best method (Baker, 1962; Greiner and Christie, 1975; Halnan, 1976b,1976c).

REFERENCES

ANDERSON, R.K. (1984). Anal sac disease and its related dermatoses. *Compendium on Continuing Education and the Practicing Veterinarian* **9**, 829.

ARCHIBALD J. & HORNEY F.S. (1974). Colon, rectum, and anal canal. In: *Canine Surgery* (Ed. J. Archibald). 2nd Edn. 603. American Veterinary Publications Inc., Santa Barbara.

ASHDOWN, R.R. (1968). Clinical Anatomy. In: Symposium on canine recto-anal disorders. *Journal of Small Animal Practice* **9**, 315.

BAKER, E. (1962). Diseases and therapy of the anal sacs of the dog. *Journal of The American Veterinary Medical Association* **141**, 1347.

DONOVAN, C. (1969). Canine anal glands and chemical signals (pheromones). *Journal of The American Veterinary Medical Association* **155**, 1969.

GREINER, T. & CHRISTIE, T. (1975). Removal of anal sacs. In: *Current Techniques in Small Animal Surgery*, (Ed. M.J. Bojrab) Lea & Febiger, Philadelphia.

HALNAN, C.R.E. (1976). The diagnosis of anal sacculitis in the dog. *Journal of Small Animal Practice* **17**, 527.

HALNAN, C.R.E. (1976a). The frequency of occurrence of anal sacculitis in the dog. *Journal of Small Animal Practice* **17**, 537.

HALNAN, C.R.E. (1976b). Therapy of anal sacculitis in the dog. *Journal of Small Animal Practice* **17**, 685.

HALNAN, C.R.E. (1976c). The experimental reproduction of anal sacculitis. *Journal of Small Animal Practice* **17**, 693.

HALNAN C.R.E. (1978). Canine anal sac disease. *Veterinary Annual* **18**, 225.

HARVEY, C. (1974). Incidence and distribution of anal sac disease in the dog. *Journal of the American Animal Hospital Association* **10**, 573.

KIRK, H. (1939). *Index of Diagnosis* p.4. Williams and Wilkins Co., Baltimore, MD.

NIELSON, S.W. (1953). Glands of the canine skin – morphology and distribution. *American Journal of Veterinary Research* **14**, 448.

CHAPTER TWENTY

ALOPECIA AND PRURITUS IN SMALL MAMMALS

Richard G Harvey and Martin P C Lawton

INTRODUCTION

Alopecia and pruritus are amongst the commonest presenting signs in small mammals and may be due to a variety of aetiologies such as infectious conditions, neoplasia and ectoparasites (Table 1) (Plates 68-73). Alopecia also may be due to a number of vices, both by the individual or by the cage mate. Ectoparasites account for the largest proportion of clinical cases (Table 2). In rodents for example, the mouse (*Mus* spp.), hamster (*Mesocritetus auratus, Cricetus cricetus, Cricetus griseus and Phodopus sungorus*) and guinea pig (*Cavia porcellus*), the pruritus associated with ectoparasitic infection may be intense and lead to severe self-trauma. There may be considerable variation in an individual's response to ectoparasite infection. This may reflect strain differences (particularly in mice) or differing host/parasite relationships between individuals (Friedman and Weisbroth, 1975; Weisbroth *et al*, 1976). It may also reflect an individual's tendency to manifest hypersensitivity to the presence of the ectoparasite. It is important, therefore, not to rule out ectoparasitism simply because only one individual in a group is clinically affected.

Table 1
Common Dermatoses of Small Mammals

Ectoparasitic infection	(see Table 2)
Fungal infection	
	T. mentagrophytes (mice, guinea pigs and rabbits)
	Cryptococcus neoformans (guinea pigs)
Bacterial infection	
	Staphylococcus infections such as *S. aureus* (mice and gerbils)
	Staphylococcosis (rabbits)
	Pseudomonas aerogenosa (rabbits)
Neoplasia	
	Mycosis fungoides (hamsters)
Other	
	Scurvy (guinea pigs)
	Barbering (guinea pigs)
	Sore hocks (rabbits and guinea pigs)
	Nasal dermatitis (gerbils)
	Slobbers (guinea pigs and rabbits)
	Ringtail (mice and rats)

Table 2
Common Ectoparasites of Small Mammals

Mouse

        lice: *Polyplax serrata,*

        mites: *Myobia musculi, Radfordia affinis, Myocoptes musculinus Psoregates simplex*

Rat

        fleas: *Xenopsylla* sp., *Leptopsylla* sp., *Nosopsyllus* sp.

        lice: *Polyplax spinulosa*

        mites: *Radfordia ensifera, Ornithonyssus bacoti,* (fur mites) *Notoedres muris,* (biting mite)

Mongolian gerbil

        mites: *Demodex meriones*

Hamster

        mites: *Demodex criceti* and *D. aurati*

Guinea pig

        mites: *Chirodiscoides caviae,* (fur mite)

              Trixacarus caviae, (sarcoptid mite)

        lice: *Gliricola porcelli* and *Gyropus ovalis,* (biting lice)

Rabbit

        mites: *Psoroptes cuniculi,* (ear mite)

              Cheyletiella parasitivorax, Listrophorus gibbus, (fur mites)

              Cuterebra spp., *Calliphora* spp. and *Sarcophaga* spp.

Ivermectin treatment has revolutionised the management of ectoparasitic disease in small mammals but it is not always curative (Sikarskie, 1986). Ivermectin is not equally effective against all stages of the life cycle of parasites, particularly if larval or adults stages are capable of surviving off the host. Where pruritus is present, the death of the ectoparasite following treatment may not be followed by immediate improvement while antigen is still present within the skin. Thus severe pruritus in guinea pigs associated with trixacarid mange may be apparent for some time after the mite has been killed. Topical therapeutics such as keratolytics may be of particular value in removing antigenic substances in superficial stratum corneum and also may have an antipruritic effect.

Notwithstanding the knowledge that has resulted from the use of many of these small mammals in the laboratory, there is much to be learned about the clinical dermatoses which affect them. All basic investigative techniques applied to dogs and cats are applicable and they should be employed in an attempt to arrive at a definitive diagnosis if at all possible. Histopathological examination of punch biopsy specimens may be indicated if the diagnosis is inconclusive or there is no response to what is considered an appropriate treatment.

APPROACH TO THE CASE

A full clinical history should be taken, although in some cases all that is available is the age, the presenting complaint and its duration. The age of the animal may suggest a likely diagnosis since dermatophytosis is commonly found in young rabbits (*Oryctolagus cuniculus*) whereas mycosis fungoides appears to be a disease of elderly Syrian hamsters (Harvey *et al*, 1992). The position of the cage in the house may be important since local environmental conditions may play a part in the pathogenesis of some dermatoses. For example ringtail in rats and mice is often associated with a low relative humidity (usually less than 40%) in concert with high temperatures and other conditions. It is especially seen in young animals where it causes one or more annular constrictions of the tail (hence "ringtail"). These subsequently interfere with the blood supply to the distal tail leading to swelling and in some case to dry gangrene which may result in sloughing of the distal part of the tail.

The majority of cases of alopecia and pruritus in small mammals are due to ectoparasites and an attempt must be made to establish whether they are involved in the case in question by careful visual examination and the use of tape strips and skin scrapings. With the exception of rabbits and guinea pigs most small mammalian pets are kept alone and this should make the occurrence of contagious dermatoses unlikely. In colonies of animals such as rabbits, guinea pigs and mice the phenomenon of latency may be encountered with *Cheyletiella parasitivorax* , *Trixacarus caviae* and the murine mange mites respectively. With latency, exceedingly small numbers of parasites remain on the host but do not cause clinical signs of disease until conditions become favourable to the parasite and they then multiply. Typical factors which might precipitate clinical disease might be intercurrent disease, population stress or poor nutritional status of the host. These stresses may also predispose to parasitic disease in other animals, for example demodectic mange in hamsters. In these individuals remission may often be obtained by correcting the underlying factors instead of instituting aggressive antiparasitic therapy.

Definitive diagnosis is hampered in cases where parasites are present only in small numbers as in mycoptic mange and some cases of trixacarid mange. The diagnosis of mycoptic mange in a mouse, for example, is further complicated because handling and adequate restraint of such very small mammals may be difficult. There is a real risk of cutting the skin if a skin scraping is taken with a scalpel blade in the normal method without sedation. In the case of gerbils (*Meriones unguiculatus*), hamsters and mice, all of which have very mobile skin, it is preferable to pull a fold of skin over the tip of the index finger with the thumb to support and tense the skin before taking a scraping. The use of tape strips and direct examination of the skin with a hand-lens or binocular loupe are useful alternative methods that may be employed. This is particularly so in mice (where demodectic mites are unlikely to be in the differential diagnosis) because the usual pathogens are the relatively large fur mites that are easily seen with a hand lens. Sedation may also be used to immobilise these often fast moving mammals in order to carry out a full clinical examination and take samples. The use of ketamine, detomidine or fentanyl/fluanisone has proved useful and at the low dosages required for sedation they are very safe.

PHYSICAL EXAMINATION

The initial examination of rats (*Rattus* spp.), mice, hamsters and gerbils is often best achieved by observing them in the cage to assess their attitude, behaviour and general condition. The cage, any furniture within the cage and the bedding should be assessed for cleanliness and examined for their potential to cause abrasions or damage. Some cases of nasal dermatitis in gerbils have been attributed to environmental abrasion; for example, if they are kept in a cage as opposed to a gerbilarium they will gnaw on the bars and the continual rubbing of the nose on the bar above the one which they are gnawing results in the lesion. The problem is rarely seen in gerbils kept in a gerbilarium where they have the opportunity to burrow. *Staphylococcus xylosus* has been implicated in some outbreaks of nasal dermatitis in gerbils but is likely to be an opportunist pathogen. A number of other staphylococci have also been isolated from gerbils (Solomon *et al*, 1990). It has also been suggested that accumulation of harderian gland secretions around the nasal and facial area may lead to the development of the dermatitis. In some cases the surgical removal of the harderian gland eliminates the condition. Another problem attributed to housing is the alopecia over the flank glands of elderly Syrian hamsters. These scent glands are used for marking territorial boundaries and alopecia may develop over them as a result of rubbing the flank against the cage. Sore hocks and pododermatitis in rabbits and guinea pigs are usually due to inadequate flooring. This is typically found to be damp, hard or rough with inadequate bedding and poor hygiene.

In those species where malocclusion is common, particularly the guinea pig and rabbit, then the teeth should routinely be examined. In severe cases of malocclusion there may be chronic dermatitis on the skin adjacent to the lips owing to ptyalism ("slobbers"). This hypersalivation will often predispose toward secondary bacterial infection and it is not uncommon for *Pseudomonas* spp. or *Staphylococcus* spp. to be associated with the moist dermatitis, particularly in rabbits. In the guinea pig hypovitaminosis C may result, producing inappetance and a dull coat with the formation of scurf and scale. In addition, even marginal hypovitaminosis C is one of the stress factors which may precipitate clinical *Trixacarus caviae* infestation.

The distribution and nature of the lesions may be helpful in suggesting a diagnosis. Thus, foul smelling exudative lesions accompanied by matted hair around the perineum of a rabbit are indicative of myiasis. The first instar larvae are very small and may easily be missed unless the region is clipped and carefully examined. Dermatophytosis in young rabbits typically affects the face or feet whereas in guinea pigs it commonly progresses from the face to the trunk. In mice and guinea pigs the typical lesions of mange are self-excoriations to the neck and scapular region.

The presence and distribution of alopecia and the nature of any surface scale should be noted as they may be helpful in making a diagnosis. Scale is frequently found in cases of cheyletiellosis in rabbits where large, soft flakes are typically found in the interscapular region and along the dorsum. In hamsters and gerbils demodectic mange is a common cause of non-pruritic alopecia, predominantly of the rump and back, and is often accompanied by a very fine scale. In guinea pigs scale may be a feature of either *Trichophyton mentagrophytes* infection or *Trixacarus caviae* infestation. *Psoroptes cuniculi* infestation will cause gross accumulation of brown scale in the external ear canal of rabbits. In ferrets (*Muscadae* spp.) and mink (*Putorius* spp.), *Otodectes cynotis* is the principle ear mite found and clinical signs are similar to those seen in the dog and cat, ie. an accumulation of brown or dark brown wax in the external ear canal and often self excoriation around the neck and ears.

ESTABLISHING THE DIAGNOSIS

Some conditions such as ptyalism, dermatitis secondary to *Pasteurella multocida* or *Mycoplasma pulmonis* conjunctivitis, pododermatitis and sore hocks are easily recognised and treatment should be directed to the underlying cause. Other conditions such as nasal dermatitis in gerbils, barbering in gerbils and guinea pigs and ringtail in rats and mice are more problematic. They are multifactorial and although the clinical signs are easily recognised the underlying aetiology is often hard to identify.

The common parasites of each species considered in this chapter are listed in Table 2 and, as with the dog and cat there are a number of techniques available for making a diagnosis. Careful examination of skin scrapings taken from affected areas is the only method by which demodicosis in hamsters and gerbils is likely to be recognised. These parasites are elongated in shape, as in the dog, but the hamster is host to two species; a short, blunt, surface inhabitant (*D. criceti*) and an elongated follicular variant (*D. aurati*). *Demodex cuniculi* may be found when taking skin scrapings from a rabbit but it is not usually associated with clinical signs (Harvey, 1990). Examination of skin scrapings is the ideal method of diagnosing *Cheyletiella parasitivorax* and *Trixacarus caviae* infestation. In the case of *Trixacarus caviae* it is advisable to scrape areas without self trauma or gross accumulations of thick scale. Scrapings from the external ear canal will confirm the presence of *Psoroptes cuniculi* or *Otodectes cynotis*, usually with little difficulty. However it can prove very difficult to confirm a tentative diagnosis of mange in mice where the relatively large fur mites are often highly mobile. It is frequently easier to examine sellotape strips or utilise a hand lens, or other form of magnification, in order to detect these parasites. Ideal sites to examine are the periorbital areas and the neck. Tape strips are also the easiest way to recover *Gliricola porcelli* and *Gyropus ovalis* from guinea pigs or *Listrophorous gibbus* from the rabbit. These last three parasites are usually regarded as non-pathogenic but they may be a cause of pruritus and in the rabbit *Listrophorous gibbus* may be associated with scale formation.

Dermatophytosis in young rabbits is often suspected from the appearance and distribution of the lesions and the age of the animal whereas in the guinea pig the lesions can be mistaken for those caused by *Trixacarus caviae* with erythema, alopecia, scale and crust being present. If a guinea pig does not rapidly respond to treatment for *Trixacarus caviae* then dermatophytosis should be considered. The commonest isolate from small mammals is *Trichophyton mentagrophytes* although other isolates may be encountered. For example *Microsporum gypseum, M. canis, M. adouini and T. schoenleini* have been isolated from rabbits with dermatophytosis. *Cryptococcus neoformis* (a monomorphic yeast) has been reported as causing cutaneous lesions in guinea pigs similar to those caused by trixacarid mange (van Herck *et al*, 1988).

Endocrine alopecia may be seen in some small mammals, particularly the ferret. Jills are induced ovulators requiring the stimulus of coitus in order to ovulate and end oestrus. The prolonged oestrus and resulting hyperoestrogenaemia can result in a number of clinical problems. Aplastic anaemia is caused by oestrogen induced bone marrow suppression but the high concentrations of oestrogen can also cause hair loss, anorexia and lethargy. The alopecia is very marked, being bilateral and often very extensive (Parrot and Parrot, 1986). Treatment with proligestone has proved successful. Ovarohysterectomy or the introduction of a vasectomised hob may be alternative solutions. Other causes of bilaterally symmetrical alopecia in the ferret include hyperadrenocorticism and telogen defluxion (Scott *et al*, 1992).

Alopecia under the dewlap may occur in rabbits, often associated with the nesting behaviour of pregnancy or false-pregnancy. The alopecia is apparent several days prior to parturition and is due to the female pulling hair in order to line her nest. A similar alopecia may be seen in intensively bred guinea pigs approaching parturition. The loss of hair is particularly noticed in the lumbosacral region and continues until the litter is weaned. If pregnancy occurs at the post-partum heat then the alopecia becomes more pronounced.

INITIAL MANAGEMENT

In those species where dermatophytosis is common, particularly the rabbit and guinea pig, then fungal culture should be considered at an early stage since zoonotic lesions are a possibility. Topical antifungal agents such as enilconazole and systemic drugs such as griseofulvin and ketoconazole may be used. For details see Chapter 30.

If ectoparasites are diagnosed then specific treatment is indicated. Ivermectin is the most widely used treatment for ectoparasite infestations in small mammals but it's use is not without problems. Great care must be taken when injecting mice with ivermectin since ulcers may develop at the site of an injection. Transient discomfort at the site of injection occurs in about 10% of rabbits. It should be borne in mind that since ivermectin is distributed systemically it has no effect on parasites if they are in the local environment and only a variable effect on ectoparasites that chew epithelial debris (as opposed to those which suck tissue fluids). Thus ivermectin should be effective in infestations with *Polyplax* spp., *Trixacarus caviae* and it is also curative in cases of *Psoroptes cuniculi* infestation in rabbits (Kurtis and Brooks, 1990). However, infestations due to *Cheyletiella* spp. and the mouse mites *Myocoptes musculinus* and *Myobia musculi* can be very difficult to eradicate, particularly in a colony situation. (Editor's note – Ivermectin is not licensed for use in small mammals in the UK). The reported efficacy of dichlovos strips in the management of mange in mice (Wiesbroth *et al*, 1976) is perhaps explained in terms of its effect on mites in the environment as well as those on the body surface.

Given that shampooing of very small creatures such as mice is difficult, it is often overlooked that shampooing larger animals such as guinea pigs is not only possible but is desirable. Specific topical therapy with enilconazole or gamma benzene hexachloride may eliminate the cause of the dermatosis and be curative but the principles of topical supportive therapy can also be applied. The use of a topical keratolytic shampoos such as tar, sulphur and salicylic acid will remove crust, scale and exudate caused by *Triaxacarus caviae* and provide some relief from the pruritus.

If these techniques fail to elucidate the aetiology or provide an empirical cure then biopsy should be considered. This is particularly important in the Syrian hamster where cutaneous neoplasia (mycosis fungoides) maybe a cause of pruritic alopecia. Taking a 4mm punch biopsy is easily achieved with local analgesia and gentle manual restraint or sedation and may help to provide a diagnosis or at least to rule out other disorders.

REFERENCES

FRIEDMAN, S. and WEISBROTH, S.H. (1975). The parasitic ecology of the rodent mite *Myobia musculi*. II. Genetic factors. *Laboratory Animal Science* **25,** 440.

HARVEY, R.G. (1990). *Demodex cuniculi* in dwarf rabbits (*Oryctolagus cuniculi*). *Journal of Small Animal Practice* **31**, 204.

HARVEY, R.G., WHITBREAD, T.J., FERRER, L. and COOPER, J.E.C. (1992). Epidermotropic T-cell lymphoma (mycosis fungoides) in Syrian hamsters (*Mesocricetus auratus*). A report of six cases and the demonstration of T-cell specificity. *Veterinary Dermatology* **3**, 13.

KURTIS, S.K. and BROOKS, D.L. (1990). Eradication of ear mites from naturally infested conventional research rabbits using ivermectin. *Laboratory Animal Science* **40**, 406.

PARROT, T. and PARROT, J. (1986). Estrogen-induced pancytopenia in a female European ferret. In: *Current Veterinary Therapy IX, Small Animal Practice* (Ed. R.W. Kirk). W.B. Saunders, Philadelphia.

SCOTT, D.W., HARVEY, H.J. and YEAGER, A.E. (1992). Bilaterally symmetric alopecia associated with an adrenocortical adenoma in a pet ferret. *Veterinary Dermatology* **2**, 165.

SIKARSKIE, J. G. (1986). The Use of Ivermectin in Birds, reptiles, and small mammals. In: *Current Veterinary Therapy IX, Small Animal Practice* (Ed. R. W. Kirk). W.B.Saunders, Philadelphia.

SOLOMON, H.F., DIXON, D.M. and POUCH, W. (1990). A survey of staphylococci isolated from the laboratory gerbil. *Laboratory Animal Science* **40**, 316.

VAN HERCK, H., VAN DEN INGH, Th.S.G.A.M., VAN DER HAGE, M.H. and ZWART, P. (1988). Dermal cryptococcosis in a guinea pig. *Laboratory Animal Science* **22**, 88.

WEISBROTH, S.H., FRIEDMAN, S. and SCHER, S. (1976). The parasitic ecology of the rodent mite, *Myobia musculi*. III. Lesions in certain host strains. *Laboratory Animal Science* **26**, 725.

FURTHER READING

COLLINS, B.R. (1987). Dermatological disorders of common small non-domestic animals. In: *Dermatology* (Ed. G.H. Nesbitt). Churchill Livingstone, New York.

DORRESTEIN, G.M. and VAN BRONSWIJK, J.E.M.H. (1979). *Trixacarus caviae* as a cause of mange in guinea pigs and papular dermatitis on man. *Veterinary Parasitology* **5**, 389.

FOX, J.G., COHEN, B.J., LOEW, F.M. (Eds.) (1984). *Laboratory Animal Medicine*. Academic Press, Orlando.

THORSON, T.E. (1983). Skin disorders of non-domesticated carnivores. In: *Current Veterinary Therapy VIII, Small Animal Practice* (Ed. R.W. Kirk). W.B. Saunders, Philadelphia.

CHAPTER TWENTY ONE

FEATHER LOSS IN BIRDS

Martin P C Lawton

INTRODUCTION

One characteristic of the class Aves is that all its members have feathers. Feathers are important for insulation, water repulsion, protection and more importantly, aiding flight.

Feathers vary at different sites of the body. Over the head, trunk and limbs they are known as general feathers, while those found over the wings and tail are flight feathers.

The feather emerges from the skin as a calamus or quill. The shaft (or rachis) is the main body of the feather. Fine branches (barbs) arise from the shaft at 45° on either side and from these barbs arise smaller branches (barbules) at an angle of 45°. Flight feather barbules are locked together by small hooks resulting in the flat but firm feather. If the barbules are not locked together then the feather will appear as a "fluffy" feather. Down powder is produced by disintegration of the tips of the powder down feathers. This powder helps to make the rest of the feathers waterproof and also helps to lubricate them.

Preening by the bird is essential for the general cleaning and protection of all the feathers as well as re-engaging any unhooked barbules to restore the normal conformation.

The growth and development of feathers are affected by light and hormones causing periodic shedding (moulting), so that new feathers (pin feathers) can grow from the feather follicle, initially in a keratin sheath with a neovascular ring. Eventually the blood vessels die back, leaving a sheath around the feather. As part of the natural grooming the bird breaks down this sheath (desheathing) to release the feather.

The plane of nutrition of the bird is important in the development of all feathers. On lower planes of nutrition, or if the bird is ill, the developing feather is affected and often there are lines running through it (fret lines). These are caused by disruption of the epidermal collar possibly due to release of natural corticosteroids during times of prolonged stress. Up to 85% of pet psittacines have deficient diets, which often result in poor feather quality.

APPROACH TO THE CASE

Feather loss is one of the most common reasons for pet birds (especially psittacines) to be presented to the veterinary surgeon (Plates 74-79). As far as possible, it is advisable for the owner to bring the pet bird in its own cage. The veterinary receptionist should always advise the owner not to clean out the cage, and particularly not to remove any feathers that may be present.

Before undertaking the physical examination of the bird or any feathers that may be in the cage, it is important to obtain a full clinical history (Table 1). Enquiries should be made as to how long the bird has been owned, whether or not it is an aviary bird or a sole pet bird (this may suggest whether or not parasitic infections are a possible cause). Other points to consider are whether the owners have recently moved (stress) and whether they are spending more or less time with the bird (stress/neurosis). The type of diet provided should be established (nutritional problems) and self remedies that have been used on the bird before presentation to the veterinary surgeon listed. It is also important to establish when the bird last moulted, and the frequency with which this occurs. It should also be established in what room the bird is kept, and approximately how many hours of light (natural and artificial) it is actually exposed to per day. The length of time that the bird has been losing feathers is important, there are some moulting abnormalities which occur where birds are exposed to long periods of light (14-18 hours per day if kept in the living room) which can cause prolonged and almost continuous moult.

The cage should be examined, particularly if there are feathers on the bottom. Check to see whether they appear normal, chewed, deformed or discoloured. Examine the cage for signs of blood, to see whether or not the bird has been chewing through or damaged any pin (blood) feathers.

Table 1
Bald Bird Examination

1. CLINICAL HISTORY

    a) When purchased?
    b) Other birds?
    c) When feather loss started?
    d) What diet?
    e) Where kept?
    f) What toys provided?
    g) Owners occupation and length of time left alone.

2. FEATHERS IN CAGE

    a) Signs of damage
        I.   Self-inflicted damage
        II.   Poor feather quality
        III. Presence of fret lines
        IV.   Barbules interlocked
        V.   New or old feather

    b) Healthy feather
        I.   Microscopy
        II.   Histopathology.

3. CLINICAL EXAMINATION

    a) Over whole of body
        I.   Consider and rule out parasitic causes
        II.   Consider and rule out folliculitis
        III. Consider and rule out viral causes
        IV.   Consider and rule out other birds feather plucking
        V.   Consider and rule out Dermatophytes
        VI.   Check for follicular activity
              1) If present whether pin feathers are normal
              2) No follicular activity - consider hypothyroidism

    b) Contour feathers loss but head normal
        I.   Go through list as per generalised feather loss
        II.   Consider neurosis.

PHYSICAL EXAMINATION

All birds should be examined; some such as psittacines, raptors and owls need to be examined with care, as their beaks and/or talons can do damage to the inexperienced handler. Even the most fractious bird may be examined easily by sedating with ketamine (5-20 mg/kg). Sedation is also useful for taking samples for laboratory investigation.

At the time of examination, establish whether or not the feather loss is throughout the body, or is located to certain areas. In particular, try to determine or establish whether there is any feather loss from the head, (often birds suffering neurosis will chew or pluck feathers from their bodies, wings, tail and legs, but cannot reach their head). In parasitic infestations, dermatophytes (rare) and dermatitis, the feather loss is more generalised and often involves the head as well.

Dermatophytes (mainly *Miscrosporum gallinae*) can affect fowl (Galliformes), ducks (Anseriforms), pigeons (Columbiforms) and turkeys (Galliformes), but are very rare. Lesions are limited to fleshy or thin skinned areas of the head and are seen as scabs, crust or alopecia. *Candida albicanas* can cause similar lesions. Microscopical examination of skin scrapings gives a definitive diagnosis.

The areas which are showing signs of feather loss must be carefully examined for signs of damage or deformity to the remaining feathers. Signs of trauma to the feathers or the skin are often associated with neurosis and self-inflicted mutilation. However, deformation of the feathers can be associated with viral infection or nutritional problems. Where there is damage to the skin this should be assessed as to whether it is self-inflicted or due to parasitic or infectious causes. Sometimes cage mates may be pecking at a submissive companion bird.

At the time of clinical examination samples should be taken. If parasitic infection is considered (or needs to be ruled out) then feathers from the cage are examined under the microscope, together with one or two fresh feathers plucked direct from the bird.

Biopsy samples are often helpful and should always be full thickness and include one or two feather follicles. Although routine H & E staining, and light microscopical examination is helpful, electron microscopy is invaluable for diagnosing viral causes (Psittacine Feather and Beak Disease).

At the time of examination check for the presence of new growing feathers. If they are present, then it is unlikely that a hormonal disturbance is the cause of the feather loss. New growing feathers show that the normal feather growth cycle is active following feather loss or moults.

ESTABLISHING THE DIAGNOSIS

It is often possible to establish a definitive diagnosis after taking the case history and making the clinical examination. If the bird is showing classic self-inflicted trauma, with the presence of perfect feathers on the head, while there is loss over the body, then it is nearly always a behavioural problem. However, owners are often convinced that their bird is not suffering from such a problem, but has a parasitic infestation; this should always be ruled out by routine microscopy, examination of the bird and environment. A bird which is failing to have a normal moult (growth cycle) can be identified by the condition of the feathers. The retained feathers become dull, dirty and often of ragged asymmetrical appearance, there is also a lack of pin feathers. Often feathers are missing, these have been moulted and not yet replaced. This may be associated with hypothyroidism and although blood samples may be taken they are often difficult to interpret.

Generalised feather loss with deformed feathers in psittacine birds (especially Cockatoos [*Cacatua* spp.]) which also involves the head, should always make one suspicious of the polyomavirus associated with Psittacine Feather and Beak Disease (PFBD). Diagnosis is a specialised technique and requires electron microscopy of a plucked feather. It is important that epithelial tissue remains attached to the feather follicle. Definitive diagnosis is based on the demonstration of the viral internuclear inclusion bodies measuring approximately 17-23 nm.

The parasite *Cnemidocoptes piliae* produces classic hyperkeratosis of the skin and excessive scaliness, usually around the beak and eyes or legs and feet, and results in substantial feather loss. Passerines may be infested with *Cnemidocoptes mutans* or *Cnemidocoptes jamaicensis*.

C. laevis is the depluming mite of parrots (especially Macaws [*Ara* spp.]). This mite is found within the feather follicle. Quill mites (*Csyringophilus bipectinatus* and *Dermoglyphys elongatus*) destroy feathers early in development by entering the feather shaft. They may also cause dermal cysts. The mites are easily seen as they are quite large, living on the bird, their eggs being deposited along the feather shaft. Although definitive diagnosis can be made on a biopsy (a scraping is often unrewarding as it is difficult to actually demonstrate the mite), a final diagnosis is often made retrospectively on response to treatment. *C. piliae* spends its life cycle of 3 weeks in the skin of the host. There is often a carrier state which produces clinical signs during times of stress such as poor nutrition, poor husbandry or infectious disease.

Dermanyssus gallinae is the red mite, which only feeds at night. During the day it is within the cage in recesses or even under droppings. Diagnosis during the day requires very careful examination of the cage. Nocturnal examination of the bird may demonstrate the mite. Even without seeing the mite, there is often signs of pruritus and restlessness in the bird.

Bacterial skin infection or folliculitis is less common, however, it can be diagnosed on examination of biopsy specimens, or a Gram stain of the feather pulp.

INITIAL MANAGEMENT

Parasitic Disease

If a red mite (*Dermanyssus gallinae*) infection is the cause (usually in a aviary situation) then the environment has to be treated as these mites tend to live off the bird in the aviary or cage. Treatment of the environment with Vapona (Dichlorovos; Shell) for 3 days, repeating each 2 weeks usually eliminates the mites.

Cnemidocoptes spp. are now easily treated by the use of ivermectin injection (200 mcg/kg) although repeated doses on a fortnightly basis may be required (Ed. note – This drug is not licenced for use in birds in the UK). The use of benzyl benzoate is now not recommended as firstly, it does not penetrate the thickened skin to the mite and secondly, it is toxic.

Endocrine Disease

Cases of true hypothyroidism, where there is a failure to moult, may be treated with thyroxine 0.025mg daily; this usually causes the bird to moult within 30 days of treatment. Thyroxine therapy should be continued until the bird has moulted out. Continued therapy with thyroxine (as in the norm in mammals) can cause continuous moulting.

Viral Disease

Psittacine Feather and Beak Disease (PFBD). Previously considered to be due to a parvovirus or papovavirus-like organism, but it is now thought to be caused by a polyomavirus. The treatment is supportive, to make the bird comfortable. Unfortunately, there is no cure for this disease. There is also evidence to support a vertical transmission to offspring, via the egg. In contact birds can be screened to see whether or not they are likely to develop the disease by electron microscopy of a biopsy sample. In the USA there is a DNA probe for the detection of PFBD in blood samples or swabs of the environment (Avian Research Associates Laboratory, Milford). There has also been some reported success of the use of autogenous vaccines in affected birds, although this author has had no such success with this technique. The outcome will depend on which species of bird is actually affected. It is usually fatal in cockatoos (*Cacatua* spp.) (in which it was first reported) and parakeets (*Agapornis* spp.). In budgerigars (*Melopsittacus undulatus*) it is rarely fatal, just interfering with ability to fly. Affected birds are often referred to as "creepers" or "crawlers" to reflect their mode of transport. Although PFBD has been reported in other psittacine birds, it usually has a lower mortality than in cockatoos.

Bacterial Disease

Bacterial dermatitis or folliculitis can be treated with an appropriate antibiotic (such as cephalexin 10 mg/kg orally tid or doxycycline 10 mg/kg PO sid).

Behavioural Problems

Neurosis and other behavioural problems result in feather chewing or feather plucking and are the most difficult feather loss conditions to manage. Initially, if the cause of the neurosis is established, appropriate measures should be taken in order to eliminate it. Often there are many factors involved in the original neurosis. If the bird has been recently moved from a site in which it was previously happy, then it should be moved back. This is less easy if the owners have recently moved house or flat. Birds being within sight or sound of other birds but not having contact with them may also be a causal factor. Sometimes the introduction of another bird will stop the vice, at other times it may cause the new bird to learn the vice and the result will be two feather plucking birds.

In all cases it is a good idea to advise the owner to allow the bird to have access to water, and either to have regular baths or be sprayed on a daily basis. This is particularly important for African gray parrots (*Psittacus erithacus*) that tend to produce a large amount of down powder, and are therefore prone to developing an irritant dermatitis which results in over grooming which may become excessive, and later on may develop into feather plucking.

Nervous birds should be provided with some sort of "hide" and if necessary be given a "quiet time" during some stage of the day. Birds that are left alone for long hours during the day, should either have the radio or television left on to give them company, or be given new toys on a regular basis; older toys should be removed at the same time. In this way a new stimulus for them to play with or explore is provided. Change feeding regimes to make the bird work for its food by (a) not giving *ad libitum* food and (b) adding stones or marbles (too big to be eaten) will make the bird hunt for food leaving less time for feather plucking.

If more than 12 hours of daylight (including artificial light) are provided, then it is advisable to reduce this to about 12 hours of light, 12 hours of darkness.

The bird that is feather plucking in front of the owner for attention is more difficult to deal with. This involves convincing the owner that they must not rush up to the bird and scold it (or pay any other form of attention) when it plucks a feather, as this positively reinforces the behaviour by rewarding the bird for pulling out feathers, thus making the problem worse. It is good policy to develop a reward and punishment regime, punishment involves walking up to the bird (without speaking to it), and either covering it up with a very thick blanket or curtain, or putting it under the stairs, in a cupboard, or another darkened area. Initially do this for five minutes, on subsequent occasions gradually increase by a minute each time, up to a maximum of 15 minutes. Isolating the bird out of the client's "love", or putting it into a darkened area, is a big punishment, especially to the attention seeking bird.

If attempting to stop the feather plucking by the above methods fails, then it is possible to use medication, although the author rarely uses this option. The use of hormonal therapy with megoestrol acetate (2.5 mg/kg daily to start with) has been reported to be of value in some cases. Thyroxine (100 mcg/kg each 48 hrs for 2 weeks) can induce moulting. However, hypothyroidism usually presents as dyspnoea with change of voice and strange head posture well before any clinical signs associated with feathering is noted. The use of diazepam (at 5 mg/ml, 2 drops per 30mls drinking water) or phenobarbitone (0.3 mg/100g bid) has also been reported as helpful to control neurosis, although as in humans it is possible that this could cause long term harmful effects to the bird. The use of methyl prednisolone acetate (Depomedrone; Upjohn) has also been advocated.

If environmental and managemental methods do not improve the condition, this author favours the use of an Elizabethan collar to physically prevent the bird from chewing and plucking its feathers. Often this has to be left in place for at least 3-4 months (sometimes substantially longer). However, unless changes are made to the management and environment of the bird, and the neurosis controlled, then as soon as the collar is taken off the bird can revert to the previous vice.

FURTHER READING

ALTMAN, R.V. (1977). Parasitic diseases of caged birds. In: *Current Veterinary Therapy VI, Small Animal Practice* (Ed. R.W. Kirk). W.B. Saunders & Co., Philadelphia.

FUDGE, A.M. and HEIGHTS, C. (1987). Dermatological conditions seen in avian practice. *Californian Veterinarian* September/October 9-12.

GALVIN, C. (1983). The feather picking bird. In: *Current Veterinary Therapy VIII, Small Animal Practice* (Ed. R.W. Kirk). W.B. Saunders & Co., Philadelphia.

HARRISON, G.J. (1986). Disorders of integument. In: *Clinical Avian Medicine and Surgery* (Eds. G.J.Harrison and L.R. Harrison). W.B. Saunders & Co., Philadelphia.

JACOBSON, E.R. (1986). Cockatoo beak and feather disease syndrome. In: *Current Veterinary Therapy IX, Small Animal Practice* (Ed. R.W. Kirk). W.B. Saunders & Co., Philadelphia.

LAFEBER, T.J. (1977). Feather disorders of common cage birds. In: *Current Veterinary Therapy VI, Small Animal Practice* (Ed. R.W. Kirk). W.B. Saunders Co., Philadelphia.

LAWTON, M.P.C. (1988). Behavioural problems. In: *Manual of Parrots, Budgerigars and other Psittacine Birds* (Ed. C.J. Price). BSAVA, Cheltenham.

LAWTON, M.P.C. (1988). Nutritional diseases. In: *Manual of Parrots, Budgerigars and other Psittacine Birds* (Ed. C.J. Price). BSAVA, Cheltenham.

MCLELLAND, J. (1990). *A colour atlas of avian anatomy.* Wolfe Publishing Ltd., Aylesbury.

PERRY, R.A. (1987). Avian dermatology. In: *Companion Bird Medicine* (Ed. E.W. Burr). Iowa State University Press, Iowa.

RANDALL, C.J., LEES, S. and INGLIS, D.M. (1987). Papovavirus-like infection in budgerigars (*Melopsittacus undulatus*). *Avian Pathology* **16**, 623-633.

STEHLIK, M. (1987). Entomology. In: *Companion Bird Medicine* (Ed. E.W. Burr). Iowa State University Press, Iowa.

TURNER, W.T. (1988). Skin, feathers, beak, cere and uropygial gland. In: *Manual of Parrots, Budgerigars and other Psittacine Birds* (Ed. C.J. Price). BSAVA, Cheltenham.

CHAPTER TWENTY TWO

SKIN DISEASE IN REPTILES AND AMPHIBIA

Martin P C Lawton

INTRODUCTION

The species in the classes of Reptilia and Amphibia are known jointly as Herpetiles and, although they have much in common, similarity does not extend to their skin. In general, reptiles have thick scaly skin. Some species of reptiles either have an osseous dermal shell (Chelonia) or have dermal bone known as osteoderms (Crocodilians and some lizards), giving an even harder external exterior. Amphibians have thin, moist, permeable skin often covered with a layer of mucous. There are, however, a number of toads and a few adult salamanders that do not have moist slimy skin (Marcus, 1981).

Amphibians mainly live in damp terrestrial environments or are aquatic, therefore the skin, being thin and moist, plays a major part in gaseous exchange and electrolyte balance. The amphibian skin also has a number of glands. The two most important types are mucous glands which allow skin to be kept moist at most times and granular glands. The latter are responsible, in some species, for producing toxins as a means of defence to make them less attractive as prey. Some of these toxins can be highly dangerous, while others can be hallucinogenic (*Bufo* spp.). In toads, the granular glands are often concentrated in masses seen as "warts".

The openings to the granular glands of poison arrow frogs (*Phylobates* spp.) are dispersed among the opening of mucous glands, thus the two secretions are often mixed. The granular glands are most active when the amphibian is subject to stress, at which time *Phylobates terrabilis* produces a very potent nerve toxin (batrachotoxin) which can cause death by muscular and respiratory paralysis, and is thus of concern to owners of this species. However, it has been shown that *P. terrabilis* kept in captivity, after a time, have a reduced toxicity, and after several generations the toxicity actually decreases to be almost ineffective (Heselhaus, 1992). Two of the granular toxins (bufotoxins) produced by Bufo toads are bufotalin and bufogin, both of which resemble digitalis and affect the function of the heart (Noble, 1955). Some salamanders can produce toxins, such as samandarin, which although a weak alkaloid, can produce respiratory effects in dogs that eat them.

Reptilian skin usually lacks glandular tissue and is hard, although it varies in thickness. Scent glands are present in a number of families. Iguanidae tend to have femoral pores, which are especially advanced and developed in the males and located on the ventrocaudal aspects of the thighs. Crocodilians usually have scent glands located on the lower jaw and another pair located in the cloaca, in both sexes (musk glands). Dosonuchal glands are found in some snakes and appear to have chemosensory functions (Davies, 1981). Reptilian and amphibian skin are typical of vertebrates, consisting of outer epidermis derived from the embryonic ectoderm and the inner dermis derived from embryonic mesoderm. Reptiles have scales that vary in type and shape over different parts of the body. The scale pattern is often species specific and used in the classification and identification of reptiles (Marcus, 1981). In some species there is osseous dermal bone (Chelonia, Crocodilia and some lizards) and the keratinised epithelial tissue in Chelonia forms shields (or scutes) overlying the dermal bone.

The colouration of reptile and amphibian skin is usually determined by the interaction of four types of cells (iridocytes, guanophors, lipophores and melanophores). In some species (*Chamaeleo* spp.) nervous and humoral control over the melanophores allow an amoeboid increase or decrease in the cell size, which alters the colouration of the animal (Marcus, 1981).

Ecdysis

Reptilians and amphibians can shed their old epidermal layers, a process known as ecdysis (sloughing), as part of their normal physiology. This gives reptiles and amphibians a major advantage over other animals with dermatological conditions, in that in some cases it is possible for the veterinary surgeon to induce ecdysis to speed up healing and new healthy skin formation, thus eliminating some dermatological problems.

The sloughing cycle can be compared to the hair growth cycle in mammals, in that there are distinct resting, moulting/sloughing and growth stages. In reptiles, after the resting stage, there is a breakdown of tissue between the old and new generations of epithelial cells of the stratum germinatium. Leakage of lymphatic fluids containing enzymes between these two layers of epithelium further helps the break down process. In some reptiles (especially snakes) ecdysis occurs over the whole body, while in many lizards and Chelonia, it may occur piecemeal. Some species such as the leopard gecko (*Eublepharis macularius*) may not be seen to shed, as they eat sloughing skin. This ingested tissue plays an important part in digestive process, providing fibre and bacteria.

Ecdysis, although affected by the environmental temperature, nutrition and day/night length, tends to follow a set regime. In snakes, ecdysis lasts approximately two weeks (Frye, 1983). The start of the cycle is noted by a change in the colour of the spectacle (eyecap). This becomes dull and is referred to as "going opaque", although it is usually seen as a bluish hue. At the same time the snake usually refuses to eat until ecdysis is complete. The bluish discolouration of the spectacle is a temporary phenomenon due to the accumulation of fluid between the old and new spectacle layers, and usually diminishes as shedding approaches. Normally shedding occurs five days after the clearing of the spectacle. Herpetologists should be encouraged to keep records of these cycle lengths as this also aids in detecting whether any abnormalities (such as increased or decreased frequency) occur.

APPROACH TO THE CASE

Case History

A full case history should always be taken for any reptilian or amphibian case. This requires correct species identification. The suitability of diet, environment and preferred body temperature range, all vary depending on the species kept. The origins of the herpetile should be established, whether recently captured or captive bred. Recently imported species may have different endo- or ectoparasites than those encountered in captive bred species. It is not unusual for captured reptiles to be infested with ticks, both hard and soft bodied, whilst these are very rare in captive bred species (Cooper, 1992).

The other species kept may also be important, especially if they share the same vivaria/ terraria. Male lizards are very territorial and this may result in fighting and skin trauma. Organisms and parasites may not be equally pathogenic in all species. There may be a conflict in the environmental needs of the various species. Overcrowding may result in stress and predisposition to secondary bacterial infections or inadequate hygiene.

Environment

As far as possible it is important to try to see or be given information about the vivarium or terrarium within which the herpetile is housed. This allows assessment of the suitability of the environment for the species kept. The size of water bowls is an important consideration in the prevention of shedding problems. Dysecdysis is the term used to describe the inability to shed normally, this is most commonly encountered where the environmental needs are not met. The adequate provision of "furniture" assists ecdysis in snakes by allowing rubbing to shed the skin.

The material the vivarium or terrarium is constructed of may be unsuitable. An untreated wooded environment may predispose towards dermatitis due to difficulties in maintaining adequate hygiene. An all glass front may result in a snake continuously rubbing against this, resulting in damage to the nose and lips (rostral erosion). This may be prevented by painting the exterior bottom 3 inches of the glass black.

Temperature - Reptiles and Amphibia are ectothermic. They rely on external heat sources and behavioural means to regulate their core body temperature. All species have a preferred body temperature (PBT), at which their metabolism is optimum. To enable their PBT to be achieved, herpetiles must be kept within a correct temperature range (which varies between species), known as the preferred optimum temperature zone (POTZ) (Cooper and Lawton, 1992). If the POTZ is not provided, then the PBT is unlikely to be achieved. Herpetiles with a core body temperature below their PBT are more likely to have dermatological problems. Failure to maintain their PBT may result in decreased immunological competence and opportunist bacteria becoming pathogenic.

The environmental temperature of all herpetiles should be measured and recorded. Any abnormalities in the POTZ for the species kept, should be corrected. Incorrect environmental temperature should always be ruled out as a possible contributory factor for any dermatological problem.

The type of heat source provided may also directly or indirectly cause dermatological pathology. A light bulb can lead to skin damage by direct contact resulting in burns. This is more commonly seen in snakes, which may wrap themselves around the light bulb. Under floor heating may provide too much heat and predispose to ventral dermal necrosis in snakes, or shell rot in Chelonia.

Humidity - This should be correct for the species kept. Adequate humidity is essential for the successful keeping of Amphibia. A low humidity may cause dysecdysis in all herpetiles. Too high a humidity may cause blister disease in Squamata (the Order containing snakes and lizards).

Hygiene

The general standard of hygiene should be high. The frequency of cleaning the vivarium/terrarium will have a substantial influence on the prevention of bacterial dermatitis. The frequency of handling the herpetile will improve the early detection of potential problems, especially ventral lesions. Snakes kept under poor hygienic conditions and infrequently handled will be presented with a more advanced ventral dermal necrosis.

For aquatic species, establish how the water is cleaned. Inadequate filtration of the water will lead to a build up of harmful bacteria such as *Pseudomonas* spp. and *Aeromonas* spp. Skin and shell infections in aquatic species are nearly always related to water quality and bacterial contamination, as is septicaemia in Amphibia ("red leg"). Internal or external filters are usually required for herpetiles. These filters may be biological or mechanical. If the former are used then the therapeutic use of antibiotics may result in the bacteria being killed off and the filter no longer working. Under gravel filtration should be avoided for aquatic Chelonia as these species disturb the gravel and affect its working ability. Under gravel filtration may, however, be suitable for some Amphibia, depending on the volume of waste they produce.

4) Records

If the owner keeps records, these should be examined as they can indicate the normal frequency of the shedding cycles. A reduced shedding frequency may indicate inadequate temperatures, or possible endocrinological conditions. An increased shedding frequency may indicate too high an environmental temperature, iatrogenic hypervitaminosis A or endocrinological problem. A history of dysecdysis may indicate inadequate humidity, parasitism or general ill health.

PHYSICAL EXAMINATION

As for any other species, the physical examination of reptiles should be systematic. For the safe examination of potentially dangerous species, such as *Varanus* spp., Crocodilia, poisonous snakes or snapping turtles (*Chelydra serpentina*), it may be advisable to sedate the patient. The use of ketamine (10- 50 mg/kg, i/m or s/c) may be employed. It is always advisable to have an assistant to hold larger snakes (boids) and thus allow physical examination. Great care should be taken when handling Amphibia, because of their delicate skin. The use of gloves or a wet tea towel is advised, not only because it may absorb chemicals from the human hand, but also because some species excrete toxic or noxious substances,

Shed skin

Before examining the animal itself, wherever possible, examine any shed skin first. External parasites, especially mites, are more easily seen in sloughed skin than on the live animal. In snakes, the slough should be in one piece and not be piecemeal. A slough in several pieces indicates shedding problems.

Skin

On examining a reptile make sure that there is no retained skin, indicating problems with shedding (dysecdysis). Retained skin, especially in lizards and snakes, may cause a tourniquet effect around the digits or tail resulting in necrosis distal to the retained circle of skin. Areas of retained skin may also be found to harbour mites (Frye, 1983).

Trauma can result in splitting of the skin (partial autotomy) in lizards, as can handling of a snake at the time it is sloughing. Certain species (*Testudo* spp.) will bite at limbs as part of their courtship ritual, which can result in damage to the skin and secondary infection. Terrapins kept and fed together in a small tank may go into a feeding frenzy and snap and bite at each other resulting in trauma to the skin.

Shell

Hatchling and juvenile Chelonia should have a normal conformation of their shells with no "lumps or bumps" that may indicate a calcium deficiency. A "squeeze" test should be gently performed to evaluate the density of the dermal bone and to determine whether or not calcium deficiency is developing.

Cracking of the shields and necrosis of the underlying dermal bone may be associated with trauma. Chelonia may often have their shields and dermal shell damaged by falls, lawnmowers or attacks by dogs or other carnivores. Attempted hibernation under a bonfire may result in the shell being burned. Burnt shields will eventually be sloughed exposing a necrotic (white) dermal bone. The mating courtship ritual of *Testudo* spp., where the male repeatedly bashes into the females posterior carapace, causes trauma and eventually necrosis of the shields and possibly the underling dermal bone.

Petechiation

The skin of reptiles and Amphibia should be carefully checked for any discolouration especially of a pinkish or haemorrhagic nature. Infectious dermatoses may often be seen initially as petichiation followed by ecchymotic haemorrhages before becoming necrotic and ulcerative. Severe infectious dermatitis (such as unnoticed or neglected ventral dermal necrosis in snakes) may be of full skin thickness (Lawton, 1991). In Amphibia particular attention should be paid to the ventral abdomen and skin over the legs, where it is not uncommon to find petechiation in the skin associated with septicaemia (*Pseudomonas* spp. or *Aeromonas* spp.) which is referred to as "red-leg".

In Chelonia, petechiation under the shields is a sign of septicaemia or trauma. Fluid accumulation underneath the shields will also cause discolouration and is associated with active "shell rot". This should be investigated further, often requiring removal of the overlying shields (sometimes under anaesthesia). Sometimes the lesion may be deep enough to also involve the dermal bone. "Shell rot" is particularly noted on the ventral aspects (plastron) of red-ear terrapin (*Trachemys scripta elegans*) and tortoises (*Testudo* spp.).

Discolouration of the skin or shell is not only associated with bacterial infection; in aquatic species, algae may give a greenish, brown or even white tinge to the shell, scales or skin. A grey or white appearance of terrapin (*Trachemys scripta elegans*) shields are often associated with a retained shield and air between this and the underlying newer shield. This should not be considered pathological, and gentle brushing will often remove the retained shield. Retained shields are usually associated with poor environmental conditions. The terrapin that does not have a basking area to allow it to leave the water and dry out, will fail to displace the older shields. Fungal infections are often found in reptiles and Amphibia and usually cause granulation and severe inflammation.

Bruising and trauma may be noted in snakes if they are handled too roughly; this may even cause death some 7-10 days later from toxaemia due to muscle autolysis. Hospitalised Chelonia may be bruised or develop damaged skin around their neck and ears following repeated handling for stomach tubing or the treatment of stomatitis.

Blisters

Blisters may be found anywhere over the body. In lizards, such as water dragons (*Physignathus* spp.), they are more commonly found on the ventral surface. In snakes, such as garter snakes (*Thamnophis* spp.), European grass snakes (*Natrix natrix*) and dice snakes (*Natrix tesselata*), they are more frequently found on the lateral and ventral surfaces. Blisters may be associated with excessive environmental humidity, or in aquatic species, infected or poor quality water (Lawton, 1991). Bacterial or parasitic infections may also induce blisters. *Kalicephalus* spp., the hook worm, is often found to be involved in the pathogenesis of blisters in water snakes, due to percutaneous penetration which leads to inflammatory reaction or secondary bacterial infection.

Ulceration

Aquatic Chelonia are particularly prone to ulceration of the skin and shell. These ulcerations are often due to infections with Enterobacteriacae and other Gram negative bacterial infections associated with poor water quality. The soft shell terrapin (*Trionyx* spp.) is particularly prone to an ulcerative disease affecting the skin and shell, known as septicaemic cutaneous ulcerative disease (SCUD). SCUD is usually, but not always, associated with *Citrobacter frundeii*. In other aquatic species *Pseudomonas* spp., *Aeromonas* spp., *Proteus* spp., *Flavobacterium* spp. and *Proventia* spp. might also be associated with these lesions.

Any ulceration of scales or skin should be swabbed, ideally with a small paediatric or nasal swab, from the edge of the lesion for bacterial culture and sensitivity. Often skin scrapings or biopsies may also be taken to help establish a diagnosis. These can be submitted for histopathological examination, or for direct bacterial or fungal culture. Some samples, such as dermal bone, may need decalcification before examination is possible.

External parasites

Careful but systematic examination for ectoparasites should be undertaken. Magnification is advisable to look for mites and ticks, which often blend in well with the scales and for the inexperienced may be difficult to find. Often ectoparasites, such as the snake mite (*Ophionyssus natricis*) may show predisposition for particular sites. This parasite is often found in the region between the facial scales and the spectacle, within the orbital ridge. Ticks in Chelonia are found in the axillary and inguinal region. In some turtles, leeches may be found around the cloacal area.

Swellings

Cutaneous and subcutaneous swellings are not uncommonly found in reptiles. In the majority of cases these are related to abscesses. In lizards and Amphibia, where the swelling is near a limb, secondary pathological fractures or osteodystrophia fibrosa should be ruled out by radiography. Whitish nodules on aquatic Chelonia or Amphibia warrant further microscopical investigation, to establish wheather a bacterial or fungal infection is involved.

Tumours are uncommon. However, there are a number of viral diseases that may result in tumourous changes. Viral papillomata, in the European Green Lizard (*Lacerta viridis*) are found around the head in males and around the hind legs and tail in females. Viral grey patch disease or fibropapillomata in turtles (*Chelonia mydas*) causes raised plaques affecting the skin and shell. Pox virus in caiman (*Caiman crocodilus*) also causes skin lesions.

ESTABLISHING THE DIAGNOSIS

Physical examination and environment

Often a diagnosis may be established by physical examination alone. Where environmental temperatures and relative humidities are not known, the animal's keeper should be encouraged to record these. Dysecdysis is more likely to be associated with incorrect environmental temperature and humidity. Blisters may also be associated with high humidity. Without thermometers or hydrometers it may not be possible to establish wheather such environmental factors are involved.

Parasites

When external parasites are found identification should be attempted. However, the treatment is usually the same irrespective of the species of the parasite present, although some parasitic burdens (ticks, leeches and oral trematodes) may be self limiting due to improved hygiene or the lack of intermediate host. These parasites will not always require medical treatment.

Cytology

Skin lesions should initially have scrapings taken for cytological examination (stained with Gram stain and with a Romanowski type stain eg. Dif Quick) to establish whether there is bacterial or fungal involvement. Fungal infections are commonly found in aquatic Chelonia and Amphibia, where the mycelial strands are often identified on microscopical examination.

For skin blisters, fluid should be directly examined under a microscope for evidence of larvae that might be associated with percutaneous migration. A dried (or spun down sediment) sample when stained may show evidence of bacteria. In the case of Amphibia, a wet preparation of a scrape from a lesion, especially if around the cloaca, should be examined for evidence of protozoal flagyllates or ciliates.

Culture

Swabs for culture should be taken from the edge of the lesion. Where taking a swab would be difficult, fungal and bacterial culture can be performed by placing parts of shell (especially shields) directly onto the culture media.

Bacterial culture of specimens from amphibians and reptiles should be undertaken using slightly different methods to those applied to mammalian samples. Bacterial cultures should be incubated at 25°C and 37°C. Some bacteria may only grow at low incubation temperatures and after a minimum of 4 days. Mycobacteria which affect Amphibia (*M. ranae*, *M. zenopi* or *M. marinum*) are known as "cold water" mycobacteria and will only grow on appropriate media when incubated at 23°C (Anver and Pond, 1984). This is also true for many other pathogenic bacteria of ectothermic and poikilothermic species. These bacteria would be missed if the cultures were only incubated at 37°C. Microaerobic and anaerobic cultures are also helpful. Antibiotics to be tested for sensitivity should be chosen for the anticipated organisms.

Histopathology and electron microscopy

Histopathology and electron microscopy of skin and shell lesions often provides the definitive diagnosis. Keratin shields and dermal bone biopsies, may require oscillating saws and any samples should be decalcified before sections are cut. As a rule, any swelling or elevation of the skin or shell should be biopsied. Even biopsies from abscesses sometimes can prove useful. *Dermatophilus congolensis* is characterised by raised lesions and subcutaneous abscesses over the body (Cooper, 1992) and definitive diagnosis is made on histopathological examination. Similarly in Amphibia, subcutaneous nodules or ulcers may be associated with mycobacteriosis, chromomycosis, chromoblastomycosis as well as a variety of other bacterial or mucormycosis. Electron microscopy is especially useful in the diagnosis of suspected viral infections, such as green turtle fibropapilloma (GTFP) which is caused by a herpes virus (Norton *et al*, 1990) or pox in caiman (*Caiman crocodilus*).

INITIAL MANAGEMENT

Environment

The temperature and humidity should be adjusted to the appropriate levels for the species.

Dysecdysis

The old, retained skin, may be gently removed by rubbing, with firstly wet and then dry pieces of cotton wool. In most species rub in the direction of the scales, from rostrum to tail. In Squamata that have a spectacle (fused eyelids), establish whether this has already been shed. Retained spectacles may also be removed with gentle rubbing. Dysecdysis is often multifactorial but causes include the following: poor or imbalanced nutrition, dehydration, inappropriate humidity or temperature, infectious disease, parasitism, hormonal dysfunction, or trauma (Frye, 1983). Where the cause is established, this should be corrected to prevent recurrence. However, if the herpetile is scarred, then there is likely to be continuous problems with dysecdysis over this site.

Dermatitis

Infected skin lesions, whether they are bacterial or fungal, should be cleaned with an antiseptic solution such as povidone-iodine. However, the use of other topical preparations besides this will depend on the diagnosis. Bacterial infections are often Gram negative and respond well to topical applications of framycetin (Soframycin; Roussel), tobramycin (Tobralax; Alcon), or silver sulphadiazine (1% Flamazine; Smith & Nephew). In the case of fungal infections, clotrimazole (1% Canesten; Bayer) or other preparations may also be used. Where there is evidence of petichiation or ecchymotic haemorrhages and therefore septicaemia is suspected, systemic antibiotics should be prescribed. "Red-leg" in Amphibia is a systemic infection, and as such requires systemic antibiotics. It is advisable to administer these by injection rather than by immersing the amphibian into an antibiotic solution. Particular care has to be taken with tetracyclines as these can react with the water to make compounds that may be irritant to the skin.

In extensive cases of scale rot, ventral dermal necrosis or shell rot, some protective dressing may also be required. The use of Opsite (Smith & Nephew) has proved useful, particularly in Squamata. Following extensive damage to the skin, fluid therapy may also be required. Any breach of the skin may result in evaporation and fluid loss. Opsite dressing will limit the loss and prevent further contamination of the wound.

"Shell rot" should be treated initially by debridement of infected shields and if necessary dermal bone. Topical and systemic antibiotics, where appropriate, together with antiseptic povidone-iodine applications will often eliminate the problem. Once infection is totally eliminated, then the shell may be repaired if necessary (see "Shell damage").

Fungal infections in aquatic Chelonia and Amphibia can be treated topically with clotrimazole (1% Canesten; Bayer) which is useful particularly if they are semi-aquatic, and therefore can be kept out of water for a while. True aquatic Amphibia may be treated with malachite green or copper sulphate.

Shell damage

Following trauma, initial treatment should include a suitable topical antiseptic and systemic analgesics. Once bacterial infection and contamination have been eliminated, the damaged shell may be rebuilt with an appropriate epoxy resin or cynoacrylic. For aquatic species this may be made watertight with UHU glue or an aquarium sealant.

Parasites

External parasites may be successfully treated in some reptiles with ivermectin (200 ug/kg). The use of ivermectin is contraindicated in Chelonia, as it may cause paralysis or even death (Teare and Bush, 1983). The environment must also be treated to remove any residual parasites. The reptile should be injected with ivermectin and then placed into a clean hospital vivarium. The original vivarium should be treated with dichlorvos while empty (Vapona; Shell) impregnated strips, which should be left in the tank for a minimum of 28 days (the average life cycle of the mite). The reptile should be treated with ivermectin 28 days after the initial dose. At this time, it should be returned to its original, clean, vivarium. The hospital tank should be treated with dichlorvos for a minimum of 30 days. Unless the reptile is removed from its original vivarium which is then treated effectively, then it is unlikely that mites (especially *Ophionyssus natricis*) will be effectively eliminated. Treatment of the environment with dichlorvos while the reptile or amphibian is still present must be undertaken with care. This is particularly important in insectivores as this may result in their becoming intoxicated by eating insects that have themselves become poisoned with the dichlorvos.

(Editors note — Ivermectin is not licenced for use in Reptiles and Amphibia in the U.K.)

Viral infections

Attempts may be made to treat viral papillomata and pox by surgery, including radiosurgery or cryosurgery. This is often unsuccessful. Autogenous vaccines may be prepared and administered, although they are usually ineffective.

REFERENCES AND FURTHER READING

ANVER, M.R. and POND, C.L. (1984). Biology and diseases of amphibians. In: *Laboratory Animal Medicine* (Eds. J.G. Fox, B.J. Cohen and F.M. Loew). Academic Press, Orlando.

COOPER, J.E. (1992). Integument. In: *Manual of Reptiles* (Eds. P.H. Beynon, M.P.C. Lawton and J.E. Cooper). BSAVA, Cheltenham.

COOPER, J.E. AND LAWTON, M.P.C. (1992). Introduction. In: *Manual of Reptiles* (Eds. P.H. Beynon, M.P.C. Lawton and J.E. Cooper). BSAVA, Cheltenham.

DAVIES, P.M.C. (1981). Anatomy and physiology. In: *Disease of the Reptilia, Volume 1* (Eds. J.E. Cooper and O.F. Jackson). Academic Press, London.

FRYE, F.L. (1983). Epidermal shedding problems in reptiles. In: *Current Veterinary Therapy VIII, Small Animal Practice* (Ed. R.W. Kirk). W.B. Saunders Co., Philadelphia.

HESELHAUS, R. (1992). *Poison-arrow frogs, their natural history and care in captivity* (Translated by A. Mick). Blandford, London.

JACOBSON, E.R., GREINER, E.C., CLUBB, S. and HARVEY-CLARKE, C. (1986). Pustular dermatitis caused by subcutaneous Dracunculiasis in snakes. *Journal of American Veterinary Medical Association* **189** (9), 113-114.

LAWTON, M.P.C. (1991). Reptiles - Part 2. Lizards and Snakes. In: *Manual of Exotic Pets* (Eds. P.H. Beynon and J.E. Cooper). BSAVA, Cheltenham.

MARCUS, L.C. (1981). *Veterinary biology and medicine of captive amphibians and reptiles.* Lea & Febiger, Philadelphia.

NOBLE, G.K. (1955). *Biology of Amphibia.* Dover Publications, New York.

NORTON, T.M., JACOBSON, E.R. and SUNDBERG, J.P. (1990). Cutaneous fibropapillomas and renal myxofibroma in a green turtle, *Chelonia mydas. Journal of Wildlife Diseases* **26** (2), 265-270.

ROSSKOPH, W.J. (1986). Shell diseases in turtles and tortoises. In: *Current Veterinary Therapy IX, Small Animal Practice* (Ed. R.W. Kirk). W.B. Saunders Co., Philadelphia.

TEARE, J.A. and BUSH, M. (1983). Toxicity and efficacy of Ivermectin in Chelonians. *Journal of the American Veterinary Medical Association* **183**, 1195-1197.

WILLIAMS, D.L. (1991). Amphibians. In: *Manual of Exotic Pets* (Eds. P.H. Beynon and J.E. Cooper). BSAVA, Cheltenham.

Pododermatitis
(Chapter 17)

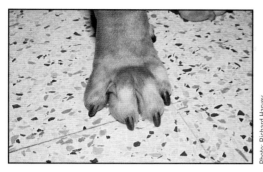

Photo: Richard Harvey

Plate 46
Demodectic pododermatitis

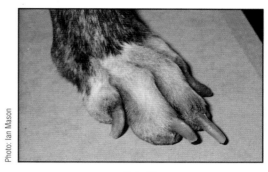

Photo: Ian Mason

Plate 47
Hookworm in a racing greyhound

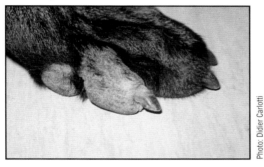

Photo: Didier Carlotti

Plate 48
Alopecia of a digit and proximal onychomycosis in a
labrador infected with *Microsporum canis*

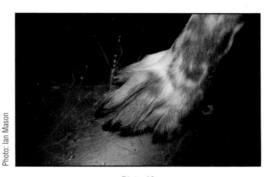

Photo: Ian Mason

Plate 49
Atopic dermatitis

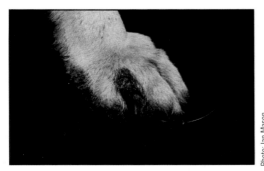

Photo: Ian Mason

Plate 50
Deep cellulitis of German shepherd dog

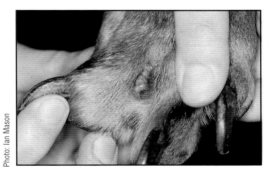

Photo: Ian Mason

Plate 51
Interdigital pyoderma

Disorders of pigmentation
(Chapter 19)

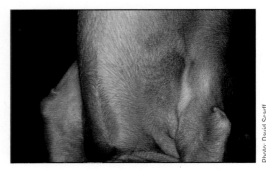

Photo: David Scarff

Plate 52
Miniature dachshund showing auxillary lichenification
and hyperpigmentation characteristic of primary
acanthosis nigricans

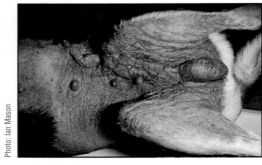

Photo: Ian Mason

Plate 53
Chronic inflammatory hyperpigmentation
due to superficial pyoderma

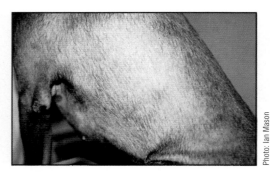

Photo: Ian Mason

Plate 54
Colour dilute alopecia in a blue doberman

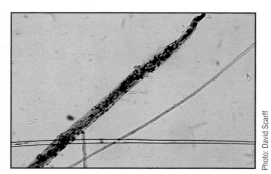

Photo: David Scarff

Plate 55
Hair from dog in plate 54.
Note macromelanosomes in the hair cortex

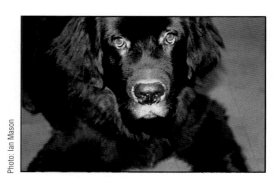

Photo: Ian Mason

Plate 56
Vitiligo

Nodular Skin Diseases
(Chapter 7)

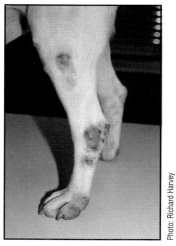

Photo: Richard Harvey

Plate 57
Deep (callus) pyoderma

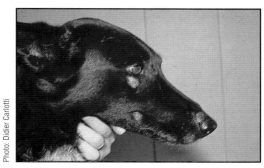

Photo: Didier Carlotti

Plate 58
Kerions of the face of a Belgian shepherd dog
infected with *Microsporum canis*

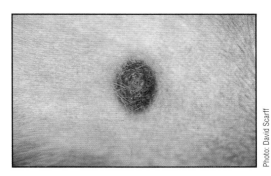

Photo: David Scarff

Plate 59
Canine Langerhans cell tumour on trunk of a crossbred dog

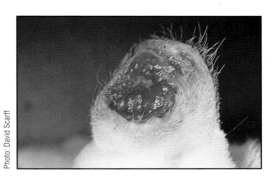

Photo: David Scarff

Plate 60
Squamous cell carcinoma on the pinna of a cat

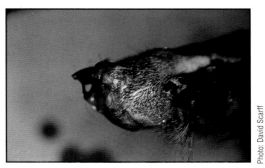

Photo: David Scarff

Plate 61
Squamous cell carcinoma on the digit
of a standard poodle

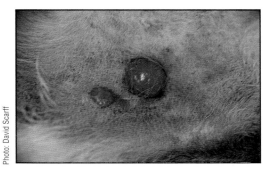

Photo: David Scarff

Plate 62
Mast cell tumour on the ventrum of a dog

Miscellaneous and unusual conditions

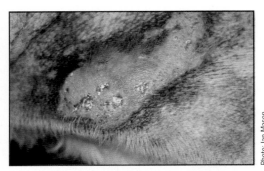

Photo: Ian Mason

Plate 63
Iatrogrenic hyperadrenocorticism.
Note calcium deposition in skin of ventral abdomen

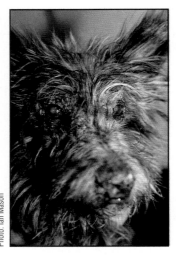

Photo: Ian Mason

Plate 64
Erythema multiforme

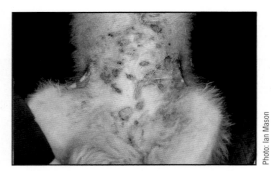

Photo: Ian Mason

Plate 65
Ulcerative dermatosis on a Shetland sheepdog

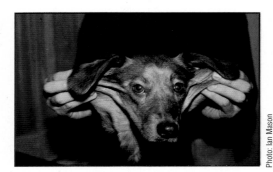

Photo: Ian Mason

Plate 66
Cutaneous asthenia
(Ehlers-Danlos syndrome, dermatosparaxis)

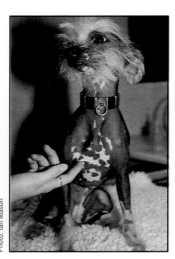

Photo: Ian Mason

Plate 67
Chinese crested dog - example of selective breeding
for a hitherto undesirable attribute

CHAPTER TWENTY THREE

SKIN DISEASE
IN ORNAMENTAL FISH

Ray L Butcher ———————————————

INTRODUCTION

The presentation of a piscine dermatosis initially may appear quite daunting to the veterinarian who is much more familiar with mammalian species. However, although there are differences, the application of the general principles of veterinary science and the adoption of a logical approach to the problem will often yield successful and rewarding results. Hopefully, this underlying consideration is highlighted throughout the following chapter.

Anatomy and physiology

The cuticle consists of sloughed cells and mucus secreted largely by the goblet cells of the epidermis (Fig. 1). It is approximately 1 μm in thickness, and its consistency varies with the species. The mucus generally contains specific immunoglobulins and lysozymes.

Figure 1
A diagrammatic section through the skin of a teleost fish

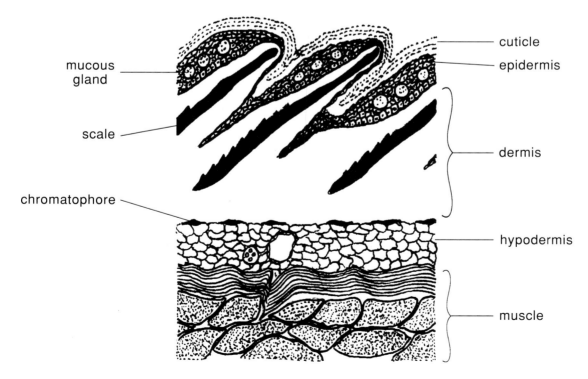

The epidermis is unlike that of mammals in that cells of all levels are living and capable of mitotic division. The thickness of the epidermal layer varies, being generally greater over the fins and in species without scales. A feature of the dermis in many species is the presence of scales. These are calcified, flexible plates that are situated in scale pockets within the dermis. These scales may be classed as ctenoid or cycloid, depending on the presence or absence of stiff spinous processes respectively. In many species, scales may show growth rings which can aid aging. The dermis may also contain specialised pigment containing cells called chromatophors, which are responsible for the colour changes seen in camouflage and sexual activity.

The skin forms a waterproof barrier which is an important part of the fish's ability to maintain it's fluid balance. Any skin lesion that causes disruption of this barrier can therefore severely impair the fish's homoeostasis. It is important to note that the scales are situated within the dermis, and hence any lesion involving loss of scales is not simply superficial. In order to repair this outer protective barrier as quickly as possible fish have developed a two phase healing process. Initially, there is a rapid epithelial covering made by migration of cells from the surrounding epithelium which results in a corresponding thinning of this layer in the surrounding skin. This is then followed by a slower, temperature dependant, reconstitution of the epithelial layer by mitotic division. The initial rapid migration of cells is inhibited by the presence of infectious organisms.

Intercurrent disease

The presence of a skin lesion may reflect some more generalised disease process, making a complete clinical examination essential in every case. Furthermore, it is well documented that many diseases, especially those caused by opportunist pathogens, only become apparent if the fish is weakened by intercurrent disease or by sub-optimal environmental factors (Snieszko, 1974). Most parasites can be regarded as normal if present in low numbers; it is only when a threshold number is reached, or another stress factor is present, that the disease is manifested. It cannot be over-stressed that any investigation of a fish problem should involve not only a full clinical examination of the fish, but also a complete appraisal of the environmental parameters such as water chemistry, stocking density, filtration etc (Butcher, 1992).

A PROBLEM ORIENTATED APPROACH TO SKIN LESIONS

An attempt has been made to group the skin diseases of ornamental fish in terms of the presenting signs. These are somewhat arbitrary and so some overlap is inevitable. The main groups are given in Table 1. Some common conditions are illustrated in Plates 86-91.

1. Grossly visible parasites/agents

Lernaea cyprinacea (the anchor worm) is a crustacean ectoparasite found on carp, although it is not host specific. It is more important in warm water and is unable to complete its life cycle below 15°C. The female anchor worm is attached to the host's body by means of a penetrating cephalic process, while the readily visible egg sacs trail in the water releasing eggs which hatch into nauplii. Even small numbers of parasites will cause serious damage to the host. As well as causing signs of generalised irritation (see below) the attachment sites are usually very inflamed, and may develop into granulomata with necrotic centres. These may be very slow to heal after removal of the parasite.

Argulus sp. (the fish louse) is another crustacean parasite, and in Europe it is generally associated with problems in freshwater fish. Unlike *Lernaea* sp., the female leaves the host to lay eggs on aquatic plants. These hatch to form free-living larvae which then find a new host to continue the life cycle, the whole process taking 40 to 100 days depending on the temperature. Egg production ceases below 16°C, and hibernation on the body of the host occurs below 8°C. The clinical signs are those typical of irritant skin disease (see below).

Piscicola sp. (fish leech) can be easily identified by the presence of large suckers. They may cause skin damage during feeding, and this may result in debility and predispose to secondary infection.

Table 1
Major presenting signs of skin disease in ornamental fish

1. Grossly visible parasites/agents

Lernaea cyprinacea (anchor worm)
Argulus sp. (fish louse)
Piscicola sp. (fish leech)
Philometra sp.(blood worm)

Fungi
Myxobacteria

2. Irritant skin lesions

3. Nodular lesions

Parasitic
Fungal
Bacterial
Viral
Neoplastic

4. Ulcerative/erosive lesions

Septicaemias/viraemias
Acute superficial bacterial disease
Myxobacterial disease
Parasitic
Fungal
Rupture of nodular lesions
Physical factors

5. Colour Changes

Generalised
Localised

6. Texture Changes

Raising of the scales
Roughening of the skin
Slime disease

An uncommon parasite, that can be seen with the naked eye, is *Philometra* sp. (blood worm). These are thin, red nematode worms up to 16 cm in length. The adult females generally migrate to the surface of the skin and the fins and protrude the posterior part of their body through the skin, releasing live larvae directly into the water.

The tufts of "cotton-wool" like material (the mycelium) characteristic of superficial fungal infections are readily seen, especially when the fish is in water. The individual long branched hyphae can be identified microscopically. The common species involved are *Saprolegnia* sp. and *Achyla* sp. which occur worldwide in both fresh and brackish water and can affect both fish and their eggs. The fungus is usually a secondary invader colonising already damaged tissue. Once infection is established the production of proteolytic enzymes causes further damage such that the disease can progress to skin ulceration or even generalised disease. Once an infection is present within an aquarium or pond however, the concentration of infective material may increase dramatically to the point when even apparently healthy fish succumb.

Similar "cotton-wool" like lesions can be found in association with myxobacterial infections. Specific identification of the organism by microscopy is therefore essential to differentiate these two conditions.

2. Irritant skin lesions

The typical symptoms associated with irritant skin disease include behavioural changes such as 'flashing' where fish suddenly dart through the water, often turning on their side showing their lighter underside (the 'flash'). Affected fish may also rub against objects and break the surface of the water. An excess of mucus is produced giving the fish a dull grey colouration and a slimy feel (Slime disease). Damage to the fins or gills (either directly by the parasite, or secondarily due to rubbing) can lead to secondary infection by fungi or bacteria. Long standing disease may result in the exhaustion of the mucus secreting cells such that the skin becomes roughened.

Skin irritation is most commonly associated with ectoparasites, although pollutants and chemicals could be involved. The larger parasites such as *Argulus*, *Lernaea*, and *Piscicola* can be readily identified, although microscopical examination of skin scrapings is necessary to identify the protozoal parasites and flukes that may be involved.

Protozoal parasites include *Ichthyophthirius multifiliis* (see below), and *Ichthyobodo* sp.(costiasis). *Chilodonella* sp. can affect all species of freshwater fish, while *Brooklynella* sp. is a marine equivalent.

The Trichodinids (including *Trichodina* sp., *Trichodonella* sp., and *Tripartiella* sp.) are found worldwide and can affect the skin and the gills of all species of marine and freshwater fish. *Scyphidia* sp., *Epistylis* sp., and *Vorticella* sp. are generally regarded as commensals, but rapid multiplication can occur when there is a high organic loading in the water leading to skin irritation.

Monogenean flukes have a worldwide distribution, although are probably more common in fresh water. Most species are host specific although some cross infection may occur. *Dactylogyrus* sp. (gill fluke) are most commonly found on the gills although they can affect the skin. Eggs are produced which fall from the host and hatch into free swimming larvae. *Gyrodactylus* sp. (skin fluke) are more commonly found on the skin. They are viviparous and juveniles develop within the body cavity which are then released directly onto the host. Often these juveniles themselves contain further juveniles and so parasite numbers can build up very rapidly under the right conditions.

3. Nodular lesions

Parasitic

The life cycles of a number of protozoal and trematode parasites are characterised by a developmental phase within the skin of fish resulting in small, discrete, proliferative lesions due, in part, to the growth of the parasite and in part to the host's tissue reaction. These are visible to the naked eye, and if present in large numbers may result in widespread skin changes.

Ichthyophthirius multifiliis is a ciliate protozoa that is extremely common worldwide and produces a disease called 'white spot' or 'ich'. The infective stage is the tomite which penetrates the epidermis of the skin or gills and develops into the trophont. The mature trophonts may reach 1 mm in diameter producing the characteristic and readily visible 'white spot'. Once mature, the trophont leaves the fish, encysts and produces approximately 2000 tomites. The speed of the life cycle is temperature dependent, taking 6 days at 27°C, but 15 days at 15°C. As well as the characteristic 'white spot', the disease signs are those typical of irritant skin disease (see above). *Cryptocaryon* sp. produces a marine equivalent of the disease.

Chronic boil-like lesions, usually seen in individual fish, can result from infection by the intracellular parasites belonging to the microspora group. When they occur below the skin they appear as grey swellings which may rupture leaving an open wound. Terminal cases may become emaciated, lethargic and show abnormal colouration. *Pleistophora hyphessobryconis* is the causal agent of Neon Tetra disease which normally presents as a loss of colour with milky white areas under the skin along the dorsum.

The metacercariae of the digenean fluke *Neascus* sp., seen most commonly in cyprinids, produce cysts in the skin up to 0.5 mm in diameter. These become melanised, and hence the common name of the condition is "black spot". The metacercariae of *Clinostomum* sp. (yellow or white grubs) produce large nodules (0.5 cm in diameter) which, if near the surface, may ulcerate.

Fungal lesions

Ichthyophonus sp. results in a systemic granulomatous disease. Heavy infection can result in a "sandpaper-like" effect of the skin. These lesions may become melanised or may rupture leaving small ulcers. Extensive growth can result in abscess formation with the presence of grey/white/yellow nodular lesions in the internal organs. Mortality levels will depend on the degree of infection and the organs affected. The 'sandpaper' effect produced should be differentiated from that due to lymphocystis and to chronic irritation.

Dermocystidium sp. can form cysts anywhere in the body, but are commonly seen in the skin or gills. These cysts are usually smooth, yellowish/white, and can be up to 1 cm in diameter. Low levels of infection cause little harm although heavy infestations may be debilitating, especially if present on the gill.

A number of other fungal species have been associated with skin granulomas in fish. *Verticillium piscis* has been described in goldfish, whereas *Exophiala pisciphila* has been isolated from skin lesions in a variety of marine aquarium fish.

Bacterial lesions

These are generally insidious in onset with the formation of granulomata in many organs as well as the skin. Rupture may result in ulceration at the surface.

The commonest organisms involved are *Mycobacterium* sp., and these produce a chronic to sub-acute disease in all water conditions. They are especially associated with over stocking. Oral transmission is most usual, although infection through wounds or via ectoparasites may occur. The incubation period is about 6 weeks and all imported fish are potential carriers. Affected fish are generally listless and emaciated, and abdominal swelling together with exophthalmos are not uncommon.

A similar disease can result from infection by *Nocardia asteroides*. However, in this case infection is thought to be principally via wounds or injuries. *Flavobacterium* sp. have been associated with a chronic granulomatous disease in Black Mollies and other aquarium fish, and *Pasteurella* sp. are involved in the chronic condition known as pseudotuberculosis.

Viral lesions

Carp pox results in epidermal hyperplasia and is found in a number of carp species. It is thought to be the result of infection with a herpes virus, and presents as characteristic discrete "candle-wax" lesions. It is seasonal in incidence, epidemics occurring in the spring but disappearing in late summer as the temperature drops. Immunity to infection is not thought to be strong and recurrence can occur in subsequent years.

Lymphocystis has been described in many species of fresh water and marine fish and is due to infection by a DNA virus. The disease is chronic in nature and results in the development of small circumscribed skin nodules (described as "pearl-like"). These may be single or multiple, and when present in very large numbers on the skin may give a "sandpaper" effect. Eventually, an inflammatory reaction produces necrosis and sloughing leaving an intact epidermis. The condition, although unsightly, is rarely fatal.

Neoplastic lesions

Papillomata are common in many species of fresh water and marine fish. They are benign, and can vary in form from a slightly raised area of hyperplastic epidermis to very obvious papillary projections.

Melanomata occur in the skin as pigmented masses. Lymphosarcomata have been described, often taking the form of ulcerating subcutaneous lesions, with metastasis to other organs.

Subcutaneous masses, whether neoplastic or granulomatous, may present as an apparent skin lesion.

4. Ulcerative/erosive lesions

Acute systemic disease

This can be caused by a primary pathogen, but is more commonly due to secondary infection of a fish that is weakened by intercurrent disease, stress or immunosuppression. The clinical signs reflect generalised septicaemia with inappetence and lethargy, together with erythema and petechiation of the skin and fins. Ulceration of the skin may be present. The internal organs may be congested and show haemorrhage. Ascites and exophthalmos may be present. Peracute infections can occur. The organisms most commonly associated are Gram-negative rods such as *Aeromonas* sp., *Pseudomonas* sp., *Vibrio* sp., *Flavobacteria* sp., *Yersinia* sp. and *Edwardsiella* sp. although streptococcal septicaemia can occur as epizootics in warm water. Some of these organisms are associated with specific diseases - *Yersinia ruckeri* is the causative agent of Enteric Red Mouth (ERM) that can affect goldfish, whereas Hole-in-the-Head in young catfish results from an infection by *Edwardsiella ictaluri*.

Aeromonas sp. are often seen in fish suffering from Spring Viraemia of Carp (SVC). This is the most important viral disease of ornamental, as well as wild and farmed carp, usually occurring in the spring as the water temperature rises. It is caused by the virus *Rhabdovirus carpio* and is notifiable in the UK under the Diseases of Fish Act, 1937.

Superficial bacterial disease

Some bacteria may directly invade the epithelium causing damage to the fins, skin ulceration or gill damage whereas others may simply secondarily infect areas already damaged by other means. Skin ulceration can progress to systemic invasion and can result in severe osmoregulatory imbalance.

Carp erythrodermatitis (also called Goldfish Ulcer disease or Ulcer disease) is caused by *Aeromonas salmonicida achromogenes*, a variant of the bacterium that causes furunculosis in salmonids. The ulcers are said to have a characteristic "punched-out" appearance, having a red centre surrounded by a white rim, the latter being surrounded by an erythematous area.

Myxobacterial disease is the name given to the disease caused by the cytophagaceae (Slime bacteria). These are generally secondary pathogens or opportunist invaders, and the commonest example is *Cytophaga* sp. (previously called *Flexibacter* sp.). The common skin conditions are attributed to these organisms are Columnaris Disease and Cold Water Disease.

Columnaris disease is usually associated with stress, nutritional imbalances or other husbandry problems. It is also called Cotton Wool disease and Mouth Fungus, the latter being especially common in livebearers, such as Black Mollies. It seldom occurs below 10°C, and can occur as an explosive epidemic above 18°C. This condition may present simply as the presence of the 'cotton wool'-like tufts when it needs to be differentiated from fungal lesions.

Cold Water disease (Fin Rot, Peduncle disease) also requires the presence of predisposing factors, although once established the bacteria will spread to healthy tissue. The lesions generally begin as fin rot, but progressively spread to involve the base of the tail (the peduncle). It is a chronic condition, usually seen in cold water from 4-10°C. The causative organism is usually *Cytophaga psychrophila* and this does not grow above 12°C. A form of peduncle disease may, however, occur in warm water above 25°C.

Hole-in-the-Head disease described in cichlids is thought to be associated with *Hexamita* infection, although nutritional factors are probably also involved.

Tetrahydena corlissi and *Uronema* sp. are discussed in the section on colour changes in relation to 'Tet disease'. Discrete white patches are visible on the skin, but as the parasite multiplies and spreads through the body, these tend to ulcerate and rapid death occurs.

A number of fungal species, including *Aphanomyces* sp., *Rhizopus* sp. and *Phoma* sp. have all been associated with ulcerative lesions in fish.

Physical factors

Traumatic injuries can occur, for example, during spawning or as a result of attacks by predators such as cats or herons. Superficial skin lesions may also be a sequel to exposure to excessive ultra-violet irradiation in unshaded ponds.

5. Colour changes

Generalised

It must be remembered that colour changes may occur in some species as a normal behavioural response or as part of their normal sexual cycle.

Hyperaemia and reddening may be a symptom of a generalised septicaemia/viraemia, or can occur as the result of stress such as with handling or transport. The viraemia associated with SVC is said to cause darkening of the skin.

Pallor and 'washed-out' colours may result from anaemia, chronic nutritional deficiencies, or chronic systemic disease (eg. tuberculosis). Loss of colour, with milky white areas under the skin along the dorsum, is a common presenting sign of Neon Tetra disease which is caused by *Pleistophora hyphessobryconis*.

Dullness of the skin colouration could also be a sequel to ectoparasite infestation where the irritation results in an increase in the surface covering of mucus. This will often give a blue-grey sheen to the skin which is especially apparent over the darkly pigmented areas. Widespread infection with *Amyloodinium* sp. (marine) and *Oodinium* sp. (freshwater) will impart a gold or rust coloured, velvet-like appearance (hence the common names of the disease are Velvet, Gold Dust, or Rust disease). The colour is due to the fact that the parasitic trophont stage,which attaches to the skin and the gills causing necrosis, contains chlorophyll.

Discrete localised areas

Discrete localised areas of colour change may be a symptom of parasitic disease. Milky white areas under the skin along the dorsum are a feature of Neon Tetra disease.

Tetrahymena corlissi occurs in warm waters; guppies and other livebearers being the most susceptible (hence the common names of 'Tet disease' and 'Guppy Killer'). The parasites may swarm in localised areas of the skin, producing discrete white patches. There may be no obvious predisposing cause and, generally, only stressed or debilitated individuals are affected. Females show a higher incidence than males. The parasite can invade most tissues and organ systems leading to rapid mortality. Deep ulcers may be visible with invasion of the organism into the musculature. *Uronema* sp. causes a marine form of this disease.

Some of the small nodular lesions discussed above have a distinct colour. Small white nodules 1mm in diameter are associated with *Ichthyophthirius multifiliis* infection. Larger (0.5cm diameter) white or yellow nodules are produced by the metacercariae of the digenean fluke *Clinostomum* sp. whereas those of *Neascus* sp., seen most commonly in cyprinids, become melanised, producing black spots of up to 0.5mm in diameter. Large white "candle-wax" lesions are characteristic of carp pox.

Melanomata in the skin may present as localised pigmented patches or nodules. The scales in these areas are often raised due to the underlying mass. The pigment cells are under neurological control, and so damage to the nerve supply can cause localised pigment changes.

6. Textural changes

Raised scales

The scales can become raised due to the presence of swelling beneath. This can become generalised as a sequel to abdominal swelling ('dropsy') when the fish develops a characteristic 'pine-cone' appearance. Localised areas of raised scales may indicate an underlying tumour or granuloma.

Dry rough 'sandpaper' effect

This appearance may result from infection with *Ichthyophonus* sp. or the viral infection lymphocystis. The constant irritation due to chronic ectoparasites may lead to an exhaustion of the mucus secreting cells giving a similar rough texture to the skin.

'Slime disease'

Irritation of the skin, most commonly by parasites, stimulates the production of excess mucus, giving a slimly texture to the skin. The mucus will cause a dulling of the skin colours and the fish will exhibit characteristic behavioural changes as a result of the irritation.

ESTABLISHING THE DIAGNOSIS

Clinical Examination

It is important to stress that the investigation of any disease problem in fish should be associated with a complete appraisal of the environmental and water quality conditions. Ideally, individual fish are examined in the aquarium or pond so that their general behaviour can be assessed. Closer examination, whilst maintaining the fish in the water, is facilitated by using a polythene bag as this allows examination from all angles when more accurate assessment of colour changes can be made. The latter may not be easily seen once the fish is out of the water. Examination of the fish out of water is generally performed in an anaesthetised/sedated fish. The common agents used are tricaine methanesulphonate (MS222, Sandos Ltd.) and ethyl - 4 amino benzoate (benzocaine), although MS222 is the only licensed product available in the UK. These drugs are added to the water and the suggested dosages are given in Table 2.

Great care should be taken when calculating the dose to allow for species variation in tolerance as well as the fact that the efficacy/toxicity will be influenced by variations in water quality. A full discussion of anaesthesia in ornamental fish is given by (Brown, 1992).

Table 2
Dose Rates of anaesthetic agents

Tricaine methanesulphonate (MS222)

A 1:10,000 solution is considered an anaesthetic dose
A 1:20,000 solution is considered a tranquillising dose

Benzocaine

Either the same concentration as for MS222 or make a stock solution of 100 g benzocaine in one litre of ethanol and store in a dark glass container. This is added to the water containing the fish a few drops at a time until the desired effects are noted.

Sampling/laboratory analysis

A more detailed account of the methods of sampling and laboratory analysis is given by Southgate and Branson (1992). Scrapings of mucus can be obtained from normal or anaesthetised fish and examined for the presence of parasites. Although the process is easier in anaesthetised fish the anaesthetic agent may affect the viability of the parasite and hence hinder identification. Scrapings can be taken from post mortem material, although this needs to be extremely fresh since rapid autolysis will make the samples useless. Samples of mucus transferred to a microscope slide are best suspended in a drop of water from which the fish has come.

Impression smears from ulcerated lesions can be made and usefully stained with Gram and Ziel-Nielson stains for the identification of bacteria. For specific identification of bacterial pathogens, together with antibiotic sensitivity testing, culture is required. This may require the use of specialist media (eg. Tryptone Soya Agar, TSA) with generally longer incubation times, at lower temperatures, than those of mammalian pathogens (Frerichs, 1984).

Additional impression smears can be stained using the rapid Wright's stains (Diff-Quik) and examined to identify the cellular elements present. This may indicate the nature of any inflammatory response or may indicate abnormal cells associated with specific conditions, such as the large cells seen with lymphocystis infection (Stoskopf, 1992).

Biopsy samples can be taken from an anaesthetised fish and fixed in 10% formal saline and submitted for histological analysis. No attempt is made to suture the biopsy site which is then left as an open ulcer and treated with local applications of antibiotic together with a barrier cream such as Orabase (Squibb). For correct interpretation samples are best sent to a laboratory with experience in fish histopathology.

INITIAL MANAGEMENT

A full review of the therapeutic agents used to treat the diseases of ornamental fish is given by (Scott, 1992)

Individual fish species have adapted to a wide range of environments and so have varying preferences for water pH, temperature, hardness, and salinity etc. This makes the calculation of drug dosages extremely difficult since the efficacy, toxicity and solubility of the drugs themselves will vary in these different water quality conditions. The range of chemicals that are commonly used as "water treatments" is under critical review. It is likely that new legislation will dramatically reduce the availability of many of the common proprietary medications that are used at present.

Antibacterial agents

These can be administered via the water, by inclusion in the food or by injection. The widespread, uncontrolled use of antibiotics in the Far East has lead to the development of antibiotic resistance reported in imported tropical and coldwater fish (Shotts et al., 1976). Ideally the choice of antibiotic used should be based on laboratory isolation of the infectious agent followed by "sensitivity testing". However, since it may not be wise to delay the onset of treatment until the laboratory tests are complete, the initial choice of antibiotic is often made empirically. This may then be modified in the light of laboratory results.

1. Administration via the water.

This is the least effective method but may be the only practical option if the fish are not eating. A separate treatment tank in which the water quality can be controlled by partial water changes is essential since the antibiotics are likely to impair a bacterial filter. Calcium present in hard water areas will often chelate certain antibiotics reducing their availability (Gratzek, 1981). A list of those antibiotics commonly administered via the water is given in Table 3.

2. Administration via the food.

The four most common antibiotics used are oxytetracycline, oxolinic acid, amoxycillin and the potentiated sulphonamides. These are generally used by mixing the antibiotic into the food or simply coating the surface of food particles. Manufactured, medicated foods are preferable since the availability of the drug is more uniform. The currently available medicated flake foods are Aquaflake and Oxyflake (PH Pharmaceuticals) containing oxolinic acid and oxytetracycline respectively. Specialist manufacturers of flake or pelleted foods (King British) will supply medicated foods on receipt of a veterinary written direction (VWD).

The dosages used for marine fish may be different from those used in freshwater fish (Scott, 1992) as there is a reduced uptake of oxolinic acid and oxytetracycline in the former. Sulphonamides may be dangerous due to the potential formation of crystals in the more concentrated urine of marine fish (Wood and Johnson, 1957).

3. Administration by injection.

This is the best method when fish are of a sufficient size. Suitable drugs and dosages are given in Table 4.

Treatments for ectoparasites

A variety of medications have been used, generally by using a concentrated solution as a short dip, or, in a more dilute solution, as a permanent bath. Care should be taken in the latter case if the system incorporates a biological filter since the chemicals could destroy the bacteria that

Table 3
Dosages of antibiotics administered via the water (Scott, 1992)

Oxytetracycline	13 - 120 mg/litre (chelated in hard water)
Doxycycline & Minocycline	2 - 3 mg/litre
Chloramphenicol	20 - 50 mg/litre
Potentiated sulphonamide	(80 mg trimethoprim & 400 mg sulphadiazine per ml) used at 1 ml/100 - 120 litres
Nifurpirinol	0.1 mg/litre
Metronidazole	7 mg/litre (double for *Oodinium* sp.)
Dimetridazole	5 mg/litre (said to inhibit spawning)
Neomycin	50 mg/kg (used in seawater)
Gentamycin	4 - 5 mg/kg (used in seawater)
Kanamycin	50 - 100 mg/litre
Nitrofurazone	1 - 3 mg/litre

Table 4
Dosages of antibiotics given by injection (Scott, 1992)

Ampicillin	10 mg/kg daily
Chloramphenicol succinate	40 mg/kg daily
Gentamycin	3 mg/kg every other day
Oxytetracycline	10 mg/kg daily
Potentiated sulphonamide (48%)	1 ml/16kg every other day
Enrofloxacin	5 - 10 mg/kg daily

are responsible for the metabolism of nitrogenous waste products. These chemicals are generally fairly toxic and it should be remembered that weak, debilitated fish are more susceptible to their adverse effects. Great care should also be taken when handling these chemicals in their concentrated forms, and adequate protective clothing should be worn. A list of the more commonly used chemicals is given in Table 5.

In addition to the traditional water treatments ivermectin (Ivomec, MSD) has been used by intramuscular injection for the treatment of *Lernaea* sp. in goldfish (Hyland and Adams, 1987).

General antimicrobial agents

A number of agents have been used widely as water treatments and may be a useful supplement to antibiotic therapy. Benzalkonium chloride (Ark-Klens, Vetark) is a blend of quaternary ammonium compounds and is used as a permanent bath at 0.1-0.5 mg/litre, although the dose should be halved in soft water. It is useful against myxobacterial infections. Chloramine-T (Vetark) is also useful for myxobacterial infections, although it also has an effect against *Costia*, white spot, and *Gyrodactylus* sp. Its action is based on a slow breakdown of hypochlorous acid, releasing oxygen and chlorine, and it should not be used at the same time as other chemicals. Acriflavine is a fairly popular disinfectant used in koi. Other species have a variable tolerance to it and plants are often adversely affected.

Salt

The use of salt has already been mentioned in relation to the treatment for leeches. Its most useful role, however, is to reduce osmotic stress, and hence metabolic requirements, in freshwater fish with gill damage or ulcers. Concentrations of 0.15% (1500 mg/l) are increased over a 3 day period to 0.6% (3000 mg/l).

Local applications

It is be possible to anaesthetise fish and treat lesions individually. Adult *Lernaea* are best removed in this way, although treatment of the water is still necessary to kill the larvae.

Ulcers require thorough debridement followed by application of antibacterials such as povidone iodine or topical antibiotics. The ulcer is then packed with a barrier cream, such as Orabase (Squibb), to reduce the osmotic stress on the fish. Parenteral antibacterial agents are usefully given at the same time.

Care should be taken to disinfect nets and other equipment between handling each fish and benzalkonium chloride is useful in this regard.

Vaccination

Recently Aquavac Cyprivac CE (AVL) has become available in the UK. for the vaccination of cyprinids against erythrodermatitis and ulcer disease caused by *Aeromonas salmonicida*.

Table 5
Common water treatments for ectoparasites

Medication	Method of administration	Target pathogen
Formalin	30-60 minute dip (250 mg/litre) Permanent Bath (15-25 mg/litre)	Protozoa Flukes
Malachite green	30 minute dip (2 mg/litre) Permanent Bath (0.1 mg/litre)	Fungi Some Protozoa
Formalin & Malachite green (Leteux-Meyer mixture)	60 minute dip (25 mg/L Formalin & 0.05 mg/L Malachite) Permanent bath (15 mg/L Formalin & 0.05 mg/L Malachite)	Protozoa
Potassium permanganate	60 minute dip (1-5 mg/Litre)	Protozoal parasites Bacterial gill disease (Not recommended)
Methylene blue	1-2 mg/litre	Protozoal Parasites (Harmful to filters)
Copper sulphate	0.1 mg/litre	Protozoa in marine and freshwater aquaria (Important to monitor copper levels)
Trichlorphon (Diptrex 80, Bayer) (Masoten, Vetark)	Permanent bath 0.2 mg/litre	*Lernaea* sp., *Argulus* sp. Flukes
Salt	15-30 min dip (20-30 g/litre)	Leeches
Freshwater	2-10 minute dip	Ectoparasites on marine fish

REFERENCES

BROWN,L.A.(1992) Restraint, handling and anaesthesia. In: *Manual of Ornamental Fish.* (Ed. R.L.Butcher) BSAVA Publications.

BUTCHER,R.L.(1992) (Ed.) *Manual of Ornamental Fish.* BSAVA Publications.

FRERICHS,G.N. (1984) The isolation and identification of Fish Bacterial Pathogens. *Institute of Aquaculture, Stirling,* Scotland.

GRATZEK,J.B.(1981). An overview of ornamental fish disease and therapy. *Journal of Small Animal Practice* **22**:345.

HYLAND,K. and ADAMS,S. (1987). Ivermectin for use in fish. *Vet. Record* **120**:539.

SCOTT,P.W.(1992) Therapeutics. In: *Manual of Ornamental Fish.* (Ed. R.L.Butcher) BSAVA Publications.

SHOTTS, E.B., KLECHNER, A.C., GRATZEK, J.B. and BLUE, J.C. (1976). Bacterial flora of aquarium fishes and their shipping waters imported from South East Asia. *Journal Fish Research Bd,* Canada **33**:732.

SNIESZKO,S.F. (1974). The effects of environmental stress on outbreaks of infectious disease in fish. *Journal of Fish Biology* **6**:197.

SOUTHGATE,P.J. and BRANSON,E.J.(1992) Autopsy Procedures and Laboratory Techniques. In: *Manual of Ornamental Fish.* (Ed. R.L.Butcher) BSAVA Publications.

STOSKOPF,M.K. (1992) *Fish Medicine.* W.B.Saunders Company, Philadelphia, Pennsylvania.

WOOD,E.M. and JOHNSON,H.E. (1957) Acute sulphamethazine toxicity in young salmon. *Progressive Fish Culturist* **19**:64.

FURTHER READING

ANDREWS,C.,EXCELL,A. and CARRINGTON,N.(1988). *The Manual of Fish Health.* Salamander Books,London.

BROWN,L.A. (1981) Anaesthesia in Fishes. *Journal of Small Animal Practice* **22**:385.

HOFFMAN,G.L. and MEYER,F.P.(1974). *Parasites of Freshwater Fishes.* T.F.H. Publications, New York.

LAGLER,K.F.,BARDACH,J.E.,MILLER,R.R. and PASSINO,D.R.M.(1977). *Ichthyology.* 2nd Edition J. Wiley and Sons, New York.

PESUT,A.P. and GOLDSCHMIDT,M. (1983) Selected Integumentary Diseases of Tropical Freshwater Fish. *The Compendium of Continuing Education* **5**:343.

POST,G. (1987). *Textbook of Fish Health.* T.F.H. Publications, New York.

RIBELIN,W.E. and MIGAKI,G. (Eds.) (1979). *The Pathology of Fishes.* The University of Wisconsin Press.

RICHARDS,R.H.(1977) Diseases of aquarium fish - Skin Diseases. *Veterinary Record* **101**:132.

RICHARDS,R.H.(1977) Diseases of aquarium fish - Treatment. *Veterinary Record* **101**:166.

ROBERTS,R.J.(1989) *Fish Pathology.* Baillière Tindall.

SCOTT,P.W.(1991) Ornamental Fish. In: *Manual of Exotic Pets.* (Eds. P.H.Beynon and J.E.Cooper) BSAVA Publications.

SNIESZKO,S.F. and AXELROD,H.R. (Eds.) (1970 to 1976) *Diseases of Fishes, Books 1-5,* T.F.H. Publications, New York.

STUART,N.C. (1983) Treatment of fish disease. *Veterinary Record* **112**:173.

STUART,N.C. (1988) Common skin diseases of farmed and pet fish. *In Practice* **10**:47.

VAN DUIJN,C. (1973) *Diseases of Fishes.* 3rd Edition Iliffe Books, London.

UNTERGASSER,D.(1989) *Handbook of Fish Diseases.* T.F.H. Publications, N.J. 07753.

SKIN DISEASE IN INVERTEBRATES

John E Cooper

"...the poor beetle that we tread upon,
In corp'ral sufferance finds a pang as great
As when a giant dies."

William Shakespeare: *"Measure for Measure"*.

INTRODUCTION

In recent years the veterinary profession has begun to concern itself with the health and welfare of captive invertebrates (Cooper, 1991; Frye, 1986; 1992). These animals may be kept as pets, for display (zoos), for educational purposes, for research and as a source of food for humans and animals.

The invertebrates comprise millions of species, ranging from single-celled protozoa to multicellular arthropods, molluscs, worms, leeches, sponges and corals. Although many species are kept in captivity, those likely to be of particular relevance to the small animal practitioner are members of the Phylum Arthropoda and the Phylum Mollusca. The emphasis in this chapter will, therefore, be on members of these two groups. Mention will, however, be made of other invertebrates where they serve to illustrate important points. Much of the research in this field has been performed on invertebrates of economic importance (for food or because they are pests) rather than those that are kept as "companion" animals.

Throughout the chapter the terms "integument" and "skin" will be used interchangeably, but others, such as "cuticle" only in their correct sense.

Useful comparative data on the structure of invertebrates, including their integument, are to be found in Fretten and Graham (1976), Laverack and Dando (1987), Leake (1975) and Wigglesworth (1984).

Although the investigation of diseases of invertebrates appears novel to veterinary surgeons, this does not mean that the subject is a recent one. The normal skin of many species was studied in detail centuries ago (Cole, 1949) and some investigators coupled this with an interest in pathology. For example, the 18th century anatomist and surgeon, John Hunter, who is closely linked with the development of the veterinary profession, studied wound healing and other processes and examples of normal and pathological material from invertebrates still feature in the Hunterian Museum at the Royal College of Surgeons of England (Figure 1). A century later, Metchnikoff (1892) observed amoebocytic cells in invertebrates and described their response to insults: his research paved the way to our understanding of inflammation and the immune processes (Turk, 1991). For many years invertebrate pathology has been studied, mainly by biologists, and there is now a wealth of literature on this subject, some of which is listed in the "References and Further Reading". Of necessity, therefore, this chapter must be general in its approach, the prime aim being to familiarise the veterinary practitioner with the normal features of certain invertebrates and to introduce some of the conditions that may adversely affect their integument.

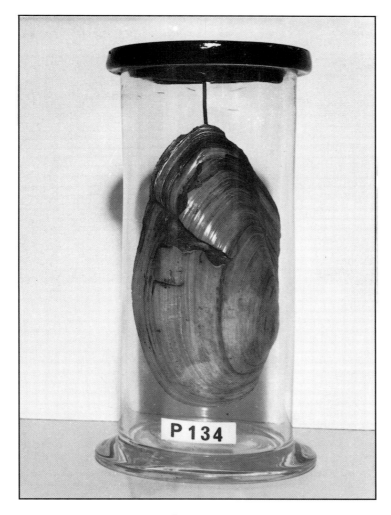

Figure 1
The integument of invertebrates has long attracted interest amongst scientists.
This healed shell in a bivalve is one of the surviving 18th century specimens housed
in the Hunterian Museum in London

Normal biology

The Phylum Arthropoda consists of several classes of animals of which the following are the most relevant to this chapter:

1.   Class Insecta (insects)
2.   Class Arachnida (spiders, scorpions, ticks and mites)
3.   Class Diplopoda (millipedes)
4.   Class Chilopoda (centipedes)
5.   Class Crustacea (crabs, lobsters, shrimps, woodlice)

Arthropods are characterised by a chitinous exoskeleton which has played a key role, partly because it hampers fluid loss and partly because of the support it offers, in the success of these creatures in colonising the land. Scientific study of the chitinous exoskeleton, a unique structure, goes back to the work of Odier in 1823 (Miller, 1980). In recent years, work on the arthropod integument has largely been prompted by the need to develop insecticides that can penetrate chitin or impair its formation but it is also of relevance to a better understanding of skin diseases in these animals. The structure of two types of arthropod cuticle is depicted in Figure 2.

Fig 2A
Insect integument

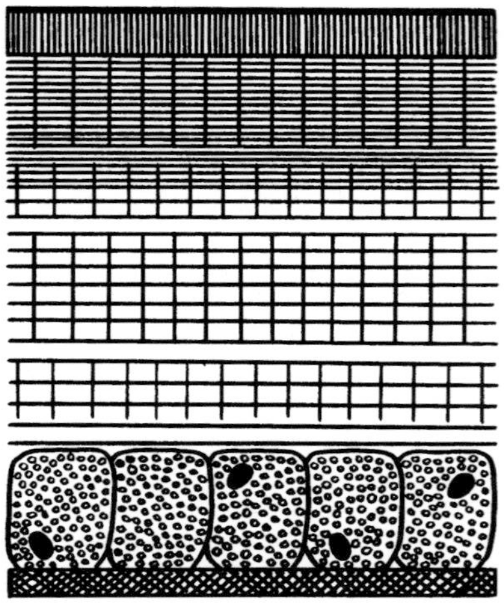

Epicuticle

Exocuticle

Endocuticle

Epidermis

Basement
membrane

Fig 2B
Crustacean integument

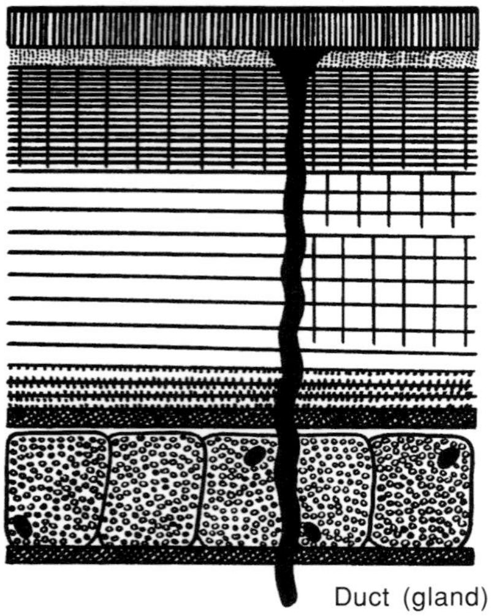

Epicuticle

Pigmented
layer

Calcified
layer

Non-calcified
layer

Epidermis

Basement
membrane

Duct (gland)

The Phylum Mollusca also consists of several classes, of which the following three are at present of most veterinary importance:

1.   Class Gastropoda (slugs and pulmonate snails)
2.   Class Bivalvia (bivalve snails eg. oysters and mussels)
3.   Cephalopoda (octopuses, squids, cuttlefish)

Molluscs do not have a chitinous exoskeleton. Their skin is soft (the name is derived from the Latin "mollis") and some species have a specialised protective covering ("shell") of calcium carbonate. The structure of the mollusc (gastropod) integument is depicted in Figure 3.

Table 1 lists some of the features of the Arthropoda and Mollusca, with particular reference to the integument. Standard references should be consulted for detailed information on the physical and chemical features of the arthropod cuticle and the mollusc shell.

Figure 3
Mollusc integument

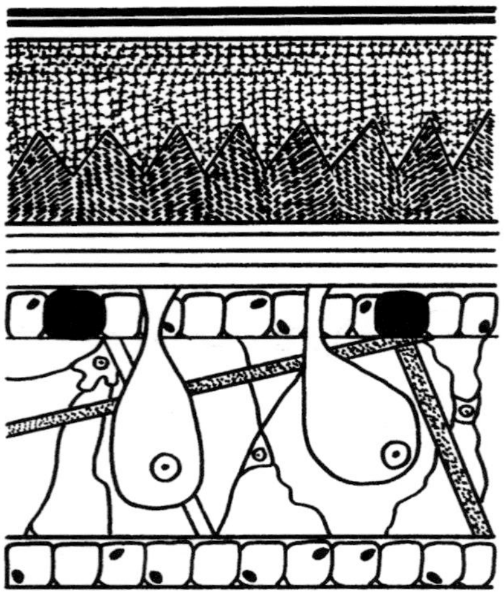

Periostracum

Layer I

Layer 2

Layer 3

Epidermis

Mantle

Epidermis

200

Table 1
Some features of the Arthropoda and the Mollusca

	Arthropoda	Mollusca
Habitat	Terrestrial, aquatic (freshwater and marine), many insects aerial. Often tolerant of dry conditions.	Terrestrial, aquatic (freshwater and marine). Occasionally aerial (squids). Some species can tolerate dry conditions but only by protective behaviour (aestivation).
Basic morphology	Segmented and bilaterally symmetrical. Paired jointed appendages - limbs, sensory structures and feeding organs.	Unsegmented. Essentially bilaterally symmetrical but gastropods show torsion of the body.
Skeleton	A hard cuticular exoskeleton, made of chitin (see below).	Some species (snails) secrete a calcareous shell to protect visceral hump. Many molluscs use blood (haemolymph) in haemocoel as a hydrostatic skeleton.
Organ systems	A tubular gut. Nervous system consists of chains of ganglia. Respiration by tracheae, gills, lungs, gill books, lung books etc., rarely across body surface. Cardiovascular system of adult consists of heart and haemocoel (body cavity). Separate sexes.	A tubular gut. Nervous system consists primarily of circumoesophageal ring containing ganglia. "Brain" in cephalopods. Respiration by gills or lungs, often also across body surface. Cardiovascular system consists of heart, arteries, veins, haemocoel and haemolymph.
Integument	Essentially a chitinous exoskeleton, secreted by epidermis, divided into hard plates with flexible joints. The cuticle is waterproof and relatively impermeable but a breach in it can result in loss of haemolymph. Thickness and composition of cuticle varies. In many Crustacea it is calcified: in some insects it is thin and pliable. Often there are invaginations of the cuticle forming respiratory organs and lining the fore and hindgut. Sometimes the integument is protected by setae (hairs) - hollow outgrowths of the cuticle - or other morphological adaptations. The wings of Lepidoptera bear coloured scales. Some arthropods protect their integument by constructing or adopting a protective "home" eg. the case that is made and carried by caddis fly larvae (*Trichoptera*) or the empty shell that is occupied by a hermit crab. If such "homes" are lost the animal is vulnerable. The cuticle is shed at intervals (ecdysis). A new cuticle forms and hardens (sclerotisation): the animal is particularly vulnerable to damage or predation immediately following ecdysis.	Essentially a thin, mucous epidermis, often ciliated. No cuticle, setae or other appendages. A muscular foot and tentacles present in many species. A calcareous external shell, secreted by epidermis in many gastropods and bivalves: this is often ornate and sculpted. Shell is internal in modern cephalopods eg. cuttlefish. Some species of pulmonate gastropod can tolerate dry conditions by aestivation -sealing the shell with a mucous (sometimes calcareous) epiphragm and accompanying physiological changes. In some gastropods the body wall is perforated by the partner during copulation. Molluscs do not shed their skin. Soft tissue and bone grow gradually.

It is important to note that both arthropods and molluscs are ectothermic, ie. the majority have no internal (physiological) control over their body temperature and must use behavioural strategies in order to raise or lower it. Most processes in these animals are temperature dependent including growth, regeneration and repair of the integument. As in other species the outer layers play an important part in maintaining homoeostasis: since most invertebrates are small and thus have a large body surface area in relation to their mass, this function is vital. It therefore follows that these animals can easily be adversely influenced in captivity by suboptimum conditions, especially too high or too low temperature and relative humidity (RH).

Defence mechanisms in invertebrates have attracted considerable attention in recent years as well as being of historical interest (see earlier). Phagocytes in haemolymph and other body fluids play an important part in most species, as do agglutination, coagulation and bactericidins (Dales, 1979). These and other factors, including free fatty acids on the body surface (Smith and Grula, 1982), or lysozyme-like secretions (Canicatti and D'Ancona, 1990) may contribute to an invertebrate's ability to resist or deal with integumentary infection or damage, as may ecdysterone, which is secreted/generated by injured cells (Wigglesworth, 1984). Wound responses in insects were reviewed by Yeaton (1983).

Diseases of the skin (integument)

Many pathological conditions of the skin are recognised in invertebrates. Some are well defined diseases or syndromes but others are probably non-specific and related to physical and other insults. In this chapter, skin diseases of invertebrates are assumed to include "any impairment of normal physiological function" and will therefore be covered under two main headings:-

a)   Non-infectious
b)   Infectious

In fact there is often overlap since (for example) an injury to the skin can provide a portal of entry for bacteria or fungi. Likewise, neoplasms (tumour-like conditions), may or may not be due to living organisms. Nevertheless, the two headings above provide a useful division for discussion. Invertebrate pathologists often refer to non-infectious diseases as "non-communicable" and infectious as "communicable" but these terms will not be used here.

As in vertebrates, many diseases of invertebrates manifest themselves by skin lesions or produce changes that may be visible by external examination. Some, such as colour changes in honeybee larvae due to brood diseases, are of economic importance. In this chapter, examples are given in which skin lesions are of primary rather than secondary importance.

APPROACH TO THE CASE

Invertebrates may be presented singly for examination (for example, the pet "tarantula" spider) or the veterinary surgeon may be asked to advise on a group of animals kept in a school, zoo or laboratory. The basic approach is the same and in many respects resembles that adopted for more conventional animals. The important steps are given in Table 2.

Handling and examination of invertebrates are covered in a number of texts (Cooper, 1991). The skin of poisonous or delicate species can be examined through a glass or plastic container. A hand-lens will facilitate examination.

Samples for laboratory investigation can be taken in a variety of ways. Non-living material, such as chitin or shell, can be removed by scraping or brushing. Deeper lesions may require excision but care must be taken to minimise damage which may lead to loss of haemolymph. Anaesthesia should be used (Cooper, 1991; Smith, 1991); hypothermia is not acceptable.

Surface lesions can also be swabbed (a moistened swab is recommended) for microbiological examination. Touch preparations (impression smears) can be taken and stained with Giemsa. Scanning electron microscopy (SEM) has been used to study the normal and pathological skin of many species but is unavailable in general practice.

Table 2
Approach to invertebrate skin disease

Presentation of case / request for assistance

↓

Which species is(are) involved?
Has it been accurately identified?
Do I have data on normal biology
and likely requirements in captivity?
Is it a toxic or dangerous species?

↓

What history is available?
Is the animal captive bred or imported?
How experienced is the owner?
Are his/her records accurate and up-to-date? (CHECK).
Why is assistance being sought?

↓

Is the management satisfactory?
(The cage or enclosure should be inspected, if necessary by visiting the owner's premises).
What other animals are kept? Is the food adequate/appropriate?
Are there any environmental factors that may be relevant eg. high temperatures,
high/low relative humidity, ultraviolet light, vibration, use of potentially toxic chemicals?
Do the client's records provide any clues?

Table 2
(continued)

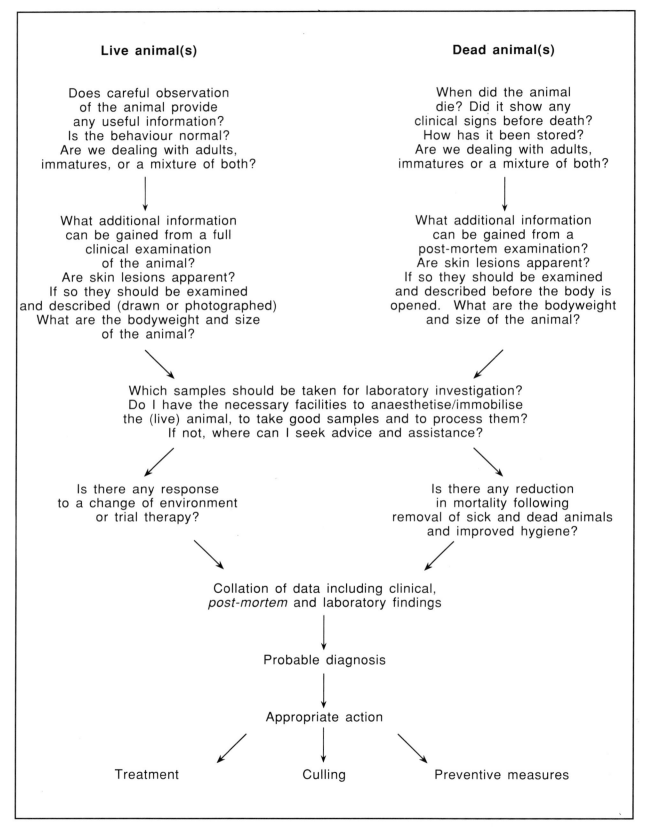

Live animal(s)

Does careful observation
of the animal provide
any useful information?
Is the behaviour normal?
Are we dealing with adults,
immatures, or a mixture of both?

↓

What additional information
can be gained from a full
clinical examination
of the animal?
Are skin lesions apparent?
If so they should be examined
and described (drawn or photographed)
What are the bodyweight and size
of the animal?

Dead animal(s)

When did the animal
die? Did it show any
clinical signs before death?
How has it been stored?
Are we dealing with adults,
immatures or a mixture of both?

↓

What additional information
can be gained from a
post-mortem examination?
Are skin lesions apparent?
If so they should be examined
and described before the body is
opened. What are the bodyweight
and size of the animal?

Which samples should be taken for laboratory investigation?
Do I have the necessary facilities to anaesthetise/immobilise
the (live) animal, to take good samples and to process them?
If not, where can I seek advice and assistance?

Is there any response
to a change of environment
or trial therapy?

Is there any reduction
in mortality following
removal of sick and dead animals
and improved hygiene?

Collation of data including clinical,
post-mortem and laboratory findings

↓

Probable diagnosis

↓

Appropriate action

Treatment   Culling   Preventive measures

Post-mortem sampling of invertebrates is discussed in detail by Cooper and Cunningham (1991).

Shed skins and discarded eggs or cocoons can provide valuable information and should be stored in airtight containers or plastic bags pending examination.

Aids to clinical and *post-mortem* diagnosis include radiography. Other imaging techniques (Figure 4) are proving useful but are likely in the immediate future to be restricted to research establishments or work with invertebrates of considerable economic value. Scanning electron microscopy is of great value when investigating *post-mortem* material.

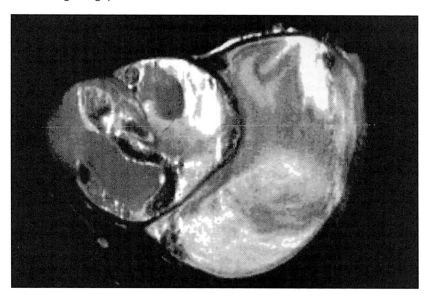

Figure 4
Nuclear magnetic resonance scan of a live anaesthetised *Achatina* snail.
The calcareous shell is virtually invisible but the underlying soft tissue,
including the integument, is clearly seen.

NON-INFECTIOUS DISEASES

Introduction

Non-infectious diseases of invertebrates may be due to trauma, changes in atmospheric pressure, adverse temperature/RH, chemicals, toxins or ionising radiation (Sparks, 1972). In addition, nutritional and endocrinological disorders occur. All of these can be considered together since invertebrates generally respond in a similar way to different insults.

Establishing the diagnosis

Diagnosis of non-infectious disease is based on the flow diagram given Table 2. Careful investigation and analysis of the environment are of great importance since many non-infectious lesions of the integument are due to, or exacerbated by, poor management or an unsatisfactory environment.

Some features of non-infectious disease in molluscs and arthropods are given in Table 3.

Initial management

The aim in managing non-infectious diseases of the skin should be:

a)   to attempt treatment of any affected animals, or to kill them humanely, and

b)   to prevent further cases.

Table 2
Some non-infectious skin diseases of molluscs and arthropods

Aetiology	Effect *	Clinical features	Comments
Trauma, including predation	Various types of tissue damage, sometimes followed by infection	Penetrating wounds in soft tissue, cracks or holes in shell or cuticle. Cuticular wounds usually associated with loss of haemolymph. Crushing wounds can also occur with no penetration of body wall but damage ("bruising") to underlying tissue. Setae and other appendages may be damaged or lost.	Wound healing is well recognised in invertebrates (Sparks, 1972) but may take several days and is influenced by temperature and other factors. Bacterial or fungal infection may supervene or animal may die as a result of haemorrhage, fluid loss or (freshwater aquatic species) fluid intake. Some species may show signs similar to those seen in secondary shock in vetebrates. Wild caught cephalopods appear particularly prone to skin damage and "bruising" (Boyle, 1991). The loss of setae from the body of some arthropods eg spiders, hairy caterpillars, is normal and can be a defensive mechanism in that they are often irritant. Regeneration of the appendages of arthropods and the tentacles of molluscs often occurs but may take some time. The degree of regeneration may be age-related. In stick insects, for example, regeneration of a lost limb is complete if this occurs before the first moult, incomplete if it occurs after the first moult and absent after the final moult (P. Zwart, pers. comm.) Healed fractures are relatively common in molluscs. (Brandwood et al, 1986).
Changes in atmospheric pressure (shock wave)	Tissue damage	Sometimes none, sometimes severe tissue damage as above. Soft bodied species are less resistant than those with a chitinous cuticle or calcareous shell.	Mainly of relevance in aquatic species exposed to explosions or violent changes in pressure.
Ionising radiation	Tissue damage	Skin lesions may occur including, in certain molluscs and planarians, "abscesses". Generalised disease leading to death.	Rarely seen except experimentally or when invertebrates are inadvertently exposed to X-rays or other radiation.
High temperature (often complicated by an adverse relative humidity)	Burns and "heat stress" Dysecdysis	Wounds in soft tissue, often leading to necrosis and formation of a "weal". Inactivity leading to death.	If given a temperature gradient most invertebrates will select their optimum (preferred) temperature. High temperatures are generally not lethal so long as they are within the "zone of thermal tolerance" for the species (Fry, 1947).
Low temperature (often complicated by an adverse relative humidity)	Tissue damage including "frost bite" Dysecdysis	Skin lesions which include necrosis (sloughing) of epidermis and underlying tissues, sloughing of limbs and other appendages. Epithelial proliferation is often a characteristic part of healing.	There is much variation in the response of invertebrates to cold. A few species eg. winter moths, are able to raise their body temperature and thus tolerate sub-zero conditions.
Chemicals	Local or generalised tissue damage	Skin lesions including necrosis. Generalised signs especially following absorption through skin of insecticidal agents.	Various liquid and gaseous chemicals can adversely affect invertebrates and some produce skin lesions. Low levels in water can affect aquatic species.

* In most cases the effect can also be death

Table 2
(continued)

Aetiology	Effect *	Clinical features	Comments
Toxins	Usually internal tissue damage	Occasionally skin discolouration or other superficial changes, usually systemic signs/lethal.	See Sparks (1972).
Nutritional deficiencies	Local or generalised disease	Snails show characteristic signs of calcium deficiency - soft shells which easily crumble and break. Calcium deficient snails nibble the shells of others.	Other nutritional deficiencies affecting the integument are not well documented but probably occur. Imbalances may also be significant.
Neoplasms	Localised tissue proliferation	Some skin neoplasms/ hyperplastic lesions have been reported.	A fertile field for research! Suspect neoplasms should be submitted for histological evaluation. See various papers eg. Harshbarger (1972).

* In most cases the effect can also be death

Insofar as treatment is concerned, the following points are important:-

(a)   The animal should be maintained at its preferred body temperature (PBT). If this is not known, a temperature gradient should be provided so that the invertebrate has a choice.

(b)   The environment (whether terrestrial or aquatic) must be kept as clean as possible (but with minimal use of chemical disinfectants) in order to reduce the risk of secondary infection; sterilisation of bedding (preferably by irradiation) is recommended for laboratory and zoo collections (P. Zwart, personal communication.).

(c)   Where possible, the environment should be manipulated in order to promote healing of the skin and to reduce adverse secondary effects eg. dehydration. Thus, for example, the RH may be increased so as to reduce fluid loss.

(d)   Invertebrates with skin lesions are liable to dehydration: water (or saline) will usually be readily taken by mouth if offered in a spoon or from a syringe. Aquatic species may suffer overhydration (freshwater species) or dehydration (marine species) and these are difficult to control.

(e)   Specific therapy will depend upon the lesion and the species. The following are examples:-

Traumatic lesions: the exoskeleton of arthropods can be closed or plugged to prevent loss of haemolymph. Emergency treatment can be carried out using icing sugar, talcum powder, paraffin wax, beeswax and celloidin, plasticine or sticky tape (Cooper, 1987a). If time permits a more permanent seal can often be achieved using tissue adhesive, for example "Vetbond" (Alfred Cox, Coulsdon), "superglues" (cyanomethacrylate) or fine sutures.

The "shell" of molluscs can be repaired using sticky tape, adhesive plastic film ("Op-Site": Smith and Nephew), liquid bandage ("New Skin": Medtech Laboratories) (F.L. Frye, pers. comm.) or a tissue adhesive (Cooper and Knowler, 1991).

Dysecdysis (retained slough) will often resolve if the relative humidity is raised and outer layers of skin are loosened with glycerine.

Other lesions: irrigation with normal saline will help to remove chemicals, toxins and necrotic material. Repair as above may or may not be possible or advisable. Lesions should be irrigated regularly with saline to keep them clean and damp.

Supportive treatment will consist of provision of dietary additives (eg. calcium for the shell of molluscs) and changes to management in order to encourage normal behaviour.

Test therapy, on a small group of animals, is often advisable.

Prevention of further cases is best achieved by attention to the environment (Cooper, 1987b).

INFECTIOUS DISEASES

Introduction

A wide range of infectious organisms can cause or be associated with disease in arthropods and molluscs (Cantwell, 1974; Cooper and Knowler, 1991; Lésel, 1990; Poinar and Thomas, 1978; Weiser, 1977). They range from viruses to metazoan ectoparasites and endoparasites. Some organisms appear to be part of the normal flora and fauna and the role of these has attracted interest in recent years (Lésel, 1990).

Establishing the diagnosis

Reference should again be made to Table 2. If an infectious disease is suspected, particular attention should be paid to microscopical examination of skin lesions and the taking of samples for laboratory investigation. Differentiation between pathogens, normal fauna/flora and contaminants from the environment is often not easy (Austin and Austin, 1989; Cooper and Cunningham, 1991).

Some features of infectious disease in molluscs and arthropods are given in Table 4.

Initial management

The aims of management are as for non-infectious disease, as are the first four points ((a)-(d)) regarding treatment. Insofar as specific therapy is concerned (e), there is a paucity of published information on the use of medicines in invertebrates other than a certain amount on bees (Bailey, 1981), mealworms (Wallach, 1972) and shellfish (Sindermann, 1990). Nevertheless, the following points may prove helpful:

Samples for diagnosis should be taken before treatment commences. Pending diagnosis, irrigation of skin lesions with saline will help to minimise dehydration and secondary infection and may, *per se*, effect a cure.

Mild disinfectant agents, such as dilute quaternary ammonium compounds, can be used with caution, to treat infections. Phenolic and halogenated disinfectants should be avoided. Tetracyclines and sulphonamides can be used, again with caution, in many species, both topically and orally.

Some chemical agents have proved useful, as dips, for the control of skin diseases in aquatic species - for example, nifurpirinol for bacterial ulcerative lesions in octopuses (Hanlon *et al*, 1984).

Pyrethroid-based sprays have proved safe in the control of ectoparasites in terrestrial snails (Goode and Hird, 1988).

Some pathogens of insects, especially viruses, can be carried on the outside of eggs. The eggs can be treated with 0.1% sodium hypochlorite followed by rinsing, immersion in 10% formaldehyde and washing (C.F. Rivers, cited in Cooper, 1980).

Test therapy is again always advisable.

Prevention of infectious diseases is based largely on hygiene and other managemental factors. It is clear that many infectious diseases of invertebrates are due to an interaction between facultative pathogens and "stressed" hosts. It is difficult to eliminate facultative pathogens but their numbers can be kept to a minimum by removing uneaten food, shed skins and faeces and by providing fresh food and water. Use of chemical disinfectants should be minimised, partly because they may prove toxic to the invertebrates and partly because normal (sometimes beneficial)

Table 4
Some infectious skin diseases of molluscs and arthropods

Aetiology	Effect	Clinical features	Comments
Viruses	Occasionally cause skin lesions eg Chesapeake Bay virus (CBV) and gill virus in crustaceans and cytoplasmic polyhedrosis virus in insect larvae (eg. "jaundice" in silkworms)	The two examples in crustaceans cause necrosis of gill epithelium while insect larvae may show a thin, corrugated, sometimes oily skin or (silkworms) yellow lesions on the abdomen.	Other viruses can probably also be associated with skin lesions in different hosts. See Smith (1967), Sindermann (1990) and Rivers (1972).
Rickettsiae	Gill and shell lesions in certain marine molluscs	Lethargy and abnormally thin shells.	
Bacteria eg. *Beneckia chitinovona*	Shell disease of crustaceans, skin diseases of other invertebrates	Erosions, pitting and other damage to exoskeleton. Discharge from wounds. Snails with generalised bacterial infections sometimes show colour changes to foot.	Chitinovorous bacteria, including *Vibrio* spp., are able to destroy the exoskeleton of arthropods. Injuries may predispose to these and other infections – for example, in locusts (Jennings, 1971). Bacterial infections delay healing in some species eg. cephalopods (Bullock *et al*, 1987).
Fungi	Various syndromes in aquatic species including "maladie du pied" in oysters and "burn spot disease" and "black mat disease" in crustaceans. Mycoses of insects eg stick insects (Jennings, 1971) and other arthropods	Abnormal shells in molluscs, colour changes and degeneration of cuticle in crustaceans. Eggs of crustaceans may be destroyed by fungi. Arthropods become covered with hyphae and the chitin may darken.	Many fungi eg. *Leptolegnia* and *Saprolegnia* are opportunistic and will colonise skin lesions in aquatic invertebrates. Terrestrial arthropods are infected when fungus breaches the cuticle at the joints of limbs or penetrates the epicuticle. Overcrowding and poor hygiene may predispose to fungal infections in insects.
Protozoa	Various conditions including bonamiasis of oysters and "gray crab disease" of crustaceans	Affected oysters show ulceration of skin. In "gray crab disease" there is a marked colour change to the ventral exoskeleton.	Some protozoa are obligate parasites but others are facultative pathogens. Injured hosts are more susceptible.
Microsporidia	Various conditions including dry, hard skin and lethargy in buffalo-worms (*Alphitobius diaperinus*) and dysecdysis in locusts (*Locusta migratoria*) (P. Zwart, pers. comm.)	As on left plus other clinical features, a number involving the skin, in different species (P. Zwart, pers. comm.)	Attempt to break life-cycle by disinfecting the eggs of the invertebrate - for example, with formalin or hypochlorite.
Helminths (trematodes, cestodes, nematodes)	Various conditions	Lesions of integument are usually restricted to holes in chitin where parasites have entered or foreign body reactions such as pearl formation in oysters. Pigmented scars may be a feature of old parasitic lesions.	Few helminths are of major importance insofar as dermatology is concerned.
Leeches (Hirudinea)	Local and generalised lesions	Attachment of leeches to skin of various aquatic invertebrates, associated lethargy or death.	Wild caught aquatic invertebrates should be carefully checked for evidence of leech infestation.

Table 4
(continued)

Aetiology	Effect	Clinical features	Comments
Mites (Acarina)	Accumulations on body and (pulmonate snails) in mantle cavity	Usually no specific lesions. Small numbers of mesostigmatid mites are normal on certain terrestrial invertebrates eg. tropical millipedes, dung beetles. Large numbers or infestation with pathogenic species can be associated with lethargy and death. This is a particular threat to breeding colonies of insects (eg. *Gryllus* spp.).	Examine incoming invertebrates as above. Also check food and substrate. (See Goode and Hird (1988) and Wallach (1972). Create dry areas in cages where invertebrates can clean themselves (P. Zwart, pers. comm.).
Hymenoptera Diptera	Internal parasitism with exit of larvae through body wall	Common arthropods. Initially no lesions but when parasites leave host they make holes in chitin and clusters of pupae of parasites may be found attached to body surface.	Exclude from captive colonies by a) quarantining incoming stock and b) using insect-proof netting.

flora may be destroyed. Relative humidity is also significant: if captive invertebrates are kept under damp conditions fungal and other infections can occur. On the other hand, too low a relative humidity can result in deformed wings and other abnormalities (Cooper, 1980). "Stress" in invertebrates can be initiated by overcrowding, excessive handling or exposure to adverse stimuli such as chemicals, bright lights or vibration. Attention to all these will help to prevent disease.

CONCLUSIONS

Despite interest for many years in the integument of invertebrates, study of skin diseases has been largely restricted to species of economic importance. As a result, the veterinary dermatologist who is presented with an invertebrate patient must usually extrapolate from the available data and apply basic principles based upon his/her knowledge of the animal's anatomy, physiology and behaviour. Veterinary surgeons will increasingly be faced with requests for advice on invertebrates and it is therefore most important that cases are seen, samples collected, therapy attempted and results recorded. In addition, material should be submitted to laboratories and authorities for examination or an opinion. Collation of data on skin diseases of invertebrates will further enhance the standing and importance of veterinary dermatology.

Vaccines have been used to prevent disease in certain invertebrates. For example, for the prevention of gaffkemia (*Aerococcus viridans*) infection of lobsters, attenuated vaccines proved more effective than formalin-killed vaccines while the best results were obtained by first injecting the animals with vancomycin, followed by live *A. viridans* (Stewart and Zwicker, 1974). Vaccination possibly has potential in both aquatic and terrestrial invertebrates but its value in protecting animals against infectious diseases of the integument is largely unknown and much research is needed.

ACKNOWLEDGEMENTS

I am grateful to Dr F.L. Frye and Professor P. Zwart for reading and commenting on this manuscript, to Miss Elaine Penfold for the drawings and to Mrs C. Steel for typing many early drafts.

REFERENCES AND FURTHER READING

AUSTIN, B. and AUSTIN, D.A. (1989). (Eds) Methods for the Microbiological Examination of Fish and Shellfish. Ellis Horwood, Chichester.

BAILEY, L. (1981). Honey Bee Pathology. Academic Press, London.

BOYLE, P.R. (1991). The UFAW Handbook on the Care and Management of Cephalopods in the Laboratory. Universities Federation for Animal Welfare, Potters Bar.

BRANDWOOD, A., JAYES, A.S and ALEXANDER, R. McN. (1986). Incidence of healed fracture in the skeletons of birds, molluscs and primates. *Journal of Zoology*, **208**: 55.

BULLOCK, A.M., POLGLASE, J.L. and PHILLIPS, S.E. (1987). The wound healing and haemocytic response in the skin of the lesser octopus *Eledone cirrhosa* (Mollusca: Cephalopoda) in the presence of *Vibrio tubiashii*. *Journal of Zoology*, **211**: 373.

CANICATTI, C. and D'ANCONA, G. (1990). Biological protective substances in *Marthasterias glacialis* (Asteroidea) epidermal secretion. *Journal of Zoology*, **222**: 445.

CANTWELL, G.E. (1974). Insect Diseases. Marcel Dekker, New York.

COLE, F.J. (1949). A History of Comparative Anatomy. Macmillan, London.

COOPER, J.E. (1980). Invertebrates and invertebrate disease, an introduction for the veterinary surgeon. *Journal of Small Animal Practice*, **21**: 495.

COOPER, J.E. (1987a). A veterinary approach to spiders. *Journal of Small Animal Practice*, **28**: 229.

COOPER, J.E. (1987b). Wirbellose (Invertebraten). In Gabrisch, K. and Zwart, P. (Eds) Krankheiten der Wildtiere, Schültersche, Hannover.

COOPER, J.E. (1991). Invertebrates. In: Eds. Beynon, P.H., Lawton, M.P.C. and Cooper, J.E. *Manual of Exotic Pets*. British Small Animal Veterinary Association, Cheltenham.

COOPER, J.E. and CUNNINGHAM, A. (1991). Pathological Investigation of Captive Invertebrates. *International Zoo Yearbook* **30**: 137.

COOPER, J.E. and KNOWLER, C. (1991). Snails and snail farming: *Veterinary Record* **129**: 541.

DALES, R.P. (1979). Defence of invertebrates against bacterial infection. *Journal of the Royal Society of Medicine* **72**: 688.

FRETTEN, V. and GRAHAM, A. (1976). A Functional Anatomy of Invertebrates. Academic Press, London.

FRY, F.E.J. (1947). Effects of the environment on animal activity. *University of Toronto Biology Services* **55**. Publication of Ontario Fisheries Research Laboratory. No 68.

FRYE, F.L. (1986). Care and feeding of invertebrates kept as pets or study animals. In Fowler, M.E. (Ed). *Zoo and Wild Animal Medicine* , W.B. Saunders, Philadelphia.

FRYE, F.L. (1992). Captive Invertebrates. Krieger, Florida.

GOODE, M. and HIRD, G. (1988). Heliculture in Great Britain. Organic Snails, Cambridge.

HANLON, R.T.; FORSYTHE, J.W.; COOPER, K.M.; DINUZZO, A.R.; FOLSE, D.S. and KELLY, M.T. (1984). Fatal penetrating skin ulcers in laboratory-reared octopuses. *Journal of Invertebrate Pathology* **44**: 67.

HARSHBARGER, J.C. (1972). Descriptions of polyps and epidermal papillomas in three bivalve mollusc species. *Marine Fisheries Review*, **1209**: 25.

JENNINGS, T.J. (1971). Animals in the Home and the Classroom. Pergamon Press, Oxford.

LAVERACK, M.S. and DANDO, J. (1987). Lecture Notes on Invertebrate Zoology. 3rd Edition, Blackwell, Oxford.

LEAKE, L.D. (1975). Comparative Histology. Academic Press, London.

LESEL, R. (1990). (Ed) Microbiology in Poecilotherms. Elsevier, Amsterdam.

METCHNIKOFF, E. (1892). Lecons sur la Pathogie comparee d'Inflammation. Masson, Paris.

MILLER, T.A. (1980). (Ed) Cuticle Techniques in Arthropods. Springer-Verlag.

POINAR, G.O. and THOMAS, G.M. (1978). Diagnostic Manual for the Identification of Insect Pathogens. Plenum Press, New York.

RIVERS, C.F. (1972). Diseases. In: Heath, J. (Ed). The Moths and Butterflies of Great Britain and Ireland Volume 1. Curwen Press, London.

SINDERMANN, C.J. (1990). Principal Diseases of Marine Fish and Shellfish. Academic Press, San Diego.

SMITH, J.A. (1991). A question of pain in invertebrates. *ILAR News*, **33**: 25.

SMITH, K.M. (1967). Insect Virology. Academic Press, New York.

SMITH, R.J. and GRULA, E.A. (1982). Toxic components on the larval surface of the corn earworm (*Heliothis zea*) and their effects on germination and growth of *Beauveria bassiana*. *Journal of Invertebrate Pathology*, **39**: 15.

SPARKS, A.K. (1972). Invertebrate Pathology: non-communicable diseases. Academic Press, New York.

STEWART, J.E. and ZWICKER, B.M. (1974). A comparison of various vaccines for inducing resistance in the lobster (*Homarus americanus*) to the bacterial infection gaffkemia. *Journal of the Fisheries Research Board of Canada*, **31**: 1887.

TURK, J.L. (1991). Metchnikoff revisited. *Journal of the Royal Society of Medicine*, **84**: 579.

WALLACH, J.D. (1972). The management and medical care of mealworms. *Journal of Zoo Animal Medicine*, **3**: 29.

WEISER, J. (1977). An Atlas of Insect Diseases. W. Junk, The Hague.

WIGGLESWORTH, V.B. (1984). Insect Physiology. 8th edition. Chapman and Hall, London.

YEATON, R.W. (1983). Wound responses in insects. *American Zoologist*, **23**: 195.

CHAPTER TWENTY FIVE

ANTIBACTERIAL STRATEGIES

Ian S Mason ————————————————————————

INTRODUCTION

Mammalian skin is highly resistant to bacterial disease. Yet pyoderma in dogs is a commonly encountered phenomenon in clinical practice. There are a number of possible explanations for this apparent paradox. Part of the explanation may lie in the results of studies of the ultrastructure of canine skin which have suggested that epidermal barriers are less well developed in this species. In addition, it is generally accepted that pyoderma usually occurs as a secondary complication of another underlying disorder. It is possible that the relatively high incidence of ectoparasitic, endocrine and hypersensitivity diseases in dogs will, in turn, lead to a high incidence of pyoderma.

In this chapter, the first section will concentrate on the management of canine pyoderma. Later sections will cover the treatment of the less frequently encountered bacterial skin problems of dogs and cats.

CANINE PYODERMA

Most cases of pyoderma are associated with coagulase-positive staphylococci, usually *Staphylococcus intermedius*, which may be isolated in small numbers from normal skin. The multiplication of these bacteria is inhibited by a number of cutaneous defence mechanisms and it is likely that the underlying causes of pyoderma exert their influence by disrupting these mechanisms. Therefore, clinicians should not depend on antimicrobial therapy alone in the management of bacterial skin disease as recurrence is likely after treatment ceases unless the primary cause is identified and treated.

In Chapter 6 the underlying causes of canine pyoderma are discussed along with a practical diagnostic approach. Unfortunately, the pathogenic mechanisms of many forms of pyoderma are poorly understood at present. It is therefore impossible, in some cases, to determine the underlying cause. Such idiopathic cases are assumed to be related to defects in either innate or specific defence mechanisms although there is little evidence to support this theory. Despite the relatively high number of idiopathic cases, a careful investigation of primary causes is mandatory in pyoderma, otherwise long term or even life long antimicrobial therapy will be required. The disadvantages of symptomatic treatment in terms of cost and inconvenience to the owner are self evident. Furthermore, some medicaments may cause toxic, immune mediated or idiosyncratic reactions in patients and prolonged therapy may induce resistant bacterial strains.

Antimicrobial agents have two major roles in pyoderma; as adjunctive therapy for those cases receiving specific treatment for an identified cause or as symptomatic therapy in idiopathic cases. The selection of medicaments and treatment protocols will differ between these two groups of cases. In those cases in which a diagnosis of the underlying cause has been attained, therapy aimed at both controlling the primary condition and reversing the changes in the skin which allowed secondary bacterial disease to occur is required. For example, the treatment of canine pyoderma due to hypothyroidism requires both thyroid supplementation and adjunctive antimicrobial

213

therapy. The distinction between such a case and idiopathic cases, is that in the former, the use of antimicrobial agents can usually be permanently withdrawn after resolution of the lesions, whereas in idiopathic cases it is likely to be required throughout the life of the dog. The management of idiopathic recurrent pyoderma will be discussed more fully at the end of this section. Table 1 summarises an approach to the management of canine pyoderma.

Table 1
Recommendations for the treatment of pyoderma

*Thorough investigation to determine underlying cause, if possible

*Initiate specific treatment

*Assess depth and severity of infection

*Select appropriate systemic and/or topical medicaments

*Evaluate response regularly

*Discontinue systemic treatment 2-3 weeks after resolution of bacterial lesions

*Evaluate effect of topical therapy alone

*Gradually increase the interval between applications of shampoos

*In cases in which a cause has been identified and treated, it may be possible to discontinue antimicrobial therapy

*Idiopathic cases will need long term therapy

*Glucocorticoids are contra-indicated in almost all cases of pyoderma, except perhaps in surface pyodermas.

Systemic therapy

Canine pyoderma should be treated with the correct drug, at the correct dose for the correct duration of therapy. Table 2 shows the doses of antibacterial agents available in the United Kingdom to treat bacterial skin disease in the dog along with their advantages and disadvantages. An assessment of the depth of infection should be made (surface, superficial or deep; (Chapter 6) as this will influence nature, frequency and duration of treatment.

The value of bacterial culture and sensitivity testing in aiding selection of "the correct drug" is controversial. Many veterinary dermatologists select systemic antimicrobial agents empirically as the prevalence of resistance to these drugs among strains of *Staphylococcus intermedius* is well documented. Furthermore, it is possible that the sensitivity profile of the strain isolated from the skin is unrepresentative of all the staphylococci present. In addition, *in vitro* sensitivity does not always correlate with clinical results. Despite these limitations, sensitivity testing is indicated in chronic, deep or recurrent cases or in those instances where no clinical response is observed following therapy.

Ideally the antimicrobial agent selected for the treatment of canine pyoderma should inhibit the specific bacteria present in a bacteriocidal manner. If possible, the selected drug should be inexpensive, convenient and easy to administer, be easily absorbed and have few or no side-effects. Narrow spectrum drugs are preferred as they have little effect on the normal skin and gut flora. In theory, bacteriostatic agents are only effective if the patient is not immuno-compromised. However, it is often not possible, in practice, to achieve these ideals and the use of bacteriostatic and broad spectrum agents causes few problems. Clearly, in those cases where deep pyoderma is present, or immunological defects suspected, bacteriocidal medicaments should be used.

214

Table 2
Commonly used antimicrobial agents for treatments of pyoderma in dogs

Drug	Dose	Advantages	Disadvantages	Comments
Cephalexin	20-30 mg/kg bid	Resistance is uncommon	Expensive	Best reserved for life threatening deep pyoderma
Clavulanic acid-potentiated amoxycillin	20-25 mg/kg bid	*In vitro* resistance not reported	Expensive	Anecdotal reports cast doubt on efficacy *in vivo*
Clindamycin	5 mg/kg bid (or 11 mg/kg sid)	Good penetration into devitalised tissue	Bacteriostatic. Cross resistance with erythromycin and lincomycin	–
Enrofloxacin	2.5-5 mg/kg bid	Rapid bacteriocidal action. Little bacterial resistance. Good penetration into devitalised tissue	Can damage articular cartilage and cause lameness in young, growing dogs. Short courses recommended. Costly	Should not be used in skeletally-immature dogs
Erythromycin	10-15 mg/kg tid	Inexpensive. May have an independant anti-inflammatory effect	Bacteriostatic. Gastric irritant: may induce vomiting. Needs to be administered three times daily. Cross resistance with lincomycin and clindamycin	–
Lincomycin	15 mg/kg tid (or 22 mg/kg bid)	Can be given twice daily	Cross resistance with erythromycin and clindamycin. Bacteriostatic	Administer one hour before or after feeding
Oxacillin	20 mg/kg tid	Resistance is rare	Needs to be given three times daily. Not licenced for use in dogs and cats in the UK. Food interferes with absorption	Administer one hour before or after feeding
Trimethoprim-potentiated sulphomanide	30 mg/kg bid	Relatively inexpensive	Idiosyncratic drug reactions (polyarthropathy, cutaneous drug eruptions, ocular lesions). Possible increasing bacterial drug resistance	Recent data suggest tissue concentrations are adequate at 30 mg/kg once daily

Therapeutic failures occur if bacterial resistance is present or if the micro-organism is protected by the production of enzymes such as the beta-lactamases or if the organism has adapted to survive within host cells such as macrophages and so is not exposed to the effects of the antimicrobial agent. Inadequate tissue levels also lead to therapeutic failure. A drug which is readily absorbed and which penetrates well in cutaneous tissue should be selected. Unfortunately skin is one of the most difficult tissues in which to achieve high concentrations of antimicrobial drugs.

The correct dose should be administered and should be based on actual rather than estimated body weight. In general, doses of antimicrobial agents are doubled for skin infections so that effective tissue concentrations are more likely to be achieved. Treatment should continue until at least 2 to 3 weeks beyond the resolution of all bacterial lesions. In severe, chronic and deep pyodermas, treatment may need to continue for 2 to 3 months or longer.

Most coagulase-positive staphylococci produce beta-lactamases (penicillinases) and so antibiotics sensitive to these enzymes, such as penicillin, ampicillin and amoxycillin, are unlikely to be successful in the management of canine pyoderma and are not recommended. Some synthetic penicillins, for example oxacillin are resistant to bacterial beta-lactamases and clinically are regarded as very efficacious drugs. However, oxacillin is costly and not licenced for use in animals in the UK. Amoxycillin has been combined with clavulanic acid which inhibits beta-lactamase activity. Anecdotal reports indicate that although almost all strains of *Staphylococcus intermedius* isolated from cases of pyoderma are sensitive to this drug *in vitro*, its clinical performance is disappointing in some cases.

Clindamycin has recently been introduced to the veterinary market in the UK. It is claimed that it penetrates well into devitalised areas and fibrotic, purulent lesions. In common with lincomycin it is a lincosamide antibiotic. This group of antibiotics has features similar to those of the macrolide group of antibiotics which includes erythromycin. Resistance to one of these drugs may be associated with resistance to the others and clinicians should not switch from one of these drugs to another if the original drug is ineffective. In theory, bacteriostatic drugs such as lincomycin and erythromycin should be avoided in cases of deep pyoderma or where immunodeficiency is suspected.

Enrofloxacin is a new broad spectrum, bacteriocidal antimicrobial agent with a unique mode of action. It inhibits bacterial DNA gyrase. This enzyme is required for the maintenance of the configuration of DNA and for DNA replication. Plasmid mediated bacterial resistance has not been documented as plasmid replication requires functional DNA gyrase. Hence, resistance can only result from mutation. As a result of this no bacterial resistance has emerged so far. Although it is not yet licenced for use in dogs, preliminary studies have shown that it is highly efficacious in cases of pyoderma. However, it is recommended that it is not used on skeletally immature dogs as damage to articular cartilage and lameness may occur in such animals. The manufacturers recommend that it is not used for longer than 10 days in dogs. This limits the potential value of this agent in the management of pyoderma as prolonged courses of antimicrobial therapy are usually required, as discussed previously.

In the UK, chloramphenicol is seldom used in canine pyoderma despite being a cheap and in many instances efficacious drug. It has the disadvantages of being both broad spectrum and bacteriostatic. Toxic reactions, particularly blood dyscrasias have also been reported. Its use cannot be recommended in this country while so many alternative agents are available.

In cases of deep pyoderma with chronic scarring, the presence of free hair shaft keratin within the dermis and granuloma formation may make it impossible to achieve adequate tissue concentrations of those antimicrobials routinely employed. Rifampicin is an agent that was previously used in the treatment of tuberculosis in man but it is effective against staphylococci and is very soluble in lipid, resulting in good tissue penetration. It can kill staphylococci within cells and is useful in chronic granulomatous disease. One problem with its use is that bacterial resistance develops rapidly and so it must be administered in combination with another antibiotic. The major disadvantage is hepatotoxicity with most cases developing elevations in serum alkaline phosphatase concentration following therapy. Other side effects include thrombocytopenia, haemolytic anaemia and the development of gastrointestinal signs. It is not licenced for use in dogs in the UK and its use should be confined to those cases where euthanasia is being considered.

In summary, penicillin, ampicillin, amoxycillin and tetracyclines are usually ineffective in the management of this group of diseases. Good results are obtained with erythromycin, lincomycin and trimethoprim potentiated sulphonamides especially in those cases where antimicrobial therapy has not been previously used. Trimethoprim potentiated sulphonamides are preferred by the author in most cases of pyoderma unless the animal has previously failed to respond to the drug or if deep pyoderma is present. There is evidence to suggest that potentiated sulphonamides should not be used in dobermans as drug induced ocular and arthritic changes have been reported in this breed following their administration. Cephalexin is expensive and resistance is starting to emerge; its use should be confined to life-endangering cases where sensitivity data indicate that it is likely to be effective. It is the author's drug of choice in cases of deep pyoderma where these criteria are fulfilled. Cases of pyoderma which do not respond within 2 to 3 weeks of the onset of appropriate antimicrobial therapy should be reassessed with a view to investigating the case more fully. A number of other diseases, such as immune mediated conditions and neoplasia, may resemble cases of pyoderma. Re-evaluation of the diagnosis is likely to be more rewarding than simply changing to another antimicrobial agent.

Topical therapy

Topical antimicrobial therapy, usually in the form of shampoos, is a useful adjunct to systemic treatment. In those cases where a definitive diagnosis has not been possible, it is sometimes possible to maintain dogs in remission using shampoos alone, so avoiding the disadvantages of long term systemic therapy (see below). In mild cases of pyoderma topical therapy may be the only form of antimicrobial therapy required. In Chapter 26 topical therapy in canine pyoderma is discussed more fully.

The frequency of application of shampoos depends on the depth and severity of the disease. In some instances alternate day or even daily medication is needed. However, most cases can be managed satisfactorily with treatment once or twice weekly. Once improvement is seen the interval between shampoos can be gradually increased until a satisfactory maintenance interval is established.

Management of idiopathic recurrent pyoderma

Idiopathic recurrent pyoderma is the term used to describe those cases of pyoderma for which no primary cause has been discovered. In this frustrating condition, the prognosis is guarded to poor as long-term, usually life-long antimicrobial therapy will be required. The prognosis varies between individual cases with more extensive and deep pyodermas having a worse outlook. In many instances euthanasia may be requested by the owner of a dog with such a condition as the management may be expensive, particularly if systemic antibiotics are used for prolonged periods in larger dogs, and may be extremely time consuming if intensive topical treatment is undertaken.

The initial aim is to resolve lesions rapidly. This is usually achieved with a combination of systemic and topical agents. Systemic medicaments have been discussed in detail previously while topical agents are covered in Chapter 26. Treatment should continue for at least 2 to 3 weeks after resolution of lesions. In cases of deep pyoderma it may be prudent to continue treatment for even longer than this. Once the problem is in remission then a strategy to maintain this state is required. Often cases of superficial pyoderma can be maintained with the use of topical therapy alone. Benzoyl peroxide shampoo (Oxydex, C-Vet; Paxcutol, Virbac) is the drug of choice because of its prolonged effect on the cutaneous microflora. In some dogs irritant or allergic reactions may occur following the use of such products. If this occurs then a less irritant shampoo such as an ethyl lactate based product (Etiderm; Virbac), one containing triclosan (Kerect; C-Vet) or chlorhexidine should be substituted for benzoyl peroxide. At first, baths should be administered 2 to 3 times weekly. If remission persists then the interval between baths can be gradually increased until the optimum treatment interval is determined by the owner. This may be as infrequent as monthly, but in most cases it will be more often. In general, more treatment will be required during the warmer part of the year.

If topical therapy alone is insufficient to maintain remission, then immunostimulation with some form of bacterial product such as an autogenous vaccine or a therapeutic agent such as levamisole or cimetidine should be considered. A discussion of immunostimulants is outside the scope of this chapter. With the exception of autogenous vaccines, immunostimulatory drugs are unlicenced or unavailable within the UK.

Should the condition relapse despite intensive topical therapy, either with or without the use of immunostimulants, then long term systemic antibacterial therapy is indicated. This form of management has a number of disadvantages including the possibility that resistant bacterial strains may be encouraged and that adverse reactions may occur. Cost may be a major consideration in some cases. Dermatologists are divided as to the most effective way to use systemic antimicrobials in these patients. Some clinicians reduce the daily dose by up to 50%, while others administer them on alternate days. The author is concerned that such regimens may encourage the production of antibiotic resistant bacterial strains and so uses them at the full dose daily until 2 to 3 weeks following remission. At this stage the drug is used on a week-on week-off basis. If after 2 months no relapse has occurred then the "off treatment" period is gradually increased to find the optimum maintenance interval. Unfortunately resistance to antimicrobials is likely to occur if potentiated sulphonamides or the lincosamide and macrolide antibiotics are used in this way. Resistance is less likely to occur with the use of drugs such as cephalexin, oxacillin and clavulanate-potentiated amoxycillin. The use of these drugs may be prohibitively expensive

OTHER CANINE BACTERIAL SKIN DISEASES

In the UK, bacterial skin disease other than staphylococcal pyoderma is rare in dogs. Table 3 gives examples of bacteria isolated from dogs with such disorders. Many of these conditions are associated with fistulae (see Chapter 8).

Table 3
Non-staphylococcal canine bacterial skin disorders

Disease	Causal Agent
Actinobacillosis	*Actinobacillus ligniersii*
Actinomycosis	*Actinomyces* spp.
Borreliosis	*Borrelia burgdorferi*
Dermatophilosis	*Dermatophilus congolensis*
Mycobacterial infection:	
i) cutaneous tuberculosis	*Mycobacterium tuberculosis, M.bovis*
ii) atypical mycobacterial infection	Various mycobacteria
Nocardiosis	*Nocardia* sp
Pseudomycetoma	Variable. Includes: *Pseudomonas* spp., *Proteus* spp., coagulase- positive staphylococci, *Streptococcus* spp., *Actinobacillus* spp.

Actinobacillosis

Surgical removal or drainage followed by curettage is recommended. Systemic therapy with sodium iodide (0.2 ml/kg of 20% solution, orally twice daily), streptomycin, sulphonamides, tetracyclines or chloramphenicol has been recommended. Usually treatment is prolonged and prognosis guarded.

Actinomycosis

Therapy is usually based on long-term therapy with high doses of penicillin (100,000 U/kg daily), sulphonamides (10 mg/kg twice daily) or potentiated sulphonamides (Table 2). Treatment must continue until at least a month after remission and usually lasts for several months. Surgical debridement may augment such systemic therapy.

Borreliosis

Cutaneous borreliosis rapidly responds to oral tetracycline therapy.

Dermatophilosis

Environmental factors leading proliferation of *Dermatophilus congolensis* on the skin should be removed. Local trauma, high environmental relative humidity and biting insects are implicated as initiating causes of this rare disorder. Removal of crusts and topical therapy with povidone-iodine along with systemic anti-microbial therapy are usually curative. The organism is usually sensitive to a wide range of anti-microbial drugs, although resistance to erythromycin, sulphonamides and low doses of penicillin is reported. High dose penicillin or tetracycline therapy for 7 to 10 days is usually adequate to eliminate infection.

Mycobacteriosis

Cutaneous tuberculosis. This is a zoonosis. After a positive diagnosis has been made, euthanasia should be performed and the public health authorities notified.

Atypical mycobacterial infection. Prolonged systemic antibacterial therapy following surgical excision and or debridement may be of value. Suggested drugs are doxacycline, enrofloxacin, ciprofloxacin and potentiated sulphonamides.

Nocardiosis

Surgical drainage of infected tissue followed by systemic antibacterial therapy is recommended. High dose penicillin or potentiated sulphonamide treatment should be administered until at least a month after remission; in practice treatment for several months may therefore be required. Erythromycin, lincomycin, streptomycin and tetracyclines may also be of value in the management of this condition.

Pseudomycetoma

This granulomatous lesion is relatively impermeable to antibiotics and so treatment must be based on complete surgical excision followed by systemic antimicrobial therapy.

Abscesses and cellulitis

Surgical drainage and debridement followed by systemic antimicrobial therapy is recommended.

FELINE BACTERIAL SKIN DISEASE

Bacterial skin disease is rare in cats with the exception of abscesses and cellulitis. Pseudomycetoma, actinomycosis, nocardiosis, cutaneous tuberculosis, atypical mycobacterial infection and dermatophilosis rarely occur in cats. These disorders are managed as in the dog.

Feline leprosy

Local and circumscribed lesions should be removed surgically. In those cases where many lesions are present or where they are in sites which preclude surgical management then clofazimine (2-3 mg/kg daily) treatment for several months is recommended.

Acknowledgement

This chapter contains some sections repeated from an article by the same author recently published in the journal "In Practice". The author is grateful to the editors of "In Practice" for permission to reproduce material in this chapter.

FURTHER READING

DEBOER, D.J. (1990). Strategies for management of recurrent pyoderma in dogs. *Veterinary Clinics of North America* **20**, 1509

IHRKE, P.J. (1987). An overview of bacterial skin disease in the dog. *British Veterinary Journal* **143**, 112

MASON, I.S. (1991). Canine pyoderma. *Journal of Small Animal Practice* **32**, 381

MASON, I.S. (1992). The selection and use of antibacterial agents in canine pyoderma. *In Practice* (in press)

WHITE, S.D & IHRKE, P.J (1987). Pyoderma. In: *Dermatology. Contemporary Issues in Small Animal Practice*, volume 8. (Ed. G.H. Nesbitt) New York, Churchill Livingstone.

TOPICAL THERAPEUTICS

Kenneth W Kwochka ⎯⎯⎯⎯⎯⎯⎯⎯⎯⎯⎯⎯⎯⎯⎯⎯

INTRODUCTION

Over the last several years there have been tremendous advances in topical therapy in veterinary dermatology. Companies specialising in veterinary dermatologics have introduced many unique and innovative products to the veterinary profession. Because of the broad range of products available to the practitioner topical treatment programmes can be tailored to each animal.

The efficacy of topical treatments is difficult to evaluate objectively and application of these products is often based solely on clinical observations. Fortunately, this seems to be changing. There have recently been two quantitative studies reported, one on antibacterial (Kwochka and Kowalski, 1991) and one on antiseborrhoeic (Gordon, 1992) shampoos used *in vivo* on dogs. Such methods will be valuable in the critical evaluation of existing products and in the development of new topical therapeutics.

Topical therapy is valuable for virtually every type of dermatosis in dogs and some skin conditions in cats. Major indications include cleansing and moisturising the skin, control of scaling disorders, cutaneous infections, inflammation and pruritus, ectoparasites (especially fleas) and otitis. Shampoo therapy is the most popular form of topical treatment because of ease of administration to the entire body through the thick hair coat. This chapter will address many of the important indications for topical therapy. Treatment for fleas, other ectoparasites, dermatophytes, and otitis is found elsewhere in this manual (Chapters 29, 30 and 15, respectively). The discussion will concentrate on shampoos and topical rinses although other delivery systems will be mentioned where relevant.

GENERAL PRINCIPLES OF TOPICAL THERAPY

A definitive diagnosis of the skin condition being treated should be made as soon as possible. This will allow better selection of the most appropriate topical treatment program and, more important, proper prescription of systemic agents to better control or cure the condition. For example, a hypoallergenic or antipruritic shampoo will be helpful in controlling cutaneous inflammation and pruritus in a dog with atopy. However, the condition will not be managed properly unless the patient is allergy tested and subsequently started on a hyposensitisation program. Topical therapy is extremely important in controlling a variety of dermatoses but is only occasionally the sole answer to the problem.

Until a definitive diagnosis can be made, specific products are usually chosen on the basis of presenting morphologic characteristics such as mild or severe dry scale, greasy scale, inflammation, pruritus, presence of ectoparasites and concurrent cutaneous infections.

Several companies produce similar products. The practitioner should be cautioned to use a limited number of these but be well informed about their indications, contraindications, compatibilities, incompatibilities, time for and duration of effect, and aesthetic qualities such as fragrance, latherability, dispersibility, and rinseability.

Some of the more potent topical products, especially those used to control scaling and infections, may have undesirable side effects. Frequent re-examinations are necessary initially because of the potential for irritancy and sensitisation. Less potent agents should be employed first. If frequent observations determine that this class of product is not working, then more potent products can be chosen.

Assessment of the client and the patient should be made before initiating topical therapy since cooperation of the patient and owner is necessary because of the time and effort involved with most topical therapy programs. The characteristics of the specific products prescribed will also have an effect on owner compliance. For example, a high concentration tar shampoo may be indicated once or twice per week for a severe greasy scaling disorder. However, compliance may be a problem because such products are malodourous and can irritate skin and stain light coloured hair coats. Although a sulphur and salicylic acid shampoo may not perform as well in controlling the scale and oil, it will not have the undesirable qualities of a tar product. Thus, improved compliance would be expected with more favourable overall results.

The ability of the owner to follow instructions must also be considered. However, many problems associated with poor owner compliance are not a result of lack of intelligence but are client communication problems due to incomplete instructions. Directions must be kept as simple as possible and should be written out or provided in prepared client education handouts. Videotapes or demonstrations of proper bathing techniques are very helpful. The ability to properly involve the client in the topical therapeutic program may actually have beneficial psychological effects by making them feel that they are contributing significantly to the improvement of their pet.

Bathing

Baths are helpful therapy for focal, regionalised, and generalised dermatoses. No matter what specific products and active ingredients are used, the mechanical process of bathing with water is helpful in removing scales, crusts, debris, dirt, allergens, organisms and old medications.

Water has tremendous hydrating effects if used properly. This is especially valuable in dry scaling disorders where the stratum corneum is dehydrated. Contact time of 10 to 15 minutes must be allowed to properly hydrate the stratum corneum. If contact time is too short and baths are being given frequently, then the continual drying actually leads to dehydration of the horny layer. After bathing or soaking and while the skin is still wet, application of an emulsified bath oil will help hold externally applied water to prolong hydration. Topical use of a humectant results in attraction of water to the stratum corneum to increase hydration. Finally, use of an occlusive agent such as petrolatum physically blocks the surface of the stratum corneum to reduce transepidermal water loss through this layer to the environment. Care must be taken not to immerse the animal in water for excessively long periods because maceration of the stratum corneum with a loss of protective barrier function might result.

Contact time for medicated shampoos varies depending on the active ingredient, concentration of active ingredient, vehicle and the condition of the skin. Most of the products used to help control scaling have labels which recommend a 5 to 15 minute contact time. Owners should be encouraged to use a watch or clock to be sure the contact time is adequate. Timing should not be started until the whole body is lathered and gentle lathering should continue for the entire time for maximum efficacy. The importance of thoroughly rinsing the animal also must be stressed to avoid problems with irritation caused by shampoo residues.

SPECIFIC INDICATIONS FOR TOPICAL THERAPY

CLEANSING AND MOISTURISING AGENTS

There are a number of mildly medicated and hypoallergenic veterinary shampoos on the market. These clean the skin without the use of soap using detergent soap substitutes and surfactants. It is the balanced anionic/amphoteric surfactant systems, not necessarily the lack of medicaments, in these products which make them mild with minimal potential for irritancy and sensitisation. Some caution should be exercised since even shampoos classified as being hypoallergenic may on occasion be irritating, especially to inflamed and damaged skin.

221

Table 1
Selected hypoallergenic and medicated shampoos

Trade Name	Manufacturer	Active Ingredient(s)	Usage
Cleansing and Moisturising Shampoos			
HyLyt*efa Hypoallergenic Moisturizing Shampoo (USA) Hylashine (UK)	DVM Pharmaceuticals (USA) C-Vet (UK)	Na lactate, coconut oil, lanolin, glycerin, protein, fatty acids	Dog and Cat
Allergroom Hypoallergenic Emollient Shampoo (USA) Sebocalm Shampoo (UK)	Allerderm (USA) Virbac (UK)	NaCl, glycerin, lactic acid, urea	Dog and Cat
Anti-Scaling Shampoos			
Sebolux Shampoo (USA & UK)	Allerderm (USA) Virbac (UK)	2% sulfur, 2% salicylic acid	Dog and Cat
SebaLyt Antiseborrheic Shampoo (USA) Kerect Shampoo (UK)	DVM Pharmaceuticals (USA) C-Vet (UK)	2% sulfur, 2% salicylic acid, 0.5% triclosan	Dog and Cat
Sebbafon Dermatologic Shampoo (USA)	Upjohn	5% precipitated sulfur, 0.5% Na salicylate, entsufon Na, lanolin, petrolatum	Dog and Cat
OxyDex Shampoo (USA & UK)	DVM Pharmaceuticals (USA) C-Vet (UK)	2.5% benzoyl peroxide	Dog and Cat
Pyoben Shampoo (USA) Paxcutol (UK)	Allerderm (USA) Virbac (UK)	3% benzoyl peroxide	Dog and Cat
Sulf OxyDex Shampoo (USA)	DVM Pharmaceuticals	2.5% benzoyl peroxide, 2% sulfur	Dog and Cat
Clear Tar Shampoo (USA)	Veterinary Prescription	2% solubilized coal tar extract, collagen, lanolin, coconut oil	Dog
NuSal-T Shampoo (USA)	DVM Pharmaceuticals	2% coal tar, 3% salicylic acid, 1% menthol	Dog
T-Lux Shampoo (USA)	Allerderm	4% solubilized coal tar, 2% sulfur, 2% salicylic acid	Dog
LyTar Shampoo (USA) Tarlite (UK)	DVM Pharmaceuticals (USA) C-Vet (UK)	3% refined coal tar, 2% sulfur, 2% salicylic acid	Dog
Mycodex High Potency Tar and Sulfur Shampoo (USA)	SmithKline-Beecham	3% coal tar, 2.5% sulfur, 2% salicylic acid	Dog
Allerseb-T Shampoo (USA) Sebolytic (UK)	Allerderm (USA) Virbac (UK)	4% coal tar, 2% sulfur, 2% salicylic acid	Dog
Selsun Blue (USA) Seleen (UK)	Ross Sanofi (UK)	1% selenium sulfide	Dog
Antimicrobial Shampoos			
OxyDex Shampoo (USA & UK)	DVM Pharmaceuticals (USA) C-Vet (UK)	2.5% benzoyl peroxide	Dog and Cat
Pyoben Shampoo (USA) Paxcutol (UK)	Allerderm (USA) Virbac (UK)	3% benzoyl peroxide	Dog and Cat
Sulf OxyDex Shampoo (USA)	DVM Pharmaceuticals	2.5% benzoyl peroxide, 2% sulfur	Dog and Cat
Nolvasan Shampoo (USA)	Fort Dodge Laboratories	0.5% chlorhexidine acetate	Dog and Cat
ChlorhexiDerm Shampoo (USA)	DVM Pharmaceuticals	1% chlorhexidine gluconate	Dog and Cat
Weladol Antiseptic Shampoo (USA)	Pitman-Moore	Polyalkyleneglycol-iodine complex, 1% available iodine	Dog and Cat
Nizoral Shampoo (USA & UK)	Janssen	2% ketoconazole	Dog and Cat
Sebolyse Foam (USA)	Dermcare	Miconazole, chlorhexidine, selenium sulfide	Dog
Dermazole Shampoo (USA)	Allerderm	2% miconazole, 0.5% chlorhexidine	Dog
Antipruritic Shampoos			
Epi-Soothe Shampoo (USA & UK)	Allerderm (USA)/Virbac (UK)	Colloidal Oatmeal	Dog and Cat
Histacalm Shampoo (USA)	Allerderm	2% diphenhydramine hydrochloride, colloidal oatmeal	Dog and Cat

Some of these shampoos also contain moisturizing agents such as sodium lactate, natural essence of coconut oil, and essential fatty acids (USA, HyLyt*efa Hypoallergenic Moisturising Shampoo, DVM: UK, Hylashine, C-Vet) and sodium chloride, glycerin, lactic acid and urea (USA, Allergroom Hypoallergenic Emollient Shampoo, Allerderm: UK, Sebocalm, Virbac). The moisturising effects can be enhanced by application of a bath oil or humectant containing rinse after bathing.

These factors make the products useful for routine bathing, particularly in dogs with sensitive skin, for allergic dermatoses (especially atopy and contact allergy) and for mild dry scaling conditions. They are usually mild enough not to irritate the skin of allergic dogs and cats and they help remove surface allergens from the skin and hair coat. In dogs which have mild dry scaling such as that associated with environmental factors (dry heat), endocrinopathies, parasitism, pyoderma and certain allergies (food allergy), all that may be needed is a mild cleansing and moisturising shampoo for rehydration of the skin along with specific therapy for the primary disease.

Cleansing and moisturising shampoos may be helpful in addition to other, more potent, anti-scaling agents in primary keratinisation disorders characterised by dry scale formation such as primary seborrhoea of Irish setters and doberman pinschers, sebaceous adenitis and canine ichthyosis. They may be alternated with the drying anti-scaling agents such as tars and benzoyl peroxide to help rehydrate the skin. Finally, cleansing and moisturising shampoos are useful when a dog with more severe scaling cannot tolerate potent anti-scaling agents.

ANTI-SCALING AGENTS

Most dogs and cats presented to a practitioner for cutaneous scale formation have secondary scaling which is not associated with a primary keratinisation defect (Chapter 5). The dermatoses which may result in secondary scaling include ectoparasitism, pyoderma, dermatophytosis, endocrinopathies, autoimmune dermatoses, allergic dermatoses and environmental dermatoses. Topical therapy is important in these diseases to help control the scaling and keep the animal comfortable until the primary disease is diagnosed and treated.

Symptomatic topical therapy, especially with anti-scaling agents in shampoo formulations, is the major form of therapy used to manage most of the primary keratinisation defects. Ointments, gels, creams, and sprays are also useful in some of the localised keratinisation abnormalities.

In a dog with a scaling dermatosis and long hair coat, it may be beneficial to clip the hair and keep it fairly short during treatment. If there is a large amount of scale formation initial bathing with a detergent, prior to the use of an anti-scaling shampoo, will allow use of less of the medicated formulation, better contact with the skin surface and thus enhanced efficacy.

Bathing is instituted 2 to 3 times per week until good control of the scale and odour is achieved and then as frequently as needed for maintenance. Moderate, dry scale with no odour may be controlled after only 2 or 3 weeks and then be maintained with a bath every month. A dog with severe greasy scale and odour may take several weeks before the owners are satisfied with the response and then still need baths every 7 to 10 days for control. The maintenance program may vary depending on the season since extremes of heat and humidity may affect the amount of dryness or greasiness, scaling and secondary bacterial infection.

Anti-scaling compounds are keratolytic or keratoplastic or both. A keratolytic agent causes cellular damage to corneocytes resulting in ballooning of the cells and subsequent cell shedding. Thus the stratum corneum is softened and removed, resulting in better control of scale formation. A keratoplastic agent results in "normalisation" of epidermal cell kinetics and keratinisation, usually by cytostatic effects on the basal cell layer. Common anti-scaling agents include sulphur, salicylic acid, benzoyl peroxide, tar and selenium sulfide.

Sulphur

Sulphur is commonly incorporated into anti-scaling shampoo products. It is keratolytic and keratoplastic and has minimal antifungal, antibacterial, antiparasitic and antipruritic activity. Depending on the method of preparation, sulphur will be found in different particle sizes (Lin *et al.*, 1988). Colloidal sulphur particles are smaller than precipitated particles and these, in turn, are smaller than sublimed sulphur. The smaller the particle size, the greater the surface area for interaction between the skin and the sulphur.

The keratoplastic effect may be cytostatic or related to the reaction in which sulphur and cysteine combine to form cystine and hydrogen sulphide. Normal keratinisation is promoted since cystine is an important constituent of the stratum corneum and the amount of hydrogen sulphide is fairly low. At higher sulphur concentrations, more hydrogen sulphide is formed which breaks down keratin and results in the keratolytic effect. The antibacterial and antifungal activities are the result of hydrogen sulphide and pentathionic acid formation. Sulphur is drying and malodorous, although not in the concentrations found in shampoos. It is not a good degreasing agent. Therefore, a sulphur containing shampoo would be used more for a dry scaling condition and when a pyoderma is present. It has synergistic keratolytic activity with salicylic acid.

Salicylic acid

Salicylic acid is keratolytic, keratoplastic, mildly antipruritic and bacteriostatic. The keratolytic effect occurs by lowering the pH of the skin, resulting in an increase in hydration of the keratin and swelling of the cells of the stratum corneum. Also important in the promotion of desquamation is the solubilising of the intercellular cement substance that binds scales in the stratum corneum. The synergistic activity between salicylic acid and sulphur appears to be optimal when the products are incorporated in equal concentrations (Leyden *et al.*, 1987).

Primary scaling disorders which may benefit from the use of a sulphur and salicylic acid shampoo include primary idiopathic seborrhoea, sebaceous adenitis, ichthyosis, ear margin dermatosis and zinc responsive dermatosis. These shampoos will also be helpful as adjunctive therapy to control dry scale associated with parasitism, pyoderma, allergies, environmental factors (dry heat) and autoimmune dermatoses (pemphigus foliaceus).

Sulphur and salicylic acid are found in equal concentrations in a veterinary shampoo (USA/UK, Sebolux Shampoo, Allerderm/Virbac). Another formulation (USA, SebaLyt Antiseborrheic Shampoo, DVM: UK, Kerect, C-Vet) contains not only sulphur and salicylic acid in equal concentrations, but also the antiseptic agent triclosan at the 0.5% level, thereby making the product valuable in cases where scaling is accompanied by secondary pyoderma. Sulphur and sodium salicylate, the salt form of salicylic acid, are also found in unequal concentrations (USA, Sebbafon Shampoo, Upjohn). This shampoo has good emollient properties by use of an entsufon sodium base, lanolin, and petrolatum.

Benzoyl peroxide

Benzoyl peroxide (USA, OxyDex Shampoo, DVM; Pyoben, Allerderm: UK, Oxydex Shampoo, C-Vet; Paxcutol, Virbac) is a good keratolytic with potent antimicrobial and degreasing activities which is very useful in severe cases of greasy scale, especially with a secondary bacterial component. Part of the degreasing effect is a result of reduced sebaceous gland activity. Benzoyl peroxide also has a flushing action which enhances removal of scale, glandular secretions and bacteria from hair follicles. Sulphur has been formulated with benzoyl peroxide (USA, Sulf OxyDex Shampoo, DVM) to augment keratolytic activity.

Benzoyl peroxide may be helpful in greasy scaling conditions such as primary seborrhoea in spaniels, terriers, basset hounds, and German shepherd dogs; epidermal dysplasia of West Highland white terriers, vitamin A responsive dermatosis, canine acne, greasy ear margin dermatosis, schnauzer comedo syndrome, follicular dystrophies, demodicosis and pyoderma.

Irritancy with erythema, pain, and pruritus may be a problem in dogs and cats when benzoyl peroxide is used in concentrations over 5%. Most of the human products are 5% or higher in concentration and should not be used. Benzoyl peroxide is very drying due to its degreasing activity. Unless the animal is very greasy, benzoyl peroxide shampoo needs to be followed by an emollient bath oil rinse or alternated with a less drying product. Owners must be warned about the potential for bleaching of fabrics.

Tar

Tar is probably the most commonly utilised anti-scaling agent in veterinary and human dermatology. In fact, it is probably over used in cases with dry or mild greasy scale formation when a sulphur and salicylic acid shampoo would be equally effective and less iritant. Tar is keratoplastic, antipruritic, degreasing and vasoconstrictive. The keratoplastic effect occurs by suppression of epidermal growth and DNA synthesis in the basal cell layer of the epidermis. Tar is usually added to the treatment program when degreasing activity is desired.

Different production techniques, especially variations in temperature and type of coal, will affect efficacy of the final preparation. Because of this, and potential packaging problems, such as leaching of the coal tar through the plastic container, labels should be followed carefully and only products from reputable companies should be used. Other potential problems include irritancy, odour, staining and photosensitisation. Tar products should not be used on cats and are unnecessary since scaling in this species usually responds well to sulphur and salicylic acid shampoos. Tars are usually formulated with sulphur and salicylic acid.

Many veterinary tar shampoos are available. The primary difference between these products is the concentration of tar. Care must be used in interpreting labels with regard to tar concentration. Tar solution is not the same as tar extract or refined tar. Thus, a shampoo containing 2.5% tar solution actually contains only 0.5% tar since the solution contains only 20% tar. Also, the type of refinement used for an individual tar product may be important since the pharmacologically active components may be altered in the final products. Other differences include whether sulphur and salicylic acid are added and their concentrations.

It is generally believed that a higher tar concentration will result in superior suppression of epidermal growth and DNA synthesis and thus better clinical efficacy. However, this is not always the case and is certainly not totally predictable. Tar probably exerts its effect in many other ways than simply by suppression of DNA synthesis. The higher concentration formulations demonstrate better efficacy for the severe oily scaling disorders. Tar shampoos are usually reserved for severe, greasy, primary idiopathic seborrhoea which has not responded to products containing sulphur, salicylic acid or benzoyl peroxide.

There are three tar shampoos now available that have been formulated in an attempt to retain the desirable keratoplastic and degreasing characteristics of tar while minimising the undesirable side effects. These products lather well and have a surprisingly pleasing odour. Although products containing 3% and 4% tar may have better clinical efficacy in severe cases of greasy scaling because of better degreasing activity, the products containing less tar have better owner compliance.

A 2% solubilised coal tar extract shampoo (USA, Clear Tar Shampoo, Veterinary Prescription: UK, Clinitar, Shire) is one of these aesthetically pleasing veterinary tar formulations. This clear amber liquid has a pleasant smell, good clinical activity, and its parent tar extract has performed well in laboratory DNA synthesis suppression assays (Lowe et al., 1982). It also contains lanolin and coconut oil extract as emollients to minimise drying. Another refined tar extract shampoo (U.S.A., NuSal-T Shampoo, DVM) is equivalent to 2% crude coal tar along with 3% salicylic acid and 1% menthol. The enhanced concentration of salicylic acid is to attain greater keratolytic activity and menthol is included for cooling and antipruritic effects. A 4% solubilised coal tar shampoo (U.S.A., T-Lux Shampoo, Allerderm) also contains 2% sulphur and 2% salicylic acid for enhanced keratolytic and keratoplastic activity.

There are two 3% veterinary tar shampoos (USA, LyTar Shampoo, DVM; Mycodex High Potency Tar and Sulphur Shampoo, SmithKline Beecham: UK, Tar-Lite, C-Vet; Sebolytic, Virbac) on the market which also contain sulphur and salicylic acid. Both are dark brown opaque suspensions and have a strong odour. They are used for moderate to severe oily scaling when sulphur and salicylic acid shampoos, benzoyl peroxide shampoos and lower concentration tar products are not effective. For even more severe oily scaling and when the 3% tar products do not work, a 4% veterinary tar shampoo (USA, Allerseb-T Shampoo, Allerderm) is available.

A recent study (Gordon, 1992) compared antiseborrhoeic effects of veterinary anti-scaling shampoos using a quantitative corneocyte count assay. No statistically significant differences were found among the shampoos because of the short duration of the study. However, potentially important trends were observed. After 4 weeks of twice weekly shampoos corneocyte production was favorably decreasing from sites treated with SebaLyt, NuSal-T and LyTar. On the other hand, counts were increasing from sites treated with Sebolux, T-Lux, and Allerseb-T. Further work will be needed to better substantiate these results.

As the tar concentration increases, the chances for excessive drying, staining and follicular irritation also increase. Owners should be advised to apply the higher concentration tar products with care and to massage into the hair coat very gently and in the direction of hair growth. This should be followed by a thorough rinse. Excessive drying may necessitate the use of an emollient bath oil rinse after each shampoo or alternating with a lower-concentration tar product, a sulphur and salicylic acid shampoo, or a hypoallergenic moisturising shampoo. Follicular irritation should be considered if the client calls with the complaint that the animal has suddenly developed "hive-like" lesions with pruritus after bathing.

Selenium sulphide

Selenium sulphide is keratolytic, keratoplastic and degreasing. It works to control scale by depressing epidermal cell turnover rate and interfering with hydrogen bond formation in keratin. It is reported to have some residual adherence to the skin. This is one of the older anti-scaling products with limited uses because it is staining, drying, and may be irritating, especially to mucous membranes and the scrotum. It is usually considered only in severe cases of oily scaling which are non-responsive to sulphur and salicylic acid, benzoyl peroxide and tar. Some cocker spaniels with primary idiopathic seborrhoea seem to do surprisingly well on this product when all other forms of therapy have failed. Several veterinary selenium-containing shampoos are available but in the author's experience they are more irritating than the human product (USA, Selsun Blue, Ross: UK, Selsun, Abbot). This shampoo is available in the same concentration as the veterinary products and is in a pleasant-scented detergent vehicle.

General Recommendations for Anti-Scaling Shampoos

Mild dry scaling may simply respond to a moisturising, hypoallergenic shampoo. If the dry scaling is more severe and does not respond to a moisturising shampoo, then a sulphur and salicylic acid combination should next be considered. Bath oil rinses or humectants should be applied after the skin has been hydrated by bathing. These moisturisers may also be effectively applied between shampoos using a plant mister bottle.

If the dry scaling is severe and still non-responsive, then tar products may be necessary. However, since tars are degreasing, further drying may result even though scale formation from the epidermis is being better controlled. After bath moisturising rinses are mandatory in these dogs. Additionally, the tar shampoo may need to be alternated with a cleansing and moisturising shampoo to prevent excess drying.

For cases of oily or greasy scaling, benzoyl peroxide, benzoyl peroxide with sulfur, tars and selenium sulphide are useful alone or alternating in combination. High concentrations of these products may be irritating and very drying. Thus, after the severe problem is controlled, switching to the most innocuous agent to control the condition is indicated. For greasy scale complicated by pyoderma, alternating a tar and a benzoyl peroxide product is useful. An emollient antibacterial shampoo with 0.5% (USA, Nolvasan Shampoo, Fort Dodge), 1.0% (USA, ChlorhexiDerm Shampoo DVM) or 4% (UK, Hibiscrub skin cleaner) chlorhexidine would be preferred to benzoyl peroxide in the case of dry scaling with pyoderma.

Spaniels, basset hounds, terriers, and German shepherd dogs tend to develop a pruritic, greasy scaling disease and they seem to benefit most from benzoyl peroxide, benzoyl peroxide and sulphur, and higher concentration tar shampoos without moisturising bath oil and water rinses or soakings. Doberman pinschers usually have a heavy accumulation of dry or waxy scale and so do better with a less drying agent such as a sulphur and salicylic acid containing shampoo. The skin must be rehydrated using frequent moisturising bath oil and water rinses and moisturising sprays between bathings. Irish setters present a therapeutic challenge. Some will have very dry scaling while others will be greasy and yet others may have areas of dry and greasy scaling on the same animal. Thus, two shampoos may be needed at each bathing; a moisturising shampoo for dry areas and a degreasing product for oily areas.

Topical Formulations for Localised Scaling

Tretinoin

Topical 0.05% tretinoin cream (Retin-A, Ortho) increases epidermal turnover rate and reduces cohesion of keratinocytes, making it useful in localised follicular or epidermal hyperkeratotic scaling disorders. It has efficacy for chin acne in dogs and cats when given daily until remission and then as needed for maintenance. In some acne cases it is alternated with topical benzoyl peroxide gel (USA, OxyDex Gel, DVM, Pyoben Gel, Allerderm: UK, Oxydex Gel, C-Vet). Tretinoin will also help control idiopathic nasal hyperkeratosis when used along with an occlusive emollient such as petrolatum. Allergic or irritant cutaneous reactions may be a problem in some cases. Tretinoin is available in lower concentrations (0.025 and 0.01%) in gel formulations for these patients. Alternating the retinoid with a 1.0% hydrocortisone cream may also help control such reactions.

Lactic acid

Lactic acid has hygroscopic activity at low concentrations and is keratolytic at higher concentrations. A high concentration lactic acid lotion (LactiCare, Stiefel) is useful for idiopathic nasal hyperkeratosis, calluses and ear margin dermatosis. It should be applied daily until the condition is controlled and then as needed for maintenance. It is a non-prescription human product which is well tolerated by dogs.

Salicylic acid

In addition to shampoo formulations, salicylic acid at 6% has been formulated with 5% urea and 5% sodium lactate as a keratolytic humectant gel (USA, KeraSolv, DVM Pharmaceuticals). This is also used for idiopathic nasal hyperkeratosis, calluses, ear margin dermatosis and acne. It should be applied daily until the condition is controlled and then as needed for maintenance.

Salicylic acid (0.5%, 2%) alcohol pads (USA, Stri-Dex Pads, Regular and Maximum Strength, Glenbrook) are helpful when used daily for chin acne to remove comedones from hair follicles. These may be irritating for some animals because of the alcohol content.

Ceruminolytic agents

Some dogs with scaling dermatoses may have focal areas of severe greasy scale which are poorly responsive to degreasing shampoos such as high concentration tars and benzoyl peroxide. The best example is the cocker spaniel with idiopathic seborrhoea and severe oily scaling of the ventral neck and trunk, axillae and interdigital areas.

These problem areas may be more easily managed by application of a ceruminolytic agent before bathing. Fifteen minutes prior to each bath, a topical ceruminolytic agent such as dioctyl sodium sulphosuccinate (USA, Clear-X Ear Cleansing Solution, DVM Pharmaceuticals) is applied to the affected areas. It is then washed off during the shampoo. This results in increased removal of debris and more rapid resolution of the condition. There may also be increased control of the associated odour.

ANTIMICROBIAL AGENTS

Staphylococcal pyoderma

One of the most common clinical presentations to the veterinary practitioner is pyoderma due to *Staphylococcus intermedius*. This cutaneous infection is usually secondary to an underlying dermatosis. The key to successful management is to diagnose and control the primary disease (Chapter 6). However, antibiotics and topical therapy are needed to control infection until this can be accomplished (Chapter 25). Topical therapy is an important adjunct in the management of recurrent superficial and deep pyodermas. It is most helpful when used prophylactically to decrease the severity and frequency of recurrence of the infection.

Benzoyl peroxide. Antibacterial shampoos are the most commonly employed method of topical therapy for superficial and deep pyodermas. Benzoyl peroxide products are especially effective because of their excellent antimicrobial activity, follicular flushing action and residual effects for 48 hours (Kligman *et al.*, 1977). Benzoyl peroxide was shown in a controlled quantitative study (Kwochka and Kowalski, 1991) to have superior prophylactic activity against *S. intermedius* when compared to chlorhexidine, complexed iodine and triclosan. Human formulations should not be used, unless the benzoyl peroxide concentration is under 5%, since the higher percentage products are irritating to dog skin. Owners must be warned about the potential for bleaching of fabrics. As described above, benzoyl peroxide is also keratolytic and degreasing. Whereas these actions will be beneficial in many cases, they can inhibit long-term usage in others because of excessive drying of the skin. In these cases a bath oil or humectant rinse (USA, HyLyt*efa Bath Oil Coat Conditioner, DVM; Humilac Dry Skin Spray and Rinse, Allerderm; Alpha-Sesame Oil Dry Skin Rinse, Veterinary Prescription: UK, Humilac, Virbac, Hylashine, C-Vet) should be used after each bathing to rehydrate the skin and hair coat. Benzoyl peroxide is also manufactured in gel formulations (OxyDex Gel, Pyoben Gel) for use on localised pyodermas such as furunculosis of the chin and pressure point pyoderma.

Chlorhexidine is a synthetic biguanide with broad-spectrum antibacterial and antifungal activity. It has the qualities of rapid kill with good residual activity. Twenty-six % remains on the skin after 29 hours and the residue is in an active form (Gilman *et al.*, 1985). It is nonirritating, nontoxic and is effective in organic debris. Chlorhexidine is found in shampoo formulations at concentrations of 1% (ChlorhexiDerm Shampoo), 0.5% (Nolvasan Shampoo) and 4% (Hibiscrub skin cleanser). Although it does not have the follicular flushing activity of benzoyl peroxide, it has the advantage of being in emollient formulations for long-term use on dry skin and coat.

Complexed iodine is bactericidal, fungicidal, virucidal and sporicidal. It is found in scrub and shampoo formulations (USA, Weladol Shampoo, Pitman Moore; Betadine preparations) but is more irritating than benzoyl peroxide or chlorhexidine, has the disadvantage of staining light coloured hair coats, and has only 6 hours of prolonged activity.

Mupirocin (U.S.A., Bactoderm, SmithKline-Beecham: U.K., Bactroban, Beecham) is a topical antibiotic in a polyethylene glycol base for localised pyoderma. It has excellent activity against Gram-positive cocci, is bactericidal, works well at an acid pH, is not systemically absorbed and is not chemically related to other antibiotics. Mupirocin penetrates very well into granulomatous deep pyoderma lesions such as interdigital abscesses. Significant decrease in severity and relapse rate of superficial and deep pyodermas is possible if owners immediately apply mupirocin twice daily when they first notice early lesions developing. This is especially true of localised conditions such as chin pyoderma, pressure point pyoderma and interdigital abscesses.

***Malassezia* dermatitis.** As with *S. intermedius*, *Malassezia pachydermatis* is increasingly recognised as a cause of skin infections in dogs secondary to underlying dermatoses (Mason, 1993). It seems especially prevalent in cases with severe greasy scaling, inflammation and pruritus. The infection must be controlled with appropriate topical and/or systemic antifungal agents to give the patient relief while a definitive diagnosis of the underlying dermatosis is being pursued.

Ketoconazole. In the author's practice, the most effective topical therapy to date has been with twice weekly ketoconazole shampoos (Nizoral Shampoo, Janssen).Treatment is continued until the condition is controlled followed by maintenance therapy as needed. This shampoo is very expensive. Severe cases which do not respond to topical therapy require oral ketoconazole (Nizoral, Janssen) at 10 mg/kg, for at least 30 days.

Miconazole lotion (Conofite Lotion, Pitman-Moore) or cream (U.S.A., Conofite Cream, Pitman-Moore: U.K., Daktarin, Janssen) is valuable for locally severe lesions such as pododermatitis, cheilitis and *Malassezia* otitis externa. A miconazole, chlorhexidine, and selenium sulphide shampoo (Sebolyse Foam, Dermcare) has been effective in Australia for dogs with *Malassezia* dermatitis (Mason, 1993). Recently a 2% miconazole and 0.5% chlorhexidine shampoo (Dermazole, Allerderm) has been marketed in the United States. No clinical studies have been reported using this product for *Malassezia* dermatitis or other fungal infections. Cost is comparable with that of ketoconazole shampoo.

Benzoyl peroxide. Studies in humans have shown excellent results using 2.5% benzoyl peroxide in patients with facial seborrhoeic dermatitis due to *Pityrosporum ovale* (Bonnetblanc and Bernard, 1986). Decreased sebaceous gland activity may play as much of a role as directly killing the fungus since it has been shown in studies in humans that sebum exerts a permissive effect on the growth of *P. ovale*. Benzoyl peroxide shampoos have given variable results when used in dogs with *Malassezia* dermatitis.

Selenium sulphide 2.5% works well to control *P. ovale* in humans and *Malassezia* in dogs. It has limited clinical efficacy at 1.0% in shampoo formulations. An alternative approach is to use the 1% selenium sulfide shampoo to remove scale and sebum followed by a topical enilconazole rinse (Imaverol, Janssen) (Mason, 1993).

Chlorhexidine. A 1% chlorhexidine shampoo (ChlorhexiDerm Shampoo, DVM) may be effective against *Malassezia*. However, 2% to 4% scrubs generally have a greater efficacy.

ANTIPRURITIC AGENTS

Although by no means appropriate as sole therapy in pruritic skin diseases, topical therapy may be helpful in symptomatic relief of pruritus. If owners are willing to expend the time and effort needed for administration of topical therapy, the requirements for high levels of systemic steroids and other anti-inflammatory agents will be decreased.

The residual antipruritic activity of most of the topical agents is minimal, 1 to 3 days. Shampoos and rinses are required for regionalised or generalised pruritus. Ointments, creams, gels and lotions are used for localised areas of pruritus. The topical agents are divided into nonsteroidals and topical glucocorticoids. This sections will concentrate on the nonsteroidals. A discussion of topical glucocorticoids for pruritus is found elsewhere (Griffin, 1993).

Hypoallergenic shampoos

Bathing contributes to relief of pruritus by removing organic and inorganic debris from the skin surface (including surface allergens and bacteria), by cooling the skin surface and by hydrating the stratum corneum. The hypoallergenic, cleansing-moisturising shampoos discussed above are best for this purpose since they have less potential to irritate already inflamed pruritic skin. Mild antibacterial shampoos containing chlorhexidine may be preferred when a secondary pyoderma is present.

Oatmeal. Colloidal oatmeal (Aveeno Colloidal Oatmeal, Rydelle) cool water rinses or soaks provide short-term relief of pruritus. Oilated oatmeal (Aveeno Oilated Oatmeal, Rydelle) is available for animals with very dry skin and hair coat. The powder form is preferred to the bar form and may be used as a rinse or soaking solution. A mixture of 2 tablespoons of powder per gallon of water is usually sufficient as a rinse. For soaking, a packet of the powder should be placed in cheesecloth or nylon stockings and then placed in the soaking water. Soaks should last for at least 10 to 15 minutes.

Recently, oatmeal has been incorporated into veterinary shampoo, cream rinse and powder formulations (Epi-Soothe preparations, Allerderm/Virbac). There are no studies reported on the efficacy of these products in controlling pruritus in dogs. My clinical experience is that the shampoo is no more effective than a hypoallergenic moisturising product. The powder has comparable efficacy to the human products (Aveeno). There are anecdotal reports that the cream rinse may provide up to 3 days of relief from pruritus when applied full strength without rinsing. This would only be practical in nonhaired areas and in short-coated breeds.

Moisturising rinses

Moisturising bath oil and humectant rinses and sprays help control pruritus by rehydrating dry skin by increasing the water content of the stratum corneum. These agents are discussed in the next section.

Table 2
Selected moisturizers and antipruritic rinses.

Trade Name	Manufacturer	Active Ingredient(s)	Usage
Aveeno Colloidal Oatmeal	Rydelle	100% colloidal oatmeal	Dog and Cat
Aveeno Oilated Bath	Rydelle	43% colloidal oatmeal, mineral oil, petrolatum	Dog and Cat
Epi-Soothe Bath Treatment	Allerderm/Virbac	100% colloidal oatmeal	Dog and Cat
Epi-Soothe Cream Rinse	Allerderm/Virbac	Colloidal oatmeal	Dog and Cat
Humilac Dry Skin Spray and Rinse	Allerderm/Virbac	Lactic acid, glycerin, urea, propylene glycol	Dog and Cat
HyLyt*efa Bath Oil Coat Conditioner (USA)	DVM Pharmaceuticals	Essential fatty acids, lanolin, emulsified oils, polyvinyl polymers, Na lactate, glycerin, mineral oil, safflower oil	Dog and Cat
Micro Pearls Humectant Spray (USA)	Evsco	Encapsulated lactic acid	Dog and Cat
Sesame Oil Emulsion Spray (USA)	Veterinary Prescription	Sesame oil, vitamin E	Dog and Cat
Alpha-Sesame Oil Dry Skin Rinse (USA)	Veterinary Prescription	Cottonseed oil, lanolin, sesame oil, PEG-4 dilaurate	Dog and Cat

Localised pruritus

When pruritus is localised to smaller areas, numerous more expensive, lotions, gels, creams and ointments may be used. Most of these contain glucocorticoids, but a variety of nonglucocorticoid formulations are available. Active ingredients include camphor, menthol, and witch hazel (PTD, Veterinary Prescription; Dermacool, Allerderm/Virbac) for their cooling effects, topical anaesthetics, and topical antihistamines. A veterinary shampoo (Histacalm, Allerderm) which contains the antihistamine, diphenhydramine hydrochloride, has recently been marketed in the USA. There are no studies reported on the efficacy of this product in controlling pruritus in dogs.

MOISTURISING AGENTS

These products are used to lubricate, rehydrate, soften and moisturise the skin. There are several categories of moisturising agents (Wehr and Krochmal, 1987) including emollients, emulsifier/ emollients, occlusives and humectants.

Emollients, emulsifiers, and occlusives

Emollients smooth the roughened surfaces of the stratum corneum by filling the spaces between dry skin flakes with oil droplets. Used alone they are not occlusive (unless in very high concentrations) and provide only temporary symptomatic relief. Emollients include oils, animal fats and hydrocarbons used for their local effect in protecting and softening the skin, increasing pliability and serving as vehicles for drugs. Emollient oils include olive, cottonseed, corn, almond, peanut, persia, coconut, sesame and safflower. Lanolin is animal fat from the wool of sheep. Hydrocarbons include paraffin, petrolatum and mineral oil.

Emulsified bath oils are highly dispersible agents that have emulsifiers to distribute the emollient oil in water. Common emulsifiers include PEG-4 dilaurate, stearic acid, stearyl alcohol, cetyl alcohol, laureth-4 and lecithin. With an emulsifier/emollient combination (Alpha-Sesame Oil Dry Skin Rinse) externally applied water can be held in the stratum corneum to prolong hydration.

Petrolatum is not only an emollient but is also occlusive. Occlusive agents block the surface of the stratum corneum and reduce transepidermal water loss to the environment. This results in increased water content in the stratum corneum.

Humectants

Humectant sprays and rinses use components of the natural moisturising factor (NMF), such as carboxylic acid, lactic acid and urea, to rehydrate the skin without oil. Other humectants include sodium lactate, glycerin, propylene glycol and polyvinyl pyrrolidone. These agents hydrate the stratum corneum by attracting transepidermal water to it, not by attracting water from the environment.

Lactic acid is used in its free form and has also been incorporated into liposomes. These spherical structures are composed of concentric lipid bilayers with a central., hollow, core for drug storage. They release the active ingredient over a period of time and thus result in more residual activity. Liposomes are used in a humectant spray formulation (USA, Micro Pearls Humectant Spray, EVSCO).

Glycerin, propylene glycol and urea are humectants and are also classified as demulcent polyhydroxy compounds. A demulcent is a high molecular weight compound that forms aqueous solutions which have the ability to alleviate irritation by coating the skin surface and protecting the underlying cells from stimuli. Glycerin, a trihydric alcohol, is miscible with water and alcohol and is a popular vehicle for many cutaneous drugs.

Propylene glycol is a clear colourless viscous liquid which is miscible with water and dissolves many essential oils. In low concentrations it is an effective humectant because it is hygroscopic. At concentrations of 40 to 50% it is antibacterial and antifungal and serves as an excellent vehicle because of its ability to enhance percutaneous penetration of drugs. Above concentrations of 50% it denatures and solubilises protein and is therefore keratolytic. It is found in veterinary bath oil rinse formulations and has reported efficacy when mixed as a 75% rinse in water or a humectant (Humilac) for ichthyosis and sebaceous adenitis.

Urea promotes hydration and removal of excess keratin and is beneficial in cases with dry, hyperkeratotic skin. At concentrations below 20%, urea acts as a humectant by its hygroscopic action. Above 40% it is keratolytic due to proteolytic activity on keratin and prekeratin. It is found in a veterinary bath oil rinse formulation (Humilac).

Principles of Moisturiser Therapy

Commercial moisturisers are beneficial for cases of dry scaling and after use of drying agents such as benzoyl peroxide, tar and topical flea products. They are also important in control of pruritus by rehydration of the stratum corneum. It is impossible to determine for an individual animal with a scaling dermatosis, whether an emollient (Sesame Oil Emulsion Spray), an emollient/emulsifier (Alpha-Sesame Oil Dry Skin Rinse), or a humectant (Humilac) product will give better results. One preparation (HyLyt*efa Bath Oil Coat Conditioner) contains a combination of 3 emollients and 2 humectants. The author has found that emollients work well with all types of coat length and texture. Humectants seem to work better on dogs with short hair than on long, thick coated breeds. Some owners may not enjoy using emollient products because they perceive an oily consistency to the coat after it is dry. This is usually not a problem if there is strict adherence to the recommended dilutions. However, the oil-free humectants offer an alternative in these situations.

The maximum hydrating effect is best achieved when a rinse is applied after bathing while the stratum corneum is still moist. The rinse should be diluted with water according to label directions and then poured or sponged over the entire body and allowed to air dry. Moisturising rinses may also be diluted with flea dips to minimise the drying effects of insecticides and petroleum distillates. They may also be diluted in plant mister bottles and sprayed on the skin and hair coat between baths as needed. However, emollients are less effective than humectants when used in this manner since the stratum corneum has not been hydrated prior to their application. Finally, they may be sprayed directly from the bottle at full strength for severe local hyperkeratotic lesions such as those seen with calluses, nasodigital hyperkeratosis and ear margin dermatosis.

In addition to their emollient effects, three products are potentially beneficial when an essential fatty acid deficiency is suspected (U.S.A., Sesame Oil Emulsion Spray, Alpha-Sesame Oil Dry Skin Rinse, HyLyt*efa Bath Oil Coat Conditioner: U.K., Hylashine, C-Vet)). Topical application of essential fatty acids has been shown to be an effective way to correct epidermal changes associated with the deficiency. Four to 6 weeks of daily application is needed to assess efficacy. Such frequent application may make the skin and hair coat too oily and limit usefulness.

REFERENCES

BONNETBLANC, J.M. and BERNARD, P. (1986). Benzoyl peroxide in seborrheic dermatitis. *Archives of Dermatology*, **122**, 752.

GILMAN, A.G., GOODMAN, L.S., RALL, T.W. and MURAD, F. (1985). *Goodman and Gilman's The Pharmacological Basis of Therapeutics 7th edn*. New York, MacMillan Publishing Co.

GORDON, J.G. (1992). Corneocyte counts as a method for evaluating the effects of antiseborrheic shampoos in the dog. In: *8th Proceedings, Annual Members' Meeting, AAVD & ACVD*. p. 3, Montreal, Quebec, Canada.

GRIFFIN, C.E. (1993). Canine atopic disease. In: *Current Veterinary Dermatology: The Science and Art of Therapy*, (Eds. C.E. Griffin, K.W. Kwochka and J.M. MacDonald) Mosby Year Book, St. Louis.

KLIGMAN, A.M., LEYDEN, J.J and STEWART, R. (1977). New uses for benzoyl peroxide: a broad-spectrum antimicrobial agent. *International Journal of Dermatogy*, **16**, 413.

KWOCHKA, K.W. and KOWALSKI, J.J. (1991). Prophylactic efficacy of four antibacterial shampoos against *Staphylococcus intermedius* in dogs. *American Journal of Veterinary Research*, **52**, *115*.

LEYDEN, J.J., McGINLEY, K.J., MILLS, O.H., KYRIAKOPOULOS, A.A and KLIGMAN, A.M. (1987). Effects of sulfur and salicylic acid in a shampoo base in the treatment of dandruff: a double-blind study using corneocyte counts and clinical grading. *Cutis*, **39**, *557*.

LIN, A.N., REIMER, R.J. and CARTER D.M. (1988). Sulfur revisited. *Journal of American Academy of Dermatology*, **18**, *533*.

LOWE, N.J., BREEDING, J.H. and WORTZMAN, M.S. (1982). New coal tar extract and coal tar shampoos. *Archives of Dermatology*, **118**, 487

MASON, K.V., (1993). Cutaneous *Malassezia*. In: *Current Veterinary Dermatology: the Science and Art of Therapy*, (Eds. C.E. Griffin, K.W. Kwochka and J.M. MacDonald) Mosby Year Book, St. Louis.

WEHR, R.F. and KROCHMAL, L. (1987). Considerations in selecting a moisturizer. *Cutis*, **39**, 512.

GLUCOCORTICOIDS – USE AND ABUSE

Ewan A Ferguson

INTRODUCTION

There can be little doubt that glucocorticosteroids are amongst the most valuable therapeutic agents available to the veterinary practitioner and that they are also amongst the most frequently abused. Cortisol was first synthesised in 1948 and successfully used to treat rheumatoid arthritis in 1949. Barely three years later the first death from iatrogenic adrenocortical atrophy was reported in man. Corticosteroid-induced adrenal atrophy was described in dogs in 1961 and by 1968 the death of a dog following glucocorticoid withdrawal had been reported. In 1974 Scott and Greene drew attention to the problem of iatrogenic secondary adrenocortical insufficiency and the principles of glucocorticoid therapy have now been taught to veterinary graduates for many years. Unfortunately, deaths due to glucocorticoid abuse still occur and it has been estimated that up to half the cases of dogs recognised to be suffering from glucocorticoid excess are of iatrogenic origin. Many more animals treated with glucocorticoids develop marked adrenocortical atrophy without displaying obvious external signs.

Glucocorticoids have an extremely wide range of effects, influencing to a greater or lesser degree virtually every mammalian cell. A thorough understanding of their physiological and pharmacological actions is required if a satisfactory balance is to be struck between their desirable and adverse effects. Factors such as the appropriate dose rate, relative potency and duration of action must be considered. Intercurrent disease or medication, pregnancy and effect on other investigations such as intradermal skin testing will influence the decision whether or not these drugs should be employed. Without exception, their use should have a rational basis and they should not be administered speculatively. To do otherwise represents an abuse not only of the drug but of the veterinary profession's privilege to prescribe and dispense medication.

PHYSIOLOGY

The steroid hormones secreted by the adrenal cortex are collectively known as corticosteroids. Cholesterol is converted by a process of side chain cleavage to pregnenolone which acts as a common precursor for mineralocorticoid, glucocorticoid and androgen synthesis. The naturally produced glucocorticoids derive from the adrenal *zona fasiculata* and *zona reticularis* and comprise more than 95% of the total corticosteroid production (Table 1). Low plasma cortisol concentrations favour the release of corticotrophin releasing factor (CRF) from neurones located in the anterior portion of the paraventricular nuclei within the hypothalamus into the hypothalamo-pituitary portal system. CRF stimulates the release of adrenocorticotrophic hormone (ACTH) and other peptides from the anterior and intermediate lobes of the pituitary. The primary function of ACTH is to stimulate the secretion of the adrenal corticosteroids but it also induces adrenal steroidogenesis and controls adrenocortical cell replication. Plasma cortisol levels rise within a few minutes of ACTH release and initially exert a negative fast-feedback effect, decreasing CRF secretion and reducing further ACTH release. This initial inhibition is dependent on the rate at which plasma glucocorticoid levels rise, not the dose administered, suggesting that mediation occurs via a direct effect on the cell membrane. Delayed feedback inhibition further suppresses CRF and ACTH secretion by both dose and time-dependent mechanisms and appears to act via the classic glucocorticoid receptor. Prolonged administration of exogenous glucocorticoids leads to a profound fall in ACTH levels as the hypothalamic-pituitary-adrenal axis becomes progressively less responsive to stress or stimulation, ultimately leading to atrophy of the adrenal *zona fasiculata* and *zona reticularis*. ACTH secretion occurs as a number of episodic secretory bursts which in man occur more frequently in the early morning, giving rise to a diurnal rhythm. It is still uncertain whether or not a similar rhythm exists in companion animals. The overall level of secretion varies in response to factors including environmental stresses, feeding, photoperiod and intercurrent disease or injury. There is also considerable interspecies and individual variation.

Table 1
Secretion sites of the major endogenous corticosteroids

Hormone	Secretion rate (μ g/kg bodyweight per day)
Glucocorticoid	
Cortisol	700-800
Corticosterone	300-400
Desoxycortisol	80-90
Mineralocorticoid	
Desoxycorticosterone	5-10
Aldosterone	5-10
APPROXIMATE TOTAL	1,200 μg/kg

PHARMACOLOGY

All glucocorticoids are based on the cyclopentenoperhydrophenanthrene nucleus consisting of one pentane and three hexane rings. The rings are designated A-D and the carbon atoms numbered from 1-21. All have a hydroxyl group at the C-17 position, distinguishing them from androgenic steroids which have a 17-ketone group and a 19 carbon basic ring structure. The hepatic conversion of the C-11 keto group to an 11-hydroxyl group transforms inactive cortisone into the active form, hydrocortisone (Figure 1). For this reason C-11 keto compounds cannot be used topically. The addition of a 1,2 double bond increases glucocorticoid activity and slows hepatic degradation although 11-hydroxylation is again required to transform prednisone to the active analogue prednisolone. There is no firm evidence that hepatic disease substantially compromises this process. Methylprednisolone has slightly enhanced glucocorticoid activity produced by the addition of a 6-methyl group.

Figure 1
Structure of hydrocortisone showing basic glucocorticoid nucleus.

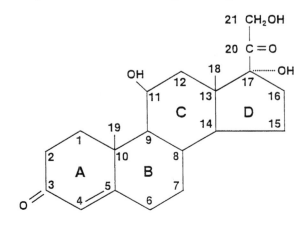

234

If fluorine is added to hydrocortisone at the 9-alpha position, both glucocorticoid and mineralocorticoid activity are increased. This compound, fluorohydrocortisone, forms the basic structure of most fluorinated steroids. The mineralocorticoid effects can be greatly reduced by methylation or masking of the C-16 or C-17 hydroxyl groups with various esters.

Further modification of 9-alpha fluorohydrocortisone is possible. The addition of a C1,2 double bond plus a 16-alpha hydroxyl group (triamcinolone), 16-alpha methyl group (dexamethasone) or a 16-beta methyl group (betamethasone) has given rise to a group of potent compounds with high glucocorticoid activity and negligible mineralocorticoid effects . All possess an 11-hydroxyl group and are therefore active forms. The relative potency and activity of the common glucocorticoids are summarised in Table 2.

Exogenous glucocorticoids administered orally are absorbed in the upper small intestine and food delays, but does not decrease, the amount absorbed. Endogenous glucocorticoid circulates bound to a specific cortisol-binding globulin or to albumin. Cortisol-binding globulin represents a high affinity, low capacity transport system whilst albumin forms a low affinity, high capacity reserve. Some 85-90% of endogenous cortisol is bound but it is the free fraction which is biologically active. In general, synthetic glucocorticoids bind less avidly than endogenous cortisol to these carrier proteins resulting in a greater active free fraction. Cortisol-binding globulin may be decreased with intercurrent disease, particularly in hypothyroidism, hepatic and renal disease. It may be increased during oestrus, pregnancy and hyperthyroidism. Albumin may also be reduced as a result of intercurrent disease or malnutrition. Glucocorticoids are inactivated by the reduction of double bonds or ketone groups at both hepatic and extrahepatic sites. Conjugation with sulphate or glucuronic acid occurs, producing water-soluble metabolites which are primarily excreted by the kidneys. Clearance may be accelerated during concurrent therapy with drugs such as phenobarbitone, phenylbutazone and phenytoin which cause the induction of hepatic enzymes.

Glucocorticoid esters must be converted to the parent drug to become biologically active. This occurs rapidly but is dependent on the solubility of the ester and the route of administration. Formulations intended for use in acute conditions must be water soluble; sodium phosphate and succinate esters are polar and highly water soluble. The bioavailability of poorly water soluble bases such as dexamethasone may be improved by presentation in solution with propylene glycol. Suspensions of poorly soluble esters such as acetates and pivalates are frequently administered by the intramuscular route in an attempt to provide long term therapy. Absorption is slow, governed by the rate of dissolution into surrounding tissue fluids which is limited by particle size. Poor

Table 2
Relative glucocorticoid (GC) and mineralocorticoid (MC)
potency and activity of the common glucocorticoids

Drug	GC potency	MC potency	Duration of effect (hrs)	Equivalent dose (mg)
Short-acting				
Cortisone	0.8	0.8	8-12	25.0
Hydrocortisone	1.0	1.0	8-12	20.0
Intermediate-acting				
Prednisone	4.0	0.25	24-36	5.0
Prednisolone	4.0	0.25	24-36	5.0
Methylprednisolone	5.0	0	24-36	4.0
Triamcinolone	5.0	0	24-36	4.0
Long-acting				
Dexamethasone	30.0	0	36-54	0.75
Betamethasone	35.0	0	36-54	0.6
Paramethasone	10	0	36-54	2

storage conditions may result in the formation of larger crystals which further slows dissolution. Although the glucocorticoids in these preparations usually have a short duration of action, the overall effect of the slow, constant release of the drug is to cause prolonged adrenocortical suppression. A single intramuscular dose of methylprednisolone acetate at the rate of 2.5 mg/kg suppresses the adrenal cortex for at least five weeks; triamcinolone acetonide at 0.22 mg/kg causes suppression for four weeks. Unfortunately, the anti-pruritic effects frequently do not last as long, prompting repetition of the therapy and thereby leading to an increased risk of adrenocortical atrophy.

MECHANISM OF ACTION

Glucocorticoids appear to affect all cells, although not necessarily in the same way. Receptors for glucocorticoids are found in most mammalian cells whilst receptors for other steroid hormones such as oestrogens or androgens are less widely distributed. The absolute number of receptors in any cell is limited and defines the degree to which each tissue responds. The sites are sensitive to changes in steroid structure and the affinity of binding closely correlates with potency. Unlike hydrocortisone, most synthetic analogues do not readily bind to mineralocorticoid receptors, thus they have little effect on electrolyte balance. Once the cell membrane is penetrated, the glucocorticoid binds to a protein aporeceptor inducing an allosteric change in the complex which exposes a site capable of binding to DNA and chromatin in the cell nucleus. Synthetic glucocorticoids have an increased duration of action due to their increased affinity for the glucocorticoid receptors and relative resistance to hepatic degradation. The majority of complexes are bound to inactive nuclear sites and only a small percentage are located at sites where the expression of specific genes can be modulated. Messenger and ribosomal RNA transcription is enhanced leading to the increased synthesis of specific proteins. The proteins produced modify the activity and response of the cell and continue to do so long after the glucocorticoid is excreted from the plasma; the duration of action of exogenous glucocorticoids does not, therefore, correlate with plasma half-life. The recovery of the adrenocortical response to exogenous ACTH administration provides a more useful measurement of the duration of the biological effect of these drugs. Cellular differentiation determines which genes are affected and, therefore, the unique response of different tissues. Quantitative differences in sensitivity exist between different tissues in the same animal and between the same tissues in different species. Changes in sensitivity may accompany differentiation, development and ageing and reflect changes in the absolute number of glucocorticoid receptors.

It is usually stated that all glucocorticoid effects are post-nuclear and whilst this appears to be true in most cases, certain steroid effects occur so rapidly that transcriptional events and *de novo* protein synthesis seem unlikely. In particular, the steroid induced inhibition of ACTH release occurs within a matter of minutes, too rapidly to reconcile with a post-nuclear mechanism. It remains possible, therefore, that some steroid effects occur through activation of non-nuclear receptors.

PHYSIOLOGICAL AND PHARMACOLOGICAL EFFECTS

Glucocorticoids are intimately involved in the maintenance of normal function of a wide variety of tissues and organs and play a central role in the physiological response to stress. The physiological effects are perhaps less varied than the pharmacological actions although this distinction is frequently difficult to make and may be based on quantitative rather than qualitative differences.

Glucocorticoids promote gluconeogenesis at the expense of muscle and fat tissue by promoting the formation of hepatic gluconeogenic enzymes. Hyperglycaemia is avoided by a concomitant increase in insulin secretion. Protein is mobilised from the majority of tissues with the exception of the liver where protein synthesis is promoted. The mobilisation and oxidation of fatty acids is enhanced and plasma cholesterol, triglyceride and glycerol concentrations increase. Not all adipose tissue is equally affected; there is an overall redistribution of fat from the extremities to the pelvis, neck, thorax and omentum giving rise to the characteristic physical appearance of animals with hyperadrenocorticism. Carbohydrate reserves are rapidly depleted following even a brief period of food deprivation in animals suffering from glucocorticoid deficiency. This results in a greatly increased sensitivity to insulin and the possibility of hypoglycaemia. Care should, therefore, be taken if the cessation of glucocorticoid therapy coincides with the introduction of unfamiliar and possibly unpalatable trial diets.

It is thought that glucocorticoids antagonise the effect of antidiuretic hormone (ADH) on the renal tubules, increase glomerular filtration and promote ADH inactivation leading to the increased diuresis that is commonly observed. Urinary potassium loss and urinary and faecal calcium loss are increased. Hypokalaemia is unlikely due to the weak mineralocorticoid effects of all the synthetic glucocorticoids except fluodrocortisone. Hypocalcaemia does not develop as long as the parathyroid glands function normally although secondary hyperparathyroidism and osteoporosis may eventually occur. Glucocorticoids may be contraindicated in renal disease.

There is an increased risk of gastrointestinal ulceration due to the effects on gastric secretion and mucosa. Pancreatic secretions become more viscous and the pancreatic duct epithelium becomes hyperplastic. Pancreatitis may be initiated or exacerbated by glucocorticoids.

The neutrophilia that accompanies glucocorticoid use results from increased production and a shift from the marginated pool and bone marrow into the circulating neutrophil pool. Egress from the circulation is also inhibited. Sequestration in the spleen and lungs and decreased efflux from the bone marrow results in a decreased circulating pool of lymphocytes, eosinophils and basophils. These effects are responsible for the phenomenon of the "stress leucogram".

Much of the information regarding the effect of glucocorticoids on the immune system derives from work in small laboratory mammals which appear to be particularly sensitive, leading to an overestimation of the suppressive effects of moderate glucocorticoid doses in the companion species. Thymic-derived (T) lymphocytes, and therefore cell-mediated immunity, are suppressed to a greater extent than bursa-equivalent (B) lymphocytes and humoral immunity. The inhibition of antigen endocytosis and presentation suggests that it would be sensible to minimise glucocorticoid therapy for a period immediately preceding and following inoculation with a novel antigen. This has particular relevance in hyposensitisation therapy as during induction, considerable pruritus persists for many animals. Glucocorticoids are probably best avoided during induction but can be administered as part of maintenance therapy without compromising the protective humoral response.

Unbound glucocorticoids pass freely through the placenta and may cause adrenocortical atrophy in the foetus. Teratogenic effects have also been reported. C-16 methylated glucocorticoids administered during late gestation can induce premature parturition in cows, sheep, horses and man. This may be a risk in cats and dogs. Foetal development may also be adversely affected.

The responses of the endocrine system are tightly integrated and exogenous glucocorticoid administration causes widespread disruption. In animals subjected to severe physiological stress the inhibitory effect of even small doses of glucocorticoid on the hypothalamic-pituitary-adrenal (H-P-A) axis may be overridden by the stimulation of ACTH secretion via suprahypothalamic neural stimuli. Pharmacological doses inhibit the secretion of many post-pro-opiomelanocortin peptides from the pituitary and decrease protein binding of thyroxine, giving rise to erroneously low serum concentrations on assay. A full review of the effects of glucocorticoids on the endocrine system is beyond the scope of this chapter. The major physiological and pharmacological effects of glucocorticoids are summarised in Table 3.

STRATEGIES FOR GLUCOCORTICOID USE

Glucocorticoids have been employed with varying success in the treatment of a wide spectrum of diseases. The major physiological indication for their use is idiopathic or iatrogenic adrenocortical insufficiency but they are far more commonly employed for their potent anti-inflammatory action. In each and every case where the use of glucocorticoids is contemplated, the potential benefits and hazards should be evaluated. There should always be a clear indication or rationale for their administration, whether alone or in combination with other drugs or treatments.

Several general therapeutic principles have emerged in the four decades since glucocorticoids were introduced:

1. Glucocorticoid therapy is palliative, not curative. These drugs are used to control symptoms associated with inflammation or for their immunomodulatory effect or, in the case of adrenocortical insufficiency, to provide physiological support either for life or until the adrenal cortex recovers.

Table 3
Major physiological and pharmacological effects of glucocorticoids

Carbohydrate, fat and protein metabolism
Promotes gluconeogenesis at the expense of muscle and adipose tissue
Mobilisation of protein from most of body except liver
Fatty acid mobilisation and oxidation promoted
Raises plasma cholesterol, triglyceride and glycerol concentrations
Redistribution of adipose tissue deposits

Water balance and electrolytes
Promotes diuresis
Increases urinary potassium loss
Increases urinary and faecal calcium loss

Gastrointestinal tract and liver
Increases gastric acid and pepsin secretion
Decreases mucosal cell proliferation
Promotes protein synthesis in liver
Increases vacuolisation with glycogen or fat and decreases mitochondria numbers in hepatocytes
Induces AP isoenzyme production by biliary endothelium, increases plasma ALT and GGT concentrations
Decreases calcium absorption leading to increased parathormone release

Musculoskeletal system
Induces muscular atrophy
Increases osteoclast activity due to increased parathormone levels leading to osteoporosis
Inhibits fibrocartilage growth and promotes catabolism of collagenous bone matrix
Inhibits Vitamin D activation

Central nervous system
Decreases seizure threshold
Mood alteration - hyperactivity, depression
Psychoses - aggression, amaurosis, disorientation, ataxia, vomiting
Stimulates appetite

Endocrine system
Suppresses ACTH secretion and hence endogenous glucocorticoid production
Reduces thyroid stimulating hormone release; decreases peripheral conversion of T4 to T3
Increases parathormone release
Antagonises receptor binding and post-receptor effects of insulin
Inhibits growth hormone and somatomedin release
Inhibits follicle stimulating hormone, luteinising hormone and prolactin release

Haematolymphatic system
Increases red blood cell production and decreases removal of old red blood cells
Increases pool of circulating neutrophils and may increase circulating monocytes
Decreases pool of circulating eosinophils, basophils and lymphocytes
Increases circulating platelets but platelet aggregation inhibited

Immunity
Inhibits neutrophil, macrophage and monocyte migration, chemotaxis and diapedesis
Inhibits phagocytosis, antigen processing and intracellular killing
Inhibits interferon production
Stabilises cell membranes and lysosomes, preventing release of lytic enzymes
Inhibits phospholipase A, blocking formation of mediators and inflammatory products derived
        from cell membrane phospholipids
Decreases capillary permeability
Reduces response to pyrogens

Dermatological effects
Inhibits anagen phase of hair growth cycle thereby promoting alopecia
Reduces sebaceous gland activity
Inhibits fibroblast proliferation and collagen synthesis, delaying wound healing and resulting in
        dermal atrophy and vascular fragility
Promotes abnormal deposition of calcium in skin (calcinosis cutis) and other tissues

AP = Alkaline phosphatase; ALT = Alanine aminotransferase; GGT = Gamma-glutamyl transpeptidase

2. There is considerable individual and interspecific variation in the dose of glucocorticoid required to achieve a desired effect. The appropriate dose for an individual must, therefore, be based to a certain extent on trial and error although general guidelines for each species will determine the initial dose administered. Where therapy is prolonged, the dose and response must periodically be re-evaluated.

3. A single dose of a short acting glucocorticoid is unlikely to have any harmful effect on the patient. Unless there are specific contraindications, two or three days of therapy with a short-acting preparation is also unlikely to be harmful unless extremely high doses are employed. However, this does not imply that glucocorticoids should be used speculatively; to do so without a specific indication for their use is poor medicine and although no harm may arise, their administration may greatly complicate or delay the diagnostic process.

4. The risk of adverse effects increases with the duration of therapy and with higher dose rates. The clinician must be alert to the development of symptoms associated with secondary problems and also be aware that some problems, such urinary tract infections, may be occult.

5. There is a significant risk of adrenocortical insufficiency manifesting if prolonged glucocorticoid therapy is abruptly discontinued. This may be life threatening.

SELECTION OF AN APPROPRIATE GLUCOCORTICOID

The decision whether or not to administer glucocorticoids is usually straightforward when the risks of therapy are outweighed by the dangers associated with the disease process. There is no qualitative difference in anti-inflammatory action between the different synthetic glucocorticoids and selection is therefore based on the route, dose rate and duration of therapy required. The most appropriate frequency of administration depends on the duration of the effect of the preparation and this varies with the compound, ester, vehicle, species and intercurrent disease.

Topical glucocorticoids are usually employed for a short period only and applied to a limited area. The delivery vehicle greatly modifies absorption with ointments, creams and lotions providing better delivery rates than foams, gels and sprays. Absorption is enhanced by occlusive dressings and modified by the integrity of the treated skin or mucous membrane. Active forms that do not require hepatic 11-hydroxylation must be used and the fluorinated glucocorticoids are a suitable choice for short term use. If long term use is contemplated, ointments or creams containing hydrocortisone at 0.25 - 2.5% should be used. Percutaneous absorption will occur with all topical glucocorticoids and significant systemic effects may be seen, up to and including iatrogenic hyperadrenocorticism. Owners should be encouraged to protect themselves from unnecessary contact by wearing gloves when administering topical agents.

Intralesional or sublesional injections may occasionally be indicated where a few small focal lesions are to be treated. The number of sites and the volume injected should be limited to minimise the systemic impact. Long acting, highly concentrated or potent glucocorticoids may cause dermal atrophy at the injection site. As with topical preparations, local injection will also lead to systemic effects.

Systemic administration can be achieved through oral or parenteral routes. The indications in veterinary dermatology for the use of parenteral glucocorticoids are extremely few and limited to the emergency treatment of acute adrenocortical insufficiency or where owner compliance or a fractious patient make oral medication impractical. Dexamethasone or betamethasone can be given orally or parenterally as a short term supportive measure if adrenocortical insufficiency is suspected as it does not cross react with most assays for endogenous cortisol and will not interfere with ACTH response tests. In all other circumstances, oral medication is the route of choice as it allows the most flexible control of the dose being administered.

Daily doses of any glucocorticoid are likely to rapidly produce profound H-P-A axis suppression but are justified in the initial stages of therapy when attempting to put a glucocorticoid-responsive disease into remission. There are numerous anecdotal reports that dexamethasone produces swifter remission of clinical signs than other glucocorticoids. This may be partly due to a longer plasma and metabolic half-life but this in turn means that adverse effects are more likely to be encountered. Dividing the daily dose produces more adverse effects than dosing once daily and for this reason as well as their low potency, short acting preparations such as hydrocortisone have little place in oral therapy. Glucocorticoids with an intermediate duration of action such as prednisolone, prednisone and methylprednisolone can be administered on an alternate day basis for an extended period without leading to significant H-P-A axis suppression and are generally considered to be the drugs of choice.

In spite of their widespread use, depot glucocorticoids have very few justifiable applications in dermatology. They should never be employed for their convenience as the risk of adverse systemic or local effects is too high when effective oral preparations are available. If oral medication is impossible and pruritus cannot be controlled by other means, the use of depot glucocorticoids may be justified but both clinician and client should be fully aware of the long term implications of this form of therapy.

CLINICAL INDICATIONS FOR GLUCOCORTICOID THERAPY

Different doses and therapeutic protocols are indicated for different dermatological conditions. These protocols fall into four main categories; physiological replacement therapy, control of pruritus, immunosuppressive and cytotoxic therapy. Inevitably, there is some overlap but in general, the principle aim of therapy will fall within one of these categories. Whilst allowance must always be made for individual variation, it is possible to provide general guidelines as to how these potent drugs should be employed.

Physiological replacement therapy

Idiopathic hypoadrenocorticism (Addison's disease) is an uncommon endocrinopathy which most full time dermatologists will encounter only rarely. Mineralocorticoid replacement therapy is required, usually for life. Glucocorticoid replacement therapy may also be required, particularly during the early stages of treatment but may not prove necessary for long term maintenance. This is in contrast to iatrogenic secondary adrenocortical insufficiency resulting from prolonged or inappropriate glucocorticoid therapy where replacement is essential to maintain health until the adrenal cortex recovers and endogenous glucocorticoids are produced in adequate quantities.

Significant suppression of the H-P-A axis is likely to occur in dogs after as little as two weeks daily glucocorticoid therapy. In cats, suppression appears to be more difficult to induce but may still occur. Restoration of normal H-P-A axis function essentially requires that exogenous glucocorticoids be discontinued. This must be achieved gradually to avoid adrenocortical insufficiency developing. Once the dose of glucocorticoid administered falls below physiological replacement levels, endogenous ACTH secretion may restart and the *zona fasiculata* and *reticularis* begin to recover. The *zona glomerulosa* is usually not affected and mineralocorticoid supplements are not required.

Prednisolone or prednisone, if not already in use, should replace other glucocorticoids and be administered at 0.1-0.2 mg/kg daily. Methylprednisolone may also be used at approximately 80% of this dose. Low dose therapy should be continued until any signs of iatrogenic hyperadrenocorticism have resolved, the duration of therapy being determined by the duration and degree of adrenocortical suppression that existed. This may take several months and maintenance doses may have to be doubled or tripled during periods of physiological stress such as surgery or serious illness. Once extra-adrenal symptoms have resolved, the daily replacement therapy should be reduced to an alternate day basis. Further gradual reduction in the alternate day dose should allow complete withdrawal after a month.

Control of pruritus

Pruritus is the single most important clinical sign reported in veterinary dermatology and the success of therapy is often determined, not least in the eyes of the client, by the success with which it is controlled or alleviated. The temptation exists to employ glucocorticoids whenever pruritus is encountered as they are cheap, easy to administer and extremely effective, providing a swift resolution or suppression of clinical signs. Frequently this symptomatic approach is a mistake as long term resolution or control of a pruritic dermatosis ultimately depends upon making an accurate diagnosis and appropriate specific therapy being directed at the underlying disease.

Used inappropriately, glucocorticoids may greatly delay the diagnostic process, perhaps for many months. They may exacerbate existing problems such as pyoderma or demodicosis and the results obtained from procedures such as biopsy, intradermal skin testing, endocrinological evaluations and biochemistry and haematology profiles will be altered, making the dermatologist's task needlessly difficult.

Glucocorticoids may justifiably be used to alleviate the intense pruritus associated with dermatoses such as sarcoptic mange or pyotraumatic dermatitis whilst specific therapy is used to treat the underlying problem. In such cases, the duration of therapy is short and provided that it does not exceed two weeks and an appropriate glucocorticoid has been used, it is not necessary to taper the dose before stopping treatment. Where significant pyoderma is present this approach is inappropriate and alternative anti-pruritics should be employed (Chapter 26).

On occasion, it may be required to control pruritus for a longer period. For atopic individuals with a strictly seasonal problem of no more than two to three months duration, alternate day glucocorticoids may be the most appropriate therapy. Some therapeutic regimes such as dietary trials and fatty acid supplementation may take several weeks before their efficacy can be properly assessed and glucocorticoids can be used to alleviate pruritus during the initial stages of treatment. If daily therapy has been used, it will be necessary to taper the glucocorticoid dose before therapy is stopped. The dose should be reduced to 1 mg/kg prednisolone (or the current dose if smaller) given on alternate days. Further tapering is achieved by halving the dose every five to seven days over two to three weeks at which point therapy can usually cease. If at any stage signs of adrenal insufficiency appear, supportive treatment should be instituted. As alternate day medication usually protects the H-P-A axis from suppression, tapering is less important but it is still a wise precaution if glucocorticoids have been administered for an extended period. It is also clearly essential to discontinue glucocorticoids well in advance of re-examination if any assessment of concurrent therapy is to be made.

Chronic glucocorticoid therapy must be administered on an alternate day basis if adverse effects are to be avoided. It is only indicated for the management of intractable severe pruritus that has proved unresponsive to alternative methods of management or where financial or practical considerations make glucocorticoids the most appropriate therapy. Compounds of intermediate duration are again indicated and the dose should be gradually lowered until the minimum effective dose is determined. It may be possible to lower the maintenance dose further by utilising the "steroid-sparing" effect reported with concurrent fatty acid supplementation. The use of antihistamines, mast cell stabilisers and other non-steroidal anti-inflammatory agents should be considered in order to achieve a similar result. Hyposensitisation may reduce the glucocorticoid requirement for part or all of the year by blunting the hypersensitivity response to seasonal or non-seasonal allergens. Topical therapy and regular ectoparasite control should not be neglected. The principle of summation of pruritus dictates that any ancillary measures that can be taken to reduce pruritus will help to minimise the dose of glucocorticoid required for maintenance.

Animals receiving long term glucocorticoid therapy may be vulnerable to opportunistic infections with bacteria, fungi or occasionally, viruses. This risk is greatly reduced with alternate day therapy. Up to 40% of such patients develop urinary tract infections and these may remain asymptomatic due to the inhibition of the inflammatory response. Ascending infections may then develop with potentially serious consequences. Urine samples should be collected by cystocentesis and screened for evidence of infection by urinalysis, cytology and culture. The febrile response to pyrogens is diminished and the clinical responses to infection such as pain and leucocytosis may be masked during long term therapy. More commonly, alterations in skin microclimate and defence mechanisms permit the development of widespread pyoderma or problems associated with other cutaneous microflora such as *Malassezia pachydermatis*. Intermittent or erratic therapy with glucocorticoids is likely to promote wide fluctuations in skin microclimate and it is probably preferable to encourage a regular, continuous therapeutic regime as this will be easier to manage and supervise. Demodicosis may arise or relapse and the development of "Norwegian" scabies, where large numbers of mites are present with minimal accompanying pruritus, has been described during glucocorticoid therapy.

Polyuria and secondary polydipsia, polyphagia and weight gain are the most common adverse effects and may be seen even on alternate day therapy. These and other less common problems may mean that glucocorticoids are unsuitable in some particularly sensitive individuals.

241

Immunosuppressive therapy

At high doses, glucocorticoids exert significant immunosuppressive actions although these are relatively weak compared to most of the other immunosuppressive agents in use today. It is common practice to combine glucocorticoids with one or more of the more potent preparations in order to induce remission of autoimmune or immune mediated disease. Non-specific immune mechanisms such as phagocytosis and intracellular killing are inhibited by anti-inflammatory doses of glucocorticoid but complement action and humoral immunity are only minimally affected. Prednisolone, prednisone or an equipotent dose of methylprednisolone are again the most appropriate glucocorticoids to employ. To suppress these aspects of the immune response, prednisolone or prednisone at 2-4 mg/kg daily is required. Cats may require even higher doses. The therapy of autoimmune and immune mediated skin disease is covered in more detail in Chapter 32.

Cytotoxic therapy

Glucocorticoids are used in the treatment of lymphoreticular neoplasia because of their anti-mitotic effects on lymphoid tissue. In some laboratory species there is a direct lytic effect on lymphoid cells but those of dogs and cats are generally resistant to this effect although some lysis of the cells of acute lymphoblastic leukaemia and lymphomas will occur. Glucocorticoids are used to treat mast cell tumours at doses up to 40 mg/m^2 daily tapering after two weeks to 20 mg/m^2 on alternate days. Initial chemotherapy usually includes other cytotoxic agents and cimetidine. A full description of the chemotherapeutic uses of glucocorticoids falls outside the scope of this chapter and further information should be obtained from a suitable oncology text.

EVALUATING PRURITUS THAT CEASES TO RESPOND TO GLUCOCORTICOID THERAPY

Not infrequently, pruritus that has been satisfactorily controlled with glucocorticoids begins to relapse. If the clinical response has altered, it is reasonable to conclude that some other factor has arisen or changed and it is essential that such cases be properly re-evaluated.

Check compliance and history

The most frequent reason for the breakdown of control is a failure to comply with the therapeutic protocol. Animals may become more difficult to administer tablets to or owners may become disillusioned. Medication may be interrupted during holidays. It is also worth confirming that the degree of pruritus reported is consistent with the clinical signs observed as different owners will assess pruritus according to individual criteria.

Eliminate secondary infection

Superficial and deep pyodermas are a very common cause of non-steroid responsive pruritus. Thorough examination, clipping the coat if necessary, will usually provide evidence for the presence of pyoderma and appropriate treatment can be instituted. The glucocorticoid dose should be lowered to the absolute safe minimum during antibiotic therapy. Dermatophytosis may also cause pruritus and if suspected, should be confirmed by fungal culture. Increased numbers of *Malassezia pachydermatis* may contribute significantly to pruritus and can best be demonstrated by cytological examination of tape strips or dry scrapes. Appropriate topical or systemic therapy can then be initiated. If any uncertainty persists, biopsy is indicated and in breeds such as the Shar-Pei or bull terrier, may be required to eliminate the possibility of demodicosis.

Eliminate other causes of pruritus

In flea allergic animals, re-infestation is a common reason for pruritus to recur. Compliance with both topical and environmental control should be checked and the possibility of a concurrent infestation with other ectoparasites such and *Cheyletiella* sp., *Sarcoptes scabiei* and *Trombicula* sp. should be considered. Therapeutic trials may be indicated.

Dietary intolerance may occur in conjunction with or subsequent to other hypersensitivity-mediated diseases and should be eliminated. Compliance with previously selected diets should be checked.

Atopic animals may develop a sensitivity to additional allergens and exceed their pruritic threshold. Repeat intradermal skin testing may be appropriate.

Steroid tachyphylaxis

A marked decline in the response seen to one form of glucocorticoid may occur, probably associated with an adaptive decrease in the numbers of nuclear receptors. An improved response can be seen on switching to an alternative glucocorticoid but the phenomenon is poorly understood. It is frequently possible to revert after some weeks to the original drug and achieve a full response once more.

Reassess diagnosis

Finally, if no progress has been made in re-establishing control, it is appropriate to re-evaluate the diagnosis. Additional problems may have developed; these may be associated with therapy, such as calcinosis cutis, or be due to entirely different pathological processes. Not all pruritus is steroid responsive and it is dangerous to assume that the original diagnosis is necessarily correct or complete.

FURTHER READING

CALVERT, C.A. and CORNELIUS, L.M. (1990) Symposium on the use and misuse of steroids. *Veterinary Medicine* Aug. p809.

CHASTAIN, C.B. (1989) Use of Corticosteroids. In: *Veterinary Internal Medicine*. (Ed. S.J. Ettinger) W.B. Saunders, Philadelphia.

FELDMAN, E.C. and NELSON, R.W. (1987) Glucocorticoid Therapy. In: *Canine and Feline Endocrinology and Reproduction* p218 W.B. Saunders, Philadelphia.

MEDLEAU, L. (1990) Symposium on managing chronic canine pruritus. *Veterinary Medicine* Mar.:p259.

MORRIS, H.G. (1980) Factors that influence clinical responses to administered corticosteroids. *Journal of Allergy and Clinical Immunology.* **66**:343.

NOXON, J.O. (1992) The effect of glucocorticoid therapy on diagnostic procedures in dermatology. In: *Current Veterinary Therapy* (Ed. J.D. Bonagura) p498 W.B. Saunders, Philadelphia.

ROMATOWSKI, J. (1990) Iatrogenic adrenocortical insufficiency in dogs. *Journal of the American Medical Association.* **196**:1144.

SCOTT, D.W. and GREENE, C.E. (1974) Iatrogenic secondary adrenocortical insufficiency in dogs. *Journal of the American Animal Hospital Association.* **10**:555.

SCOTT, D.W. et al. (1989) Dermatologic Therapy. In: *Small Animal Dermatology* (Eds. G.H. Muller, R.W. Kirk, D.W. Scott) p150 W.B. Saunders, Philadelphia.

NUTRITIONAL THERAPY

Richard G Harvey

INTRODUCTION

The skin is the largest organ in the body and is very active metabolically. It has been calculated that the growth and replenishment of hair and skin can consume as much as 30% of a dog's daily protein intake (Buffington,1987). A 30 kg labrador retriever, for example, has approximately one square metre of skin that is turning over on a regular basis and could produce in the order of 20-30 metres of hair a day. This amount of tissue synthesis requires not only proteins but also energy, essential fatty acids, minerals and vitamins. Many components of the diet have some function in one or more aspects of cutaneous homoeostasis and a few, such as vitamin C and copper, are associated with well defined cutaneous syndromes. However, in small animal practice clinical signs appear to be confined to dermatoses related to three essential fatty acids, vitamin A and zinc (Miller, 1989).

Absolute or relative deficiencies of any one of these three ingredients may produce dermatologic signs. However, because the skin has only a limited range of response and because many nutrients interact with each other the signs of nutritional deficiency are similar, whatever the ingredient implicated. Typical signs are of scale, erythema and alopecia and a greasy skin often accompanied by secondary bacterial infection. These changes reflect alterations in the process of keratinisation, the fundamental metabolic activity of the skin and the adnexae.

Although deficiencies of protein or energy are unlikely to be found in dogs or cats fed commercially prepared diets (Miller, 1989) this is not the case with essential fatty acids, vitamins and minerals. Manufacturers cater for the average dog (and cat) and the combination of a great variation in phenotype with the proliferation of available commercial diets occasionally may result in clinical signs of deficiency. Alternatively, a nutritionally balanced diet may be unbalanced by the over enthusiastic supplementation of one key nutrient by the animal's owner. An excess of one ingredient may induce the relative deficiency of another. Thus zinc competes with calcium for intestinal absorption and over supplementation with the latter may reduce absorption of the former. The calculation of a nutritionally balanced diet is complicated and if a grossly deficient diet is identified it is simpler to feed a properly balanced commercial diet than to attempt to improve one that is inadequate.

In addition to correcting signs of deficiency, nutritional therapy may be indicated in a number of other circumstances. Selected nutrients or their derivatives may be used to maximise the potential of a limiting biological process (reduced capability to absorb zinc in certain breeds of dog), circumvent a metabolic abnormality (essential fatty acid supplementation in atopy), treat a recognised and specific disorder (vitamin A responsive dermatosis) or to exploit the biological function of the ingredient (antioxidant effect of vitamin E, effect on keratinocyte differentiation by retinoids).

Table 1
Major dermatologic functions of essential fatty acids in the body

1. Precursors of eicosanoids such as prostaglandins and leukotrienes

2. Confer fluidity on cell membranes and hence affect the function of cell-bound receptors

3. Integral in the formation and maintainance of the epidermal permeability barrier

4. Help to regulate keratinocyte differentiation and desquamation

NUTRIENT REQUIREMENTS AND SIGNS OF DEFICIENCY

Essential Fatty Acids

Essential fatty acids fulfil a number of roles in the body (Table 1) and are particularly important for normal cutaneous structure and function. Fatty acids may be described on the basis of the number of carbon atoms in the molecule (thus eicosapentaenoic acid is described in shorthand as a c20 fatty acid) and on the position of the first double bond, counting from the amino end of the carbon chain (22:5n3 is the full description of eicosapentaenoic acid). The essential fatty acids are all members of the n3 and n6 families and are derived from dietary alpha linolenic and linoleic acid respectively. These parent compounds are then metabolised into more metabolically active derivatives which subserve some of the functions outlined in Table 1, particularly as sources of eicosanoids. The cutaneous signs of essential fatty acid deficiency are a dull coat, with varying amounts of scale, erythema, alopecia and pruritus. Systemic signs such as poor wound healing, reduced immunocompetance and infertility may be seen in severe cases (MacDonald et al, 1984; Buffington, 1987).

Cats require linoleic and arachidonic acids in their diet and commercial feline diets are adequately supplemented, typically with linoleic at 1% dry matter and arachidonic acid at 0.1% of dry matter. Thus essential fatty acid deficiency in cats is unlikely to occur unless the cat has a dietary idiosyncrasy and is addicted to a home prepared food that is inherently inadequate. Signs of deficiency include large flakes of scale, particularly over the sacral region and easily epilated hair. These signs do not become apparent until a diet deficient in essential fatty acids has been fed for many months (MacDonald et al, 1984).

Dogs can synthesise all essential fatty acids from dietary linoleic acid and this is typically supplied in the diet at a minimum of 2% of dietary energy or 1% dry matter (Buffington, 1987; Lewis, 1981). However the fat content of the commercial dried type is low compared to canned and moist diets and the amount of linoleic acid may fall below adequate levels if the food stored for too long, particularly in a warm, damp environment (Kelly, 1992). Signs of deficiency include a dull coat accompanied by a fine scale. Prolonged deficiency results in alopecia, a greasy skin (particularly on the pinnae and feet) and secondary pyotraumatic dermatitis.

Indications for supplementation

Defects in keratinisation such as fine scale may respond to dietary supplementation with fat (Miller, 1989; Muller et al, 1989). The underlying cause in these instances is probably an absolute or relative deficiency of fat and the traditional approach has been to administer animal fats to these animals. Recent advances in our understanding of lipid metabolism has resulted in greater stress being placed on substituting the animal fat with vegetable oil (Buffington, 1987). Increasing the amount of dietary fatty acids increases the requirement of vitamin E and, furthermore, the optimum utilisation of this added fat will depend on an adequate level of other vitamins and minerals. An attractive option to simply adding oil is therefore to administer a balanced supplement containing essential fatty acids, vitamin E and zinc (Miller, 1989). There is no evidence that supplementing with essential fatty acids is of value in the management of idiopathic defects in keratinisation such as those seen in the cocker spaniel or basset hound.

Canine atopy may be accompanied by a defect in the conversion of dietary linoleic acid to the longer chain polyunsaturated fatty acids and their derivatives, particularly the prostaglandins. This may aggravate an imbalance in the relative levels of pro- and anti-inflammatory mediators and the inflammation which results, accompanied by changes in epidermal membrane barrier function, may play a fundamental part in the aetiopathogenesis of the disease. Supplementation of the diet of atopics with essential fatty acids has proved beneficial in dogs (Lloyd and Thomsett, 1989; Miller, 1989). Clinical experience suggests that response to supplementation with essential fatty acids is associated with a time lag, often of two to six weeks, before appreciable improvement is noted. Furthermore the rate of response and the degree of improvement is dose dependent. Miller (1989) noted that 18% of atopic dogs became non-pruritic with a further 17% showing improvement when supplemented with a mixture of n3 and n6 fatty acids (Derm Caps, C-Vet). Experience in the UK with a different mixture of the same fatty acids (Efavet Regular, Efamol Vet) suggests that following supplementation of the diet with four times the manufacturer's recommended dose some 30-40% of dogs with atopy can be controlled without glucocorticoids. In a number of these cases the daily dose of supplement can be steadily reduced to the recommended dose for long-term maintainance. In animals in which the clinical signs are not completely controlled by essential fatty acids it may prove possible to reduce the daily requirement of prednisolone if combination therapy is employed (Miller, 1990).

Miliary dermatitis in cats is a frequent presenting sign and it is recognised to be the cutaneous manifestation of a number of dermatoses of which flea allergy dermatitis is the most common (Muller *et al*, 1989). Hypersensitivities, in particular atopy, other ectoparasites and dermatophytosis account for the majority of cases. Although management is best directed toward the underlying cause a number of cases will prove refractory. In these cases, supplementation with essential fatty acids may prove beneficial (Harvey, 1991).

Vitamin A and the natural retinoids

Retinol (Vitamin A) is formed by the reversible reduction of retinaldehyde, itself an oxidised product of dietary carotene (Ross, 1991). This reaction takes place in the gut. In the cat there is a dietary requirement for retinol since it cannot utilise carotenes. Retinol is transported to the liver and acts as the major transport form of vitamin A in the body. Retinaldehyde is essential for the normal development and function of the retina and is an obligate intermediate in the conversion of retinol to the final member of the natural retinoid family, retinoic acid (Ross, 1991).

Retinoic acid is considered to function as a hormone and interacts with the genome to regulate cellular growth and development (Wolf, 1990). The interaction with the genome requires the presence of zinc and results in a number of dermatological effects such as the expression of laminin (a major component of the epidermal basement membrane). Retinoic acid is important for the differentiation of the epidermis during the process of keratinisation.

Synthetic retinoids such as isotretinoin and etretinate are derivatives of these natural retinoids and have been developed to exert only one of the biological action of the natural group, thus minimising side effects (Allen and Bloxham, 1989). Currently the use of isotretinoin and etretinate is restricted to hospital pharmacies only because of their potential for teratogenicity in man.

Dogs require 5,000 IU of vitamin A per kg dry matter of diet and cats 35,260 IU/kg (Lewis, 1981) and deficiency is unlikely to occur in animals fed commercially prepared diets. Care must be taken in advising supplementation with vitamin A since toxicity can result if levels of only four times the advised requirement are fed for prolonged periods (Lewis, 1981). Toxicity produces cutaneous signs similar to those of a nutritional deficiency with pruritus, scale, erythema and alopecia being reported systemic. Signs such as anorexia and weight loss may also be seen.

Indications for supplementation

Vitamin A responsive dermatosis is a rare condition almost entirely confined to cocker spaniels. There is no evidence that affected animals have deficient diets. Signs are of a severe and more or less generalised defect in keratinisation and there may be a greasy coat, loss of hair, mild to moderate pruritus and secondary pyoderma. The condition is characterised by focal areas of follicular plugging with plaque-like accumulations of keratin projecting above the skin surface.

Histopathological examination of these areas reveals a markedly disproportionate follicular hyperkeratosis. The lesions slowly resolve with doses of 10,000 IU vitamin A daily (Ihrke and Goldschmidt, 1983; Miller, 1989). Since this is in excess of the dietary requirement care must be taken to eliminate other causes of the dermatosis before treatment is initiated although there have been no reports of vitamin A toxicity in treated dogs.

Intracutaneous cornifying epithelioma is a benign neoplasm arising from the epithelial tissue. There are breed predispositions in Norwegian elkhound, keeshond and old English sheepdog (Muller *et al*, 1989). There is a single case report of a dog with multiple intracutaneous cornifying epitheliomata in which the lesions resolved when the dog was treated with isotretinoin (Henfrey, 1991).

The term 'defect in keratinisation' characterises a number of dermatoses (Chapter 5) and there are reports that certain forms of keratinisation defect such as sebaceous adenitis, schnauzer comedo syndrome, feline acne and icthyosis will respond to retinoid therapy. Unfortunately these preliminary reports frequently contradict each other and controlled studies have not been published. Although some of the retinoids, etretinate for example, have been shown to be effective in the management of idiopathic defects of keratinisation in the dog, the cost of these products and their potential for causing toxicity to owner as well as to animal have limited their use to what are essentially clinical trials. As newer derivatives become available more veterinary applications may become apparent.

Vitamin E

Vitamin E is the generic name for a group of lipid soluble compounds known as the tocopherols, the most potent being α-tocopherol (Rice and Kennedy, 1988). These compounds are 'free radical scavengers' and protect the cells from the toxic effects of highly reactive metabolites such as peroxy and hydroxy radicals and hydrogen peroxide (Padh, 1991). A major source of potentially damaging free radicals is lipid metabolism and thus vitamin E requirement is related particularly to intake of polyunsaturated fatty acids (Putnam and Comben, 1987; Scott and Sheffey, 1987). Although other anti-oxidants such as selenium and ascorbic acid have a vitamin E sparing effect they are not as effective and cannot completely substitute for vitamin E (Putnam and Comben, 1987; Rice and Kennedy, 1988).

Dogs require 0.5 IU/kg/day of vitamin E for maintenance (Scott and Sheffey, 1987). Deficiency is rare (Miller, 1989) but may result from the feeding of poorly stored foods or foods with an excessive content of unsaturated fatty acid. Cutaneous signs of deficiency include scale formation, erythroderma, alopecia and secondary infection and these may be accompanied by muscle damage and immunosuppression (Scott and Sheffey, 1987; Miller, 1989). In cats, a relative or absolute deficiency of vitamin E and a diet high in oily fish may result in pansteatitis, inflammation of subcutaneous fat leading to pyrexia, palpable subcutaneous nodules and occasionally draining tracts (White, 1989). Deficiencies may be corrected adjusting the diet and supplementing with 25-75 IU vitamin E twice daily.

Indications for supplementation

Discoid lupus erythematosus has been reported to respond to high doses of vitamin E (Scott *et al*, 1983). The rational is that the anti-inflammatory effect of vitamin E reduces the local inflammation which results from two sources; immune mediated damage and the aggravating effect of sunlight induced actinic damage. Doses of 200-400 IU bid two hours before or after food are effective in about 50% of cases (Miller, 1989) although there is a lag period of 6-8 weeks before improvement can be expected.

Vitamin C

Ascorbic acid (vitamin C) is required for proper formation of the collagen triple helix (Miller S.J., 1989) and for the synthesis of noradrenaline (Padh, 1991). The vitamin is also a reducing agent and is thus an antioxidant (with a role similar to that of vitamin E). In addition it has a potential role in the α-amidation of several neuropeptides and hypothalamic releasing factors (Padh, 1991).

Dogs and cats can synthesise sufficient vitamin C for daily requirements but, like man, guinea pigs are dependent on dietary sources. They require 10 mg/kg/day for maintainance (Flecknell, 1991) and this is usually supplied from the diet. Problems may arise if the diet is inadequate in ascorbic acid, if it is stored for too long or if it is heat sterilised (Clarke *et al*, 1980). Sub-clinical scurvy may occur more frequently than is reported and may cause signs of decreased appetite and cutaneous scale. Decreased appetite due to dental disease, cheilitis or severe dermatoses such as *Trixacarus caviae* infestation may lead to an inadequate intake of ascorbic acid and further loss of condition.

Supplementation with 100 mg/day per guinea pig is required for treatment of clinical deficiency. Lower levels of supplementation can be achieved by increasing the provision of fresh fruit or vegetables (a quarter of an orange a day for example) or adding a soluble ascorbic acid tablet to the drinking water once or twice a week (Flecknell, 1991).

Zinc

Zinc is a co-factor for RNA and DNA polymerase (Norris, 1985). Thus zinc deficiency particularly affects rapidly dividing cells. Zinc is essential for the proper functioning of many metalloenzymes, the interaction of retinoic acid with DNA, fatty acid biosynthetic transformations and many facets of the immune and inflammatory system (Miller, S.J., 1989; Ross, 1991). Recommended levels for adult maintainance are 0.72 mg/kg/day (Buffington, 1987). Absorption of zinc from the gut is subject to competition with other minerals such as calcium and iron and hindered by dietary phytate, which chelates zinc.

Signs of deficiency in dogs may be confined to the skin with the appearance of symmetrically distributed areas of alopecia, crust and scale, particularly overlying the pressure points of the limbs, periorbitally and around the mucocutaneous junctions (Thoday, 1989) (Plate 45). In young animals there may be growth retardation, emaciation, conjunctivitis and keratitis in addition to the cutaneous signs (Miller, 1989). A hereditary, autosomal recessive disease associated with a defect in zinc metabolism has been described in English bull terriers (Jezyk *et al*, 1986).

Indications for supplementation

Defective zinc absorption or metabolism is thought to be present in some individuals of certain breeds, particularly the Alaskan malamute and Siberian husky (Miller, 1989) although similar defects have been reported in other breeds. Cutaneous signs of zinc deficiency may develop in puppies or adults, even those which are fed a high quality commercially balanced diet. Lesions consist of erythema, alopecia and scale and crust around the mucocutaneous junctions, periorbitally and overlying the joints on the lower limbs (Muller *et al*, 1989). There may be a ceruminous otitis externa. Treatment of these dogs needs to be continued for life and consists of oral zinc sulphate at a dose of 10 mg/kg daily.

Relatively, or absolutely, zinc deficient diets will also cause cutaneous signs of zinc deficiency. Typically seen in rapidly growing animals of large breeds of dog the signs are similar to those described above although in some cases stunting may occur as well (Muller *et al*, 1989). The deficiency in zinc is attributed to binding by dietary phytate or to competition for absorption in imbalanced diets or those diets which have been over supplemented, with calcium in particular. Absolute zinc deficient diets have been recorded.

These are normal animals and they respond to oral zinc supplementation. Zinc sulphate at a dose of 10 mg/kg daily is added to the food. Zinc methionate at a dose of 1.7 mg/kg once daily in food has also been advocated (Muller *et al*, 1989). Once the signs of deficiency have resolved and a properly-balanced diet is fed the supplementation can be stopped.

NUTRITIONAL STRESS

Ackerman (1987) refers to the concept that animals with extensive skin disease require increased amounts of certain nutrients to cater for the increased metabolic demand of the inflamed and hyperproliferative epidermis, even where there is no dietary deficiency or absorption defect. Thus benefit may be obtained by providing supplements of micro nutrients since these will be required in exfoliative dermatitis, for example, in amounts over and above those supplied in the diet for maintenance. Supplements typically contain zinc, vitamin A and essential fatty acids and are indicated as non-specific adjuncts to definitive therapy

REFERENCES AND FURTHER READING

ACKERMAN, L.J. (1987). Nutritional supplements in canine dermatoses. *Canadian Veterinary Journal*, **28**, 29.

ALLEN, J.G. AND BLOXHAM, D.P. (1989). The pharmacology and pharmacokinetics of the retinoids. *Pharmacology and Therapy*, **40**, 1.

BUFFINGTON, C.A.T. (1987). Nutrition and the skin. In: *Proceedings of the 11th. Kal Kan Symposium.* 11.

CLARKE, G.L., ALLEN, A.M., SMALL, J.D., LOCK, A. (1980). Sub-clinical scurvy in the Guinea pig. *Veterinary Pathology*, **17**, 40.

FLECKNELL, P.A. (1991). Guinea Pigs. In: *Manual of Exotic Pets New Edn.* (Eds, P. H. Beynon and J.E. Cooper). British Small Animal Veterinary Association.

HARVEY, R.G. (1991). The management of feline miliary dermatitis by supplementing the diet with essential fatty acids. *Veterinary Record,* **128**, 326.

HENFREY, J.I: (1991). Treatment of multiple intracutaneous cornifying epitheliomata using isotretinoin. *Journal of Small Animal Practice,* **32**, 363.

IHRKE, P.J. AND GOLDSCHMIDT, M.H. (1983). Vitamin A responsive dermatosis in the dog. *Journal of the American Veterinary Medical Association,* **182**, 687.

JEZYK, P.F., HASKIN, M.E., MACKEY-SMITH, W.E. AND PATTERSON, D.F. (1986). Lethal acrodermatitis in bull terriers. *Journal of the American Veterinary Medical Association,* **188**, 409.

KELLY, N.C. (1992). Practical evaluation and feeding of dog foods. *In Practice,* **14**, 8.

LEWIS, L.D. (1981). Cutaneous manifestations of nutritional imbalances. In: *Proceedings of the American Animal Hospital Association's 48th Annual Meeting* 263.

LLOYD, D.H., and THOMSETT, L.R. (1989). Essential fatty acid supplementation in the treatment of canine atopy. A preliminary study. *Veterinary Dermatology,* **1**, 41.

MACDONALD, M.L., ANDERSON, B.C., ROGERS, Q.R., BUFFINGTON, C.A. and MORRIS, J.G. (1984). *American Journal of Veterinary Research,* **45**, 1310.

MILLER, S.J. (1989). Nutritional deficiency and the skin. *Journal of the American Academy of Dermatology,* **21**, 1.

MILLER, W.H. (1989). Nutritional considerations in small animal dermatology. In: *Clinical Nutritional.* (Ed. F.A. Kallfelz). *The Veterinary Clinics of North America,* **19**, W. B. Saunders, Philadelphia.

MILLER, W.H. (1990). Fatty acid supplements as anti-inflammatory agents. In: *Current Veterinary Therapy* X. (Ed. R.W. Kirk). W.B. Saunders, Philadelphia.

MULLER, G.H., KIRK, R.W. and SCOTT, D.W. (1989). *Small Animal Dermatology 4th edn.* W.B. Saunders, Philadelphia.

NORRIS, D.A. (1985). Zinc and cutaneous inflammation. *Archives of Dermatology,* **121**, 985.

PADH, H. (1991). Vitamin C: Newer insights into its biochemical functions. *Nutrition Reviews,* **49**, 65.

PUTNAM, M.E. and COMBEN, N. (1987). Vitamin E. *Veterinary Record,* **121**, 541.

RICE, D. and KENNEDY, S. (1988). Vitamin E: Function and effects of deficiency. *British Veterinary Journal,* **144**, 482.

ROSS, K.A. (1991). Vitamin A: Current understanding of the mechanisms of action. *Nutrition Today,* January/February, 6.

SCOTT, D.W. and SHEFFEY, B.E. (1987). Dermatosis in dogs caused by vitamin E deficiency. *Companion Animal Practitioner,* **1**, 42.

SCOTT, D.W., WALTON, D.K. and MANNING, T.O., (1983). Canine lupus erythematosus. II. Discoid lupus erythematosus. *Journal of the American Animal Hospital Association,* **21**, 481.

THODAY, K.L. (1989). Diet related zinc-responsive skin disease in dogs: a dying dermatosis? *Journal of Small Animal Practice* **30**, 213.

WHITE, S.D. (1989). The skin as a sensor of internal medical disorders. In: *Textbook of Veterinary Internal Medicine. 3rd Edn.* (Ed. S.J. Ettinger). W.B. Saunders, Philadelphia.

WOLF, G. (1990). Recent progress in vitamin A research: nuclear retinoic acid receptors and their interaction with gene elements. *Journal Nutritional Biochemistry,* **1**, 284.

CHAPTER TWENTY NINE

MANAGEMENT OF ECTOPARASITIC DISEASE

David I Grant

INTRODUCTION

Parasitic skin diseases are common in small animal practice and there are many products available to treat them. Nevertheless many of the parasitic diseases cause problems since their management requires a high level of communication between the veterinary surgeon and the pet owner; also, successful treatment will sometimes depend on the owner's willingness and/or ability to comply with instructions. There is a need on the one hand for a knowledge of the available parasiticides, whether they are applicable for the disease in question, how best to apply them, what side effects could occur, and on the other hand an owner who can apply the parasiticides to the pet and, if necessary, the environment.

The ideal parasiticide should be:

a) effective against the particular disease being treated.

b) of minimal toxicity to the animal or to humans.

c) have no residual effect on the environment and therefore satisfy the justified concerns of increasing numbers of environmentalists.

d) inexpensive.

e) easy to use.

f) tolerated by the animal.

BASIC PRINCIPLES OF PARASITIC CONTROL

1. If at all possible accurate identification of the parasite should be made. Occasionally, as for example with *Sarcoptes scabiei var canis*, this is very difficult and a therapeutic trial may be undertaken. This is far from ideal however, as there is always a lingering doubt as to the diagnosis. In order to identify a parasite a logical step by step approach, including a full history and careful physical examination is always advisable. The majority of cases will also require laboratory investigation such as microscopical examination of coat brushings, hair pluckings and skin scrapings. The history may establish that the owner has lesions contracted from the pet. An examination of such lesions is often helpful, eg. in cases of *Sarcoptes* or *Cheyletiella* infestation.

2. A knowledge of the life cycle of the parasite is most helpful. Particular note should be made of whether a significant portion of the life cycle is spent off the host in the environment. In addition it is useful to know where the animal goes frequently as these places will also need parasiticidal treatment. Free ranging cats with several "homes" may prove difficult to rid of fleas.

3. A knowledge of what is known to be effective for each parasite is essential. Some parasites, eg. lice, are killed by most parasiticides, but others, eg. *Demodex canis* or *Sarcoptes scabiei* will need products of proven ability. In general, it is preferable to use a product licensed for the condition under treatment. Such products will have had efficacy and safety trials before being granted a licence. It is important also that the owner receives clear instructions exactly according to the manufacturers' data sheets. Side effects are then minimised.

METHODS OF PARASITICIDE APPLICATION

1. Powders

Parasiticidal powders most commonly contain pyrethroids. The powder is easy to apply but overdosage can be a problem and side effects, particularly in cats, may occur. They are not so effective as sprays, and some owners resent the appearance of the powder in the animal's coat. In general powder parasiticides are inexpensive and can also be used in the bedding and carpets.

2. Shampoos

Most present day shampoos contain synthetic pyrethroids or carbamates. They also contain emulsifiers, detergents and surfactants. They have a very high efficacy, in that they will kill fleas or lice that are present on the animal, but they have very poor persistency, because in the majority of cases the shampoo is thoroughly rinsed out of the coat after application. It is therefore necessary to emphasise the importance of environmental control in addition to the use of the shampoo. Many of the products contain conditioners and perfumes which are of value since they promote a healthy looking pleasant smelling coat, thus encouraging frequent use.

3. Dips

Unlike shampoos, dips are not rinsed off and will therefore have some residual activity.

4. Aerosols

Parasiticides delivered as a spray are a very effective means of killing fleas. Most of the licensed products will provide approximately 100% knockdown of fleas. Pyrethroid sprays will provide from 5 to 7 days residual activity, carbamates will provide from 7 to 10 days and organophosphates 10 to 14 days. Aerosols are very effective because both the parasiticide and the propellants are highly volatile and there is very fast transmission of liquid active ingredient into the vapour phase. Dichlorvos will kill fleas within an hour under laboratory conditions. The addition of fenitrothion, eg. Nuvan Top (Ciba-Geigy) adds to the residual efficacy as it has a lower volatility. Spraying should be according to the manufacturer's instructions in a well ventilated room with adequate control of the animal.

5. Collar

These products are almost exclusively employed as a means of controlling fleas. As with most of the other methods of delivering a parasiticide to an animal, they are rarely useful if used as the sole means. There is no doubt however, that they have their uses providing that a few pitfalls are avoided. The first of these is to ensure good environmental control of fleas. The second is to be aware that most owners forget when the collar was applied and frequently the collar is left on for more than double the stated length of time that the collar is said by the manufacturers to be effective, (in most cases about 3 to 4 months). More frequent application – every 2 months will increase the efficacy of many flea collars. In some instances the judicious use of flea collars offers the best chance of flea control e.g. with temperamental cats owned by old people, provided that treatment of the environment can be achieved. Under such circumstances it is useful to enlist the services of professional pest control companies to ensure that the immediate environment is properly treated.

6. Systemics

A few parasiticides are delivered to the animal's body by oral administration or by cutaneous absorption. The only oral parasiticide currently licenced in the UK is cythioate (Cyflee, Cyanamid, UK) which is discussed later. Products recently introduced are applied to the skin of the neck region. Tiguvon (Bayer) is an organophosphorus compound which having been absorbed percutaneously provides a concentration of the active ingredient (fenthion) sufficient to kill the flea when it takes a blood meal. The duration of activity is one month and during the flea season monthly applications are advised. It is also essential to continue with environmental treatment. Systemic products are not used in pregnant or sick animals or those recovering from surgery.

7. Other topically applied parasiticides

A compound applied to the skin but not systemically absorbed is the recently introduced synthetic pyrethroid product Exspot (Pitman-Moore). The active ingredient is permethrin which after being applied topically in a similar way to Tiguvon spreads across the surface of the skin. This product is effective against fleas and ticks and has a duration of activity of one month. Both Tiguvon and Exspot have the advantage of non-stressful administration, although Exspot is only for dogs.

Whatever parasiticidal delivery system is used it is advisable to consider the life cycle of the parasite and decide whether environmental control is necessary and the means to achieve this. There are some products which are specifically licensed to treat the environment, e.g. Acclaim plus (Sanofi) or Nuvan Staykil (Ciba-Geigy) and it is cost effective to use these. In general environmental control is necessary for the elimination of fleas, *Sarcoptes*, *Cheyletiella* and *Otodectes* infestations.

TYPES OF PARASITICIDES

Botanicals

Pyrethrin is derived from the *Pyrethrum* or chrysanthemum flower. It has low toxicity in mammals but has a marked toxic effect on the insect central nervous system. This effect appears to be directed at neural cell membranes rather than specific enzyme inhibition. Pyrethrins are rapidly degraded by ultra-violet light and have no residual effect in the environment. Synergists such as piperonyl butoxide are usually used with pyrethrin.

Synthetic pyrethroids have largely replaced natural pyrethrin due mainly to their lower cost. They are generally as safe and effective as pyrethrin and excellently tolerated by dogs, but may in a few cases produce unpredictable side effects in cats. These side effects (mainly hyperaesthesia) appear to be unrelated to the rates or levels of application, and in all cases appear to be reversible. Currently the third generation stable synthetic pyrethroid permethrin is the commonest of these parasiticides to be used. These products are mainly incorporated into shampoos, spot-on preparations and powders.

Chlorinated hydrocarbons

This group of parasiticides was widely used in the past. Their action on parasites is similar to the pyrethroids - inducing central nervous system paralysis. Chlorinated hydrocarbons are very stable and are therefore unsatisfactory for use in the environment. The last one to be used in veterinary medicine was gamma benzene hexachloride (Lindane) but its use has finally been phased out, even in aural preparations. Apart from the residual effect in the environment it was generally considered that chlorinated hydrocarbons were safe in animals although care was needed with the young and with cats.

Carbamates

Carbamates exert their toxicity by interfering with the activity of acetylcholinesterase, resulting in the accumulation of acetylcholine and hence continued neurostimulation. Examples of carbamates in common use are carbaryl and propoxur. They are used in shampoos, aerosols and flea collars.

Organophosphates

These are widely used compounds which also interfere with acetylcholinesterase. Products in the UK are subject to stringent safety controls and in both carbamates and organophosphates toxicity generally occurs with gross overdosage. The antidote is atropine sulphate at a dose of 0.1 – 0.2 mg/kg intravenously, as necessary. To minimise the risk of toxicity it is essential to follow the manufacturer's instructions carefully. Care should also be taken if two different cholinesterase inhibiting parasiticides are being used simultaneously in different formulations. Examples of organophosphates in current use are as follows:

a) Dichlorvos. This is a potent organophosphate with a quick knock-down parasiticidal activity. It has little residual activity but kills fleas within an hour. It is often incorporated with fenitrothion eg. Nuvan Top (Ciba-Geigy) which has a slower toxic effect but more residual activity.

b) Diazinon. This an organophosphate which is commonly incorporated into flea collars, eg. Preventef (Virbac) or Derasect (SmithKline Beecham).

c) Phosmet. An organophosphate which is an active ingredient of a dip for the treatment of ectoparasites including *Sarcoptes scabiei var canis*, eg. Vet-Kem Prolate sponge-on (Sanofi).

d) Cythioate. The active ingredient of a systemically administered formulation for the treatment of fleas in dogs and cats. The product, Cyflee (Cyanamid) is in the form of tablets containing 30 mg of cythioate. It is given by mouth and after an induction period, it is given every 2 weeks. It is relatively easy for the owner to administer and as with other products it is advisable to use in conjunction with adequate environmental control.

Formamidines

These drugs are acaricidal compounds. They exert their effect by the inhibition of monoamine oxidase. The product used in veterinary medicine is amitraz (Derasect Demodectic Mange Wash, SmithKline Beecham) which contains 5% w/v. of the drug. Amitraz is unstable and deteriorates rapidly on exposure to ultraviolet light. It is therefore necessary to dilute it from the concentrate for immediate use. The solution is used as a 0.05% concentration (1 part Derasect Demodectic Mange Wash to 100 parts of water) for the treatment of demodicosis in dogs, for which it has a product licence. The preparation is used weekly until symptoms have subsided and all skin scrapings are negative, and then for a further 3 weeks. Occasionally, there is mild transient sedation following the use of the wash. Idiosyncratic reactions have been seen in chihuahuas and the manufacturer recommends not using the preparation in this breed. Using the UK product only a small percentage of cases relapse following remission, and there is little doubt that this is the treatment of choice for demodicosis at the present time.

Miscellaneous parasiticides

Sulphur preparations are keratolytic, keratoplastic, antibacterial, antifungal and also antiparasitic. In the USA an effective and commonly used parasiticidal product is lime sulphur. In the UK several topical preparations contain sulphur, eg. 1% selenium sulphide (Seleen, Sanofi) or Tarlite (C-Vet).

Ivermectin is a member of a new class of parasiticides, the avermectins, which have a wide spectrum of antiparasitic activity. This group of compounds is believed to act by increasing the release of gamma aminobutyric acid (GABA) in nerve synapses, thus blocking GABA-mediated transmission of nerve signals. In mammals these synapses are present only in the central nervous system, whereas in parasites they are found in peripheral nerves. In general ivermectin is safe in mammals because it does not cross the blood-brain barrier. The LD50 in beagles is 80,000 μg/kg (compared to a therapeutic dose of 200-400 μg/kg). Collies, Shetland sheepdogs and their crosses are, however, susceptible to toxicity. It has been found that in these dogs adverse reactions, including death, may occur at doses of 200-600 μg/kg, presumably due to a functional anomaly of the blood-brain barrier.

Ivermectin has been found to be effective against *Sarcoptes scabiei* at a dose of 300 µg/kg given by subcutaneous injection, which may be repeated after 2 weeks. It is also effective against *Notoedres*, *Cheyletiella*, and *Otodectes* but does not have a product licence in the UK for the treatment of any of these parasites. Ivermectin is also used in many of the exotic animal parasitic conditions at a dose of 200 µg/kg (Chapter 20). In spite of anecdotal reports to the contrary, controlled studies have demonstrated that ivermectin is not an effective treatment for canine demodicosis.

INSECT GROWTH INHIBITORS

Insect growth inhibitors are products that have no effect on adult fleas, but eliminate them by interfering with the life cycle. There are three such products in wide use, methoprene and fenoxycarb, which have a similar mode of action, and lufenuron. Fenoxycarb and lufenuron are not yet available in the UK.

Methoprene

Methoprene is an analogue of insect juvenile hormone, a hormone essential for the development of the flea. During larval development the levels of this hormone are high, but later stages involving pupation and the development of the sexually mature adult require a low titre or complete absence. The presence of methoprene prevents pupation and the subsequent hatching of adults since it mimics high levels of insect juvenile hormone. It is most often applied to the environment rather than the animal, although a few products have been marketed which are for use on the animal. Because methoprene is non-toxic to adult fleas it is usually incorporated with an parasiticide, such as permethrin, eg. the product Acclaim Plus (Sanofi), which is used in the UK. for environmental control of fleas. Methoprene also has ovicidal properties. It is non-toxic to mammals or birds but it is toxic to fish. It does not persist in the environment as it is very sensitive to ultra-violet light.

Lufenuron (Program, Ciba-Geigy).

Lufenuron is a recently developed compound which has been used in some countries for the prevention and control of fleas. The drug belongs to the chemical group of benzoyl ureas. The suggested mode of action is interference with the transport process involved in the polymerisation of chitin, or in the deposition of chitin chains. Chitin is the principle component of the cuticle that forms the exoskeleton of arthropods. Lufenuron is administered orally to the animal and is absorbed into the blood stream. Adult fleas ingest the drug at feeding and pass it into the eggs. Fully developed larvae are unable to hatch because the chitinous tooth used to free the larva from the egg shell does not function. Even if larvae manage to hatch, further mortality occurs at the next moult due to impediment of the exoskeleton's function.

The drug is given once monthly. In dogs the dose is 10 mg/kg and in cats 30 mg/kg. Even at doses of 2,000 mg/kg daily for 3 months there were no side effects in clinical trials in either dogs or cats. It is evident therefore that this is an extremely safe product. In efficacy trials, elimination of fleas was achieved in all cases of severe infestation within 2 months. If the drug is given after the beginning of the flea season it may be beneficial to use additional parasiticidal environmental control to achieve quicker results.

Milbemycin oxime

Milbemycin oxime is a macrolide antibiotic produced by the fermentation of *streptococcus hygroscopicus*. It is licenced in the United States as a monthly oral heartworm preventative (Interceptor, Ciba-Geigy). Preliminary trials on dogs with demodicosis considered to be resistant to Amitraz have shown promise with a cure rate approximating 90%. Further investigations will establish whether this drug will join the small number licensed for the treatment of canine demodicosis. The mode of action of milbemycin is unknown but it is likely to be similar to the closely related compound ivermectin.

CONCLUSIONS

It is clear that ectoparasite control is undergoing much change, with the disappearance of some products and the emergence of new ones. This chapter has reviewed the principles of ectoparasite control, and discussed some of the important products available or shortly to be so. Successful elimination of parasites ultimately depends on a good understanding of these products by the veterinarian and excellent communication with the owner so that the manufacturer's recommendations are carried out. This will result in therapeutic success in most instances with minimal risk of side effects.

FURTHER READING

DRYDEN, M.W. (1989). Biology of the cat flea *Ctenocephalides felis felis*. *Companion Animal Practice*, **19**, 23.

DRYDEN, M.W., NEAL, J.J. and BENNETT, G.W. (1989). Concepts of flea control. *Companion Animal Practice*, **19**, 11.

KWOCHKA, K.W. (1987). Fleas and related disease. *Veterinary Clinics of North America: Small Animal Practice*, **17**, 1235.

Alopecia and pruritus in small mammals
(Chapter 20)

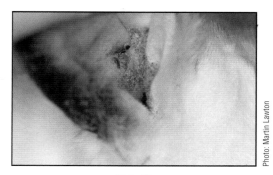

Photo: Martin Lawton

Plate 68
Psoroptes cuniculi affecting the ear of a rabbit.

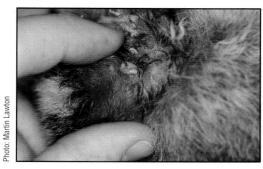

Photo: Martin Lawton

Plate 69
Maggots around the tail and vent of a rabbit

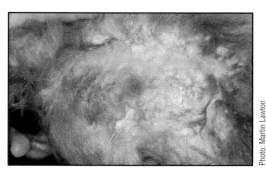

Photo: Martin Lawton

Plate 70
Cheyletiella parasitivorax infestation
on the back of a rabbit

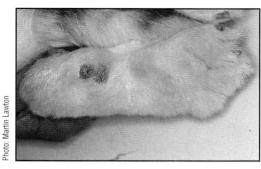

Photo: Martin Lawton

Plate 71
Pododermatitis affecting the foot of a rabbit

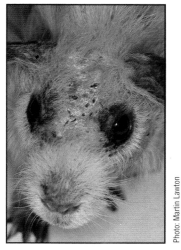

Photo: Martin Lawton

Plate 72
Trixacarus caviae infestation of the head of a guinea pig

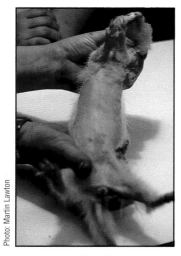

Photo: Martin Lawton

Plate 73
Hormonal alopecia of a jill (ferret)
following prolonged oestrus

Feather loss in birds
(Chapter 21)

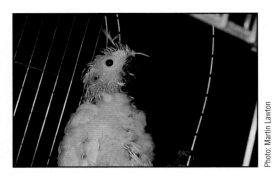

Photo: Martin Lawton

Plate 74
Feather and beak disease in a cockatoo (*Cacatua* spp.).
Note all feathers are affected, including body and head,
and the abnormal beak

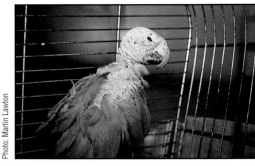

Photo: Martin Lawton

Plate 75
Feather loss in an Amazon parrot (*Amazona* spp.)
associated with chronic *Cnemidocoptes* spp. infestation.
Note the loss of feathers around the head, and
hyperkeratosis associated with response to the parasite

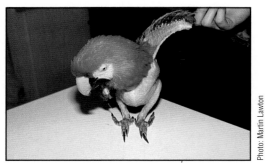

Photo: Martin Lawton

Plate 76
Nuerological feather plucking in a Scarlet macaw
(*Ara* spp.). Note the body is devoid of feathers although
the head is normal

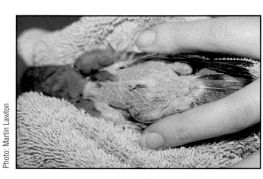

Photo: Martin Lawton

Plate 77
Physical examination of a peach faced lovebird. Feather
loss is confined to the wings and body. There is evidence
of growing feathers which rules our hormonal problems

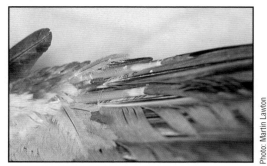

Photo: Martin Lawton

Plate 78
Growing feathers (pin feathers) with neovascular sheath
in an African grey (*Psittacus* spp.)

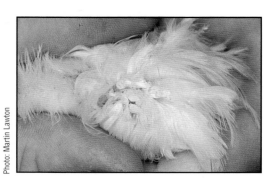

Photo: Martin Lawton

Plate 79
Multiple feather cysts affecting a canary (*Serinus* spp.)

Skin disease in reptiles and amphibia
(Chapter 22)

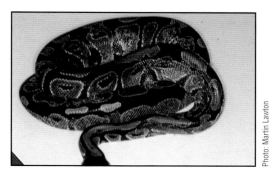

Photo: Martin Lawton

Plate 80
Dysecdysis in a royal python (*Python regis*)

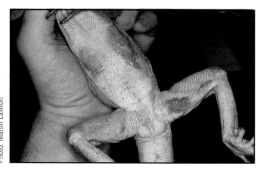

Photo: Martin Lawton

Plate 81
Blisters affecting ventral abdomen, thorax and thighs of a
water dragon (*Physignathus cocincinus*)

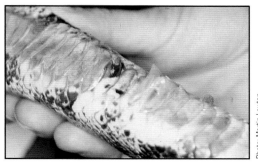

Photo: Martin Lawton

Plate 82
Ventral dermal necrosis of a royal python (*Python regis*)

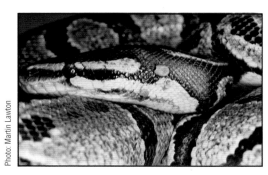

Photo: Martin Lawton

Plate 83
Two ticks on the head of a recently imported
royal python (*Python regis*)

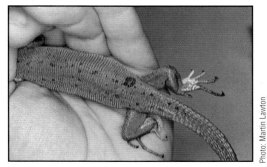

Photo: Martin Lawton

Plate 84
Viral papilloma on the back of a European
green lizard (*Lacerta* spp.)

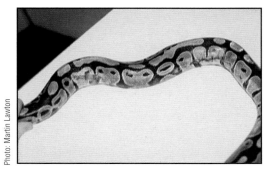

Photo: Martin Lawton

Plate 85
Light bulb trauma on the sides of a
royal python (*Python regis*)

Skin disease in ornamental fish
(Chapter 23)

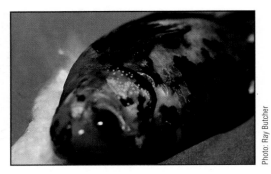

Plate 86
White spot on the gill cover of a koi carp, due to
Ichthyophthirius multifiliis infection

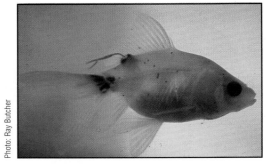

Plate 87
Anchor worm (*Lernaea* sp.) attached to
the dorsal surface of a goldfish

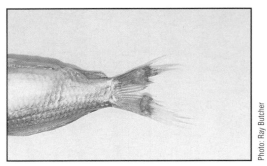

Plate 88
Fin rot due to infection by *Cytophaga* sp. (*Flexibacter* sp.)

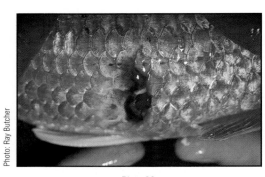

Plate 89
Localised ulceration of the skin with scale loss

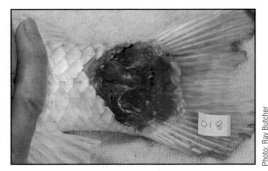

Plate 90
Extensive ulceration at the root of the tail of a koi

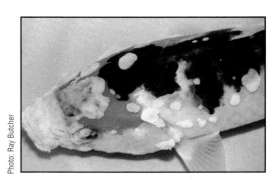

Plate 91
"Candle wax" lesions due to carp pox

MANAGEMENT OF DERMATOPHYTE DISEASE

Didier N Carlotti ────────────────────────────────────

INTRODUCTION

Skin disease due to fungi of the genera *Microsporum*, *Trichophyton* and *Epidermophyton* is termed dermatophytosis, or "ringworm" (Plates 36,40,48 and 58). Although relatively rare, dermatophytosis is important because of its zoonotic potential. Only a limited number of fungal species are associated with skin lesions in pets (Table 1).

Table 1
Dermatophytes of the small domestic mammals

Species	Status	Common host or reservoir	Other hosts
Microsporum canis	zoophilic	cat	dog, man
Microsporum gypseum	telluric	environment	cat, dog, man
Microsporum persicolor	zoophilic	bank vole	dog
Trichochophyton mentagrophytes	zoophilic	rodents	dog, cat, man, rabbit, guinea pig
Trichophyton erinacei	zoophilic	hedgehogs	dog
Trichophyton verrucosum	zoophilic	cattle	dog, man

Dermatophytes produce keratinases and live in epidermal, follicular or nail keratin. They have the capacity to infect normal hair, or skin, and are thus primary pathogens. Infection of the hair occurs only in actively growing hair shafts, although hyphae do not infect the metabolising cells proximal to Adamson's fringe. Thus, the root and the proximal portion of the hair shaft are free of infection. As the infected shaft leaves the protection of the follicle it often fractures, resulting in stubbled hair or even loss of hair. In addition to the hair shaft, dermatophytes also infect interfollicular keratin, and this results in surface scale. *Microsporum persicolor* is unusual in that it does not infect the hair, only the stratum corneum. Dermatophytes are termed **zoophilic** if they have the potential to infect animals, **anthropophilic** if they can infect man and **telluric** (or geophilic) if they are occasional or opportunistic pathogens living in the environment.

The antigenic properties of dermatophytes are poorly understood. Host defences principally involve cell mediated processes rather than the production of specific antibody. Hypersensitivity has been postulated to account for the inflammatory reaction which occurs due to the presence of a dermatophyte in the skin. The degree of inflammatory reaction varies; infection with a non host adapted species is more inflammatory than infection with a host adapted species. Thus, *Trichophyton* spp. infection in dogs, cats and guinea pigs is often very inflammatory. In contrast, *Trichophyton mentagrophytes* infection in rabbits and *Microsporum canis* in cats may be associated with minimal inflammation or asymptomatic carrier status.

The hyphae of some species of *Microsporum* produce a metabolite called pteridin. This absorbs ultraviolet light and emits visible fluorescence; the principle of Wood's light examination. The presence of fluorescence suggests dermatophytosis due to *Microsporum* species, whereas absence of fluorescence does not rule out dermatophytosis.

APPROACH TO THE CASE

Aetiology and epidemiology

Cats

Microsporum canis accounts for some 95% of dermatophytosis in cats. The remaining cases are principally due to *Microsporum gypseum* and *Trichophyton mentagrophytes*. *M. canis* is particularly well adapted to the cat and the presence of an asymptomatic carrier state is common. However, it is very rare to isolate the organism from healthy cats or from catteries with no history of dermatophytosis. In contrast, carriage rates of 100% may be expected in catteries with a history of dermatophytosis (Moriello, 1990). This poses great problems if eradication of infection is to be undertaken.

Dermatophytosis is more common in kittens, and often more severe. In adult cats, dermatophytosis is more common if there is systemic disease, immunosuppression or stress such as pregnancy or lactation. Rare cases of feline dermatophytosis due to *M. canis* could resolve although it usually takes years rather than months. However, treatment should be instituted in view of the zoonotic potential and the impact on showing and sale of kittens.

Zoonotic lesions are common. In the Ile de France region of Paris more than 90% of cases of human ringworm were due to *M. canis* contracted from cats (Badillet, 1977).

Dogs

Dermatophytosis is much less common in dogs than in cats. However, asymptomatic carriage rates of 5% have been reported (Carlotti and Couprie, 1988). A number of species of fungi can cause dermatophytosis in the dog (Table 1) although *M. canis*, *M. gypseum* and *T. mentagrophytes* account for most cases. In contrast to the cat, the proportion due to *M. canis* is only 40-80% with the other species (particularly *T. mentagrophytes*) occurring proportionally more often. Rarely, infection with *M. persicolor*, *T. erinacei* or *T. verrucosum* or even *Epidermopyton floccosum* may be encountered.

Rabbits and guinea pigs

Typically dermatophytosis in rabbits and guinea pigs is due to *T. mentagrophytes*. In rabbits, as with dermatophytosis in cats, lesions are more common in younger animals. Asymptomatic carrier status occurs in adult animals. The disease may be of major concern in breeding and commercial rabbit farms. Dermatophytosis in guinea pigs usually affects an individual rather than a colony, although this may simply reflect the fact that most are kept as solitary pets.

Clinical signs

The clinical signs of dermatophytosis are very variable and are not restricted to classical ringworm. Whilst it is true to say "if it looks like ringworm, it is probably not ringworm" (Scott, 1980), it is also true to say that if it does not look like ringworm, it could be.

In most animals the commonest lesion of dermatophytosis is nummular and peripherally expanding. The most frequent presentations, particularly in the dog, include erythema, alopecia, scale and crust and the principle differential diagnoses are listed in Table 2. As a general rule pruritus is minimal in cats and dogs unless infection with *T. mentagrophytes* is present. Less typical manifestations may be more pruritic:

- alopecia and crusting around the eyes, on the lips and on the dorsum of the muzzle.

- regional or symmetrical alopecia. In the dog, there is often a very well demarcated border between affected and unaffected skin.

- a localised, inflammatory, proliferative, erythematous, soft lesion (termed kerion) which may represent a mixed fungal and bacterial infection or a localised hypersensitivity reaction

- a draining tract associated with subcutaneous inoculation of a dermatophyte (termed pseudomycetoma)

- chronic nail infection (onychomycosis)

- crusted papules ("miliary dermatitis")

- follicular pustules

Table 2
The principle differential diagnosis of dermatophytosis

Dog	
	Superficial pyoderma
	Demodicosis
Cat	
	Flea allergy dermatitis
	Cheyletiella blakei infection
Guinea pig	
	Trixacarus caviae infection

In rabbits, lesions are of non-pruritic alopecia on the face or feet. Inapparent infections are common on adults. In guinea pigs, the infection is usually highly inflammatory and the head and trunk, rather than the extremities, are more commonly affected.

Dermatophytosis may be associated with other diseases, particularly ectoparasites; in the dog, *Demodex canis* and in the guinea pig, *Trixacarus caviae*. In catteries, *Ctenocephalides felis* and *Cheyletiella blakei* may be implicated, both in the spread of the infection and in the incidence of disease, because of the damage to the epidermis that they cause (Moriello, 1990).

ESTABLISHING THE DIAGNOSIS

Diagnosis of dermatophytosis is based upon history, clinical examination and the demonstration of fungal infection with one, or more, of the complementary aids (Chapter 3):

- Wood's light examination. Wood's light is a useful tool in the detection of dermatophytosis due to *M. canis*, provided a fluorescent strain is involved. The lamp should be allowed to warm up for 5 minutes and the examination should be performed in a darkened room (Moriello, 1990).

- Microscopical examination of hair and scale is a useful technique in skilled hands. Various chemicals may be employed to aid clearing of the keratin which allows for easier identification of ectothrix spores, the arrangement of which may help species identification (Table 3). Potassium hydroxide (KOH) in 10% or 20% solution, KOH in dimethylsulphoxide, KOH and India ink and chlorphenolac have all been advocated (Moriello, 1990).

- Fungal culture. Samples for culture may be selected with forceps or a scalpel blade. It is useful to cleanse with spirit, allowing to air dry, before taking samples as this reduces the risk of sampling surface contaminants. Rapid sampling may be achieved with the use of a Denman brush or a sterile toothbrush (McKenzie brushing) which is vigorously brushed through the entire coat and then gently pushed into the surface of the culture media. Dermatophytes are identified on the basis of colony appearance and colour, reverse pigmentation, colour changes in the medium (if Dermatophyte Test Medium is used) and the microscopical identification of macroaleurospores (Table 3) using Roth's flag technique.

Table 3
Essential microscopic and cultural features of the most common dermatophytes.

Species	Pattern of spores on hair shaft	Shape of macroaleurospores	Cultural characteristics	
			Colony morphology	Reverse pigment colour
Microsporum canis			yellow, orange with a downy surface	yellow, orange
Microsporum persicolor	N/A		peach to buff coloured when old. Powdery surface	yellow to yellow-brown
Microsporum gypseum			beige powdery to granular surface	beige
Trichophyton mentagrophytes			cream to red powdery to granular surface	cream to red

Note: Roth's flag technique: A small square of clear adhesive tape is held in forceps and touched to the surface of the colony. It is then laid over a drop of suitable stain (eg. methylene blue or lactophenol cotton blue) and examined under a microscope.

- Histopathological examination of affected skin. The use of this technique, particularly with periodic acid Schiff (PAS) stain, may allow demonstration of hyphae and arthroconidia in the hair of epidermis. This technique may allow for a more rapid diagnosis than can be achieved with fungal culture.

INITIAL MANAGEMENT

Because of the risk of zoonotic infection treatment should be instituted in all cases of dermatophytosis. The aim of treatment is to eliminate fungal infection and to reduce the risk of environmental contamination. All animals in contact with the presented animal should be identified. Animals which are Wood's lamp and/or culture positive should be housed in separate quarters and treated.

Topical therapy

Treatment of dermatophytosis solely by the application of a topical therapeutic to a localised lesion is not satisfactory. It has no effect on spores and hyphae that may be present elsewhere on the animal and therefore has little effect on environmental contamination. This is particularly relevant to the cat. The use of therapeutic agents such as miconazole and clotrimazole is best confined to "spot treatment" of clipped out localised lesions in conjunction with total body dips in 1% chlorhexidine gluconate or 0.2% enilconazole. Whole body dips should be administered twice weekly and consideration should be given to body clipping the animal since this will increase the efficacy of action.

Systemic therapy

Systemic therapy should be used in conjunction with topical therapy. Griseofulvin (microsize) at a dose of 50 mg/kg once or divided, twice daily. Absorption is maximised if given with food, particularly if a fatty meal is given. This is best achieved by adding oil (1.5 ml sunflower oil/kg) to the food. Griseofulvin is teratogenic and is contraindicated in pregnant animals. Side effects may be noted, particularly in cats. Anaemia, leucopenia, vomiting, diarrhoea, depression, jaundice and ataxia have all been noted. Although this appears to be an individual idiosyncrasy rather than dose related toxicity (Kunkle and Meyer, 1987) it is possible that pure-bred, particularly Himalayan, Abyssinian and Siamese cats, are more susceptible (Moriello, 1990).

Ketoconazole has also been used in dogs and cats (Carlotti and Couprie, 1988) in a dose of 10 mg/kg once daily. The most common side effect is anorexia. Ketoconazole depresses serum testosterone concentrations and may be teratogenic and must be used with caution in breeding catteries.

In the author's hands, the combination of topical enilconazole and systemic ketoconazole is highly effective and safe, even in the cat, although the drugs are not licenced in this species.

In apparently non-responsive cases then one should check owner compliance, reassess the diagnosis, consider underlying immunosuppression and submit samples for culture and sensitivity testing.

Guinea pigs may be treated similarly and paediatric griseofulvin suspensions may be appropriate in this species. Dermatophyte infection in rabbits may be treated on an individual basis but topical therapy of colonies with copper sulphate dips has been recommended as economical and efficacious (Franklin et al, 1991).

Cleaning of the environment

Microsporum canis can survive for up to 18 months in the environment (Moriello, 1990) and may be cultured from dust and ventilation systems. Daily vacuum cleaning must be accompanied by burning the collecting bags with their contents. Topical sodium hypochlorite, chlorhexidine gluconate or enilconazole should be applied to all surfaces on a weekly basis. In some countries (not in the UK.), enilconazole foggers are available and they are a particularly effective method of eliminating fungal elements from the environment. It is advisable to remove all bedding and soft furnishings that cannot be treated with the above since hot washing does not achieve sporicidal temperatures (Moriello, 1990). Care should be paid to the potential for cross infection if a colony is being treated and particular attention should be paid to feeding and grooming utensils as well as to the clothing of the attending personal.

Prophylaxis

When dealing with a colony infection, or when attempting to maintain an uninfected colony, every new animal should be sampled by McKenzie brushing and quarantined for at least three weeks until a negative culture is declared. The application of these measures to a cattery will effectively halt showing and exchange for breeding purposes and owners must be made aware of this.

REFERENCES AND FURTHER READING

BADILLET, G. (1977). Population Parisienne et dermatophytes transmis par les animaux. Bulletin de la *Societé Français de Mycologie Medicale*, **6**: 109.

CARLOTTI, D.N. and COUPRIE, B. (1988). Dermatophyties du chien et du chat: actualités. *Practique Médicale et Chirugicale de l'Animal de Compagnie*, **23**: 450.

FOIL, C.S. (1986). Antifungal agents in dermatology. In: *Current Veterinary Therapy IX* (Ed., R.W. Kirk). W.B. Saunders, Philadelphia.

FRANKLIN, C.L., GIBSON, S.V., CAFFREY, C.J., WAGNER, J.E. and STEFFEN, E.K. (1991). *Journal of The American Veterinary Medical Association* **198**: 1625.

GUAGUERE, E., CARLOTTI, D.N., CADOT, P. and HANNOTTE, G. (1985). Diagnostic expérimental des dermatomycoses des carnivores domestiques. *Practique Médicale et Chirugicale de l'Animal de Compagnie*, **20**: 24.

HARVEY, R.G. (1990). Fungal culture in small animal practice. *In Practice*, **12**: 11.

KUNKLE, G.A and MEYER, D.J. (1987). Toxicity of high doses of griseofulvin in cats. *Journal of the American Veterinary Medical Association* **191**: 322.

MORIELLO, K.A. (1990). Management of dermatophyte infections. In: *Advances in Clinical Dermatology. The Veterinary Clinics of North America, Small Animal Practice*, **20**: 1457.

MORIELLO, K.A. and DEBOER, D.J. (1991). Fungal flora of the haircoat of pet cats. *American Journal of Veterinary Research*, **52**: 602.

MULLER, G.H., KIRK, R.W. and SCOTT, D.W. (1989). *Small Animal Dermatology, 4th Edn.*

REBELL, G. and TAPLIN, D. (1978). Dermatophytes. Their recognition and identification. Revised Edition. University of Miami Press, Orlando.

SCOTT, D.W. (1980). Feline dermatology 1900-1978: a monograph. *Journal of The American Animal Hospital Association*, **16**: 349.

WRIGHT, A.I. (1989). Ringworm in dogs and cats. *Journal of Small Animal Practice*, **30**: 242.

MANAGING THE ATOPIC DOG

Craig E Griffin

INTRODUCTION

Long term management of atopic disease is one of the more challenging aspects of veterinary dermatology (Plates 17-21). This is because atopic disease may be controlled but not cured. Usually management is required for life and will often need to be modified at various times. Atopic disease may become more severe as the pet ages requiring adjustments to treatment. The clinician's goal should be the development of a management plan that is acceptable to the client, utilising medications with minimal side effects and good efficacy. Optimal management requires a familiarity with available treatments and a willingness on behalf of the client to follow recommendations. Often a combination of therapeutic agents is required for effective, safe control. Treatment options vary in their ease of administration, risks, efficacy, expense and monitoring required. The management plan should also include the recognition and treatment of coexisting diseases such as flea hypersensitivity or pyoderma.

APPROACH TO THE CASE

The initial stage is the education of the client about expected results and long term outlook. Initial plans may be ineffective and if clients are not well informed they may seek another opinion before an acceptable treatment is achieved. In some cases the pruritus may be reduced considerably but complete control would require additional therapy. It may be wiser in some of these cases to accept a low level of pruritus rather than increase the risk or costs of additional therapy. The following basic treatment plans are those preferred by the author for the management of atopic dogs. These plans are used in a sequence that minimises the risks to the pet over long term use. Modifications will occur based on individual patient and client circumstances. When the pruritus is localised to small areas such as the feet or pinnae then topical glucocorticoid therapy may be sufficient.

In cases that involve several body sites requiring widespread coverage then the treatment plan should include a weekly bathing program and fatty acid supplementation. Although on their own these two treatments may not achieve satisfactory control, they are usually helpful and make other treatments more effective. If the pruritus is only significant for 4 months a year or less, then antihistamines are initially recommended. Systemic glucocorticoids may be used if antihistamines are ineffective or if the client does not wish to try them. Alternate day prednisone for less than 4 months a year is not usually associated with significant serious side effects. However, increased appetite, water consumption, urination and behavioural changes can still make their use unacceptable (Chapter 27). If pruritus is present for more than 4 months each year then reliance on systemic glucocorticoids should be avoided whenever possible.

Antihistamines or hyposensitisation are the treatments of choice in cases with continuous symptoms. These may be added to the bathing program and fatty acid supplements so that the dog may benefit from the additive or synergistic effects. However, due to expense and inconvenience, some clients will prefer to use only one treatment. Avoidance of the offending allergens should be attempted whenever possible to minimise the allergenic load. In some cases, hyposensitisation or antihistamines may only result in a partial response. Some cases will have residual pruritus in a localised area. Local topical therapy may now be effective instead of increasing systemic medications. Other cases will still have significant pruritus and the addition of a treatment that was previously ineffective when used alone may now be effective. In some cases, systemic glucocorticoids may be preferred by clients because of the ease of administration, low expense and high efficacy and the perception that side effects will be slow in developing.

INITIAL MANAGEMENT

Avoidance of allergens

Avoidance requires the identification of allergens by allergy testing. Avoidance is generally impractical or unacceptable to the client. However, in some cases such as feather, tobacco and cat allergies the exposure to this part of the dog's allergies may be minimised. House dust mite allergen is difficult to control though some owners have reported that the condition is improved by keeping the dog outdoors or out of the bedrooms. Mould allergens may be partially avoided by keeping dogs indoors or away from decaying vegetation, including cut grass lawns. Controlling mildew and removing indoor plants may also help to minimise mould exposure. Most cases of atopy cannot be adequately controlled by allergen avoidance. However, whenever possible, it should be attempted as part of the therapy.

Topical therapy

The major disadvantages of topical therapy are the time and effort needed for administration. Expense may also be an important factor. Bathing the total body or use of rinses is required for regional or generalised pruritus although treatment with ointments, creams and lotions may be possible for localised areas. Topical therapy is often overlooked and not presented as an option to clients. Frequent shampooing reduces pruritus but rarely eliminates the problem. Shampooing removes surface debris and bacterial by-products that may contribute to the pruritic load. Shampooing may also remove allergens from the skin surface thereby lowering the allergenic load. It may provide temporary antipruritic effect by cooling the skin by evaporation or from the use of cool water. Soothing rinses may be used for the symptomatic relief of pruritus but their effect is short acting. These products usually contain ingredients such as colloidal oatmeal (Aveeno, Rydell Labs; Episoothe, Virbac) or aluminium acetate (Domeboro, Miles Pharmaceuticals), but just cool water may be effective. Soothing rinses are especially valuable when trying to avoid systemic drugs in preparation for diagnostic tests and managing acute exacerbations of pruritus. Rehydration of the stratum corneum helps control yet another factor which contributes to pruritus, xeroderma (dry skin). Moisturisers alleviate the pruritus associated with dry skin by increasing the water content of the stratum corneum. Emollients and moisturisers contain various combinations of oil (mineral, sesame), glycerine, lanolin, fatty acids, lactic acid, amino acids, urea, phospholipids and waxes. These ingredients are incorporated into rinses, sprays and shampoos (Chapter 26).

Occlusive (oil-based) rinses work best when applied after bathing while the skin surface is still moist. Humilac (Allerderm/Virbac) and Hylyt EFA (DVM) are marketed in pump sprayers for easy application between baths. Each may also be diluted to use as an after bath rinse. Micro Pearls Humectant Spray (Evsco) utilises a liposome technology for a delivery system. This appears to be most useful as a moisturising rinse allowing for longer term delivery of the emollient ingredients to the hair coat and skin. When pruritus is localised to smaller areas, (feet, ears, periocular, perineal, hot spots), then numerous, more expensive, lotions, gels, creams and ointments may be used. Most of these products contain glucocorticoids but a variety of non-glucocorticoid formulations are available which usually contain witch hazel (Hamamelis extract), topical anaesthetics, camphor or menthol. Topical glucocorticoids are valuable for treating localised allergic reactions such as allergic otitis externa. The anti-inflammatory potency of topical glucocorticoids is highly variable depending on the type of glucocorticoids and the vehicle.

In general, the more occlusive and moisturising the vehicle the more potent the product. Although exceptions exist, ointments are more potent than creams which are more potent than lotions assuming the glucocorticoid and its concentration are comparable. Because of their variable potency the clinician should use and become familiar with several topical glucocorticoid preparations. Therapy should usually begin with a medium to strong product applied twice daily until the inflammation is controlled. The frequency may then be reduced to once daily. The treatment should be changed to a less potent topical glucocorticoid once the disease is controlled. The objective, when long term therapy (greater than 1 month) is required, is to use the least potent drug that will effectively control the problem. Adverse effects can be seen with topical glucocorticoid use and the most serious is the development of iatrogenic Cushing's disease (iatrogenic hyperadrenocorticism) and secondary adrenocortical insufficiency. A study with otic administration of products containing triamcinolone acetonide (Panolog) and dexamethasone (Tresaderm) demonstrated adrenal suppression and elevated liver enzymes in most dogs (Morriello *et al*, 1988). Similar adrenal suppression has been seen with ophthalmic and cutaneous application.

Antihistamines

It has recently been documented that antihistamines which block H_1 receptors are beneficial in controlling pruritus associated with atopic disease in dogs. Some antihistamines have other effects. The sedative effect of many antihistamines may also contribute to the control of pruritus. Both the tricyclic piperidine antihistamine azatadin and the piperazine derivative hydroxyzine hydrochloride stabilise mast cells and decrease mediator release following antigen challenge in allergic patients. Some products also have antiserotonin, analgesic and antianxiety activity which may contribute to their effectiveness in controlling pruritus. Assessment of trial antihistamine therapy can only occur when pyoderma has been eliminated since antihistamines, unlike glucocorticoids, are not anti-inflammatory. Published reports with antihistamines have shown that 10 to 40% of atopic dogs can be managed with antihistamine therapy (Griffin, 1987; Scott and Buerger, 1988; Paradis *et al*, 1991a). The author currently utilises hydroxyzine 2.2 mg/kg/tid, diphenhydramine 2.2 mg/kg/tid, doxepin 0.5-1 mg/kg/bid and amitriptyline 1 mg/kg/bid. Since individual variation to different antihistamines is noted in humans and dogs several antihistamines from different classes should be tried.

Generally the client is asked to try 2 or 3 of these antihistamines consecutively for 7-14 days. A double blinded, placebo controlled study in 30 pruritic dogs was reported (Paradis *et al*, 1991a). Atopic disease alone was confirmed in 21 cases. Placebo was totally ineffective while clemastine (Tavegil [UK]; Tavist [USA]) at an approximate dose of 0.05 mg/kg/bid was the most effective with 30% of the cases responding. Astemizole (Hismanal) at an approximate dose of 0.25 mg/kg/sid or trimeprazine (Temaril) at a dose of approximately 0.12 mg/kg/bid were effective in 3.3% of the cases. In contrast to the author's experience doxepin at approximately 1 mg/kg/tid was not effective. When prednisone and trimeprazine were given in combination at the same doses 76.7% responded satisfactorily. The same dose of prednisone without trimeprazine was only effective in 56.7% of the cases. In 75% of the dogs that responded to prednisone alone the prednisone dose could be reduced by 30% when trimeprazine was added. This synergistic effect has also been documented with other nonsteroidal anti-inflammatory agents. A study compared the response of pruritic dogs to clemastine, a fatty acid supplement (DVM Derm Caps) or a combination of both (Paradis *et al*, 1991b) An effective response to the combination of agents was noted in 10% of the cases which failed to respond to either alone, thus indicating a synergistic effect. Another study showed a synergistic effect with DVM Derm Caps and chlorpheniramine (Miller *et al*, 1989). Sedation and anticholinergic effects are the primary side effects of antihistamine therapy. Trembling, increased pruritus and panting have also been reported whilst excitability may be seen in rare cases. Doxepin and chlorpheniramine appear to cause a higher incidence of side effects than other products in this group. Drowsiness may lessen or resolve with continued therapy but if other side effects occur or when drowsiness persists the drug should be discontinued. Once the side effects have resolved, resumption of therapy at a lower dose may still effectively control the pruritus without recurrence of the side effects. Fluoxetine (Prozac) inhibits the uptake of serotonin and, like hydroxyzine, has an antiserotonin effect. A recent pilot study evaluated response to fluoxetine at 1 mg/kg once daily and 50% of the atopic dogs demonstrated a greater than 70% reduction in their symptoms (Shoulberg, 1990). Side effects seen included lethargy, wheals and polydipsia/polyuria. Currently this is a very expensive treatment and should be reserved for cases refractory to other therapies.

Essential fatty acids

A variety of cutaneous and non cutaneous inflammatory disorders may benefit from the use of fatty acid supplements. The most important fatty acids included in such supplements are linoleic acid, alpha-linolenic acid, gamma-linolenic acid and eicosapentaenoic acid. Alpha-linolenic and linoleic acid are required in the diet. Evening primrose oil is a good source of gamma-linolenic acid while eicosapentaenoic acid is found primarily in fish oils. Free arachidonic acid released from cell membranes (mast cells, neutrophils and keratinocytes) in allergic and other inflammatory dermatoses is metabolised to pro-inflammatory mediators of inflammation and pruritus. It is believed that the pruritus associated with atopic disease may be decreased by modulation of arachidonic acid metabolism. Eicosapentaenoic acid competes with arachidonic acid for a number of enzymes and results in the formation of different classes of prostaglandins (PG) and leukotrienes (LT) which are less inflammatory. Gamma-linolenic acid is metabolised to dihomo gamma-linolenic acid which results in the production of the PG 1 series and may also interfere with the production of the PG 2 series and the LT 4 series from arachidonic acid. Since LTC4, LTD4, LTE4 are allergic mediators and PGE2 lowers the pruritic threshold, decreasing their production may help alleviate the pruritus. The importance of gamma-linolenic acid is supported by several studies utilising evening primrose oil (EPO) which showed a significant and dose related, favourable response (Lloyd and Thomsett, 1989; Scarff and Lloyd, 1989).

A number of essential fatty acid products containing gamma-linolenic acid and or eicosapentaenoic acid have been marketed for veterinary use. Studies have evaluated one such product (DVM Derm Caps) in the treatment of allergic disease or pruritus in dogs. In three trials the Derm Caps controlled pruritus to the client's satisfaction in 11.1%, 18% and 26.7% of the atopic dogs (Scott and Buerger, 1988; Miller et al, 1989; Paradis et al, 1991b, respectively). All these studies have shown that many more of the cases exhibited a moderate decrease in pruritus. Another study using EfaVet 1 (Efamol Vet), a blend of gamma linolenic acid, eicosapentaenoic acid and vitamins, showed excellent results in 18% of cases and an additional 76% of cases showed a good response (Lloyd, 1989). Fatty acid metabolites are believed to exert their effect by competing with other fatty acids, especially arachidonic acid. Since there is substrate competition for these enzymes it is possible that the diet of the animal might effect the efficacy of these supplements. There is some evidence (Harvey, in preparation) that this may be the case. If so, it may suggest that increasing the dose may result in an improved response. This was not found in a study by Scott and Miller (1990) which reported that doubling the dose of Derm Caps did not improve efficacy. However, experience in the UK suggests that dosages of 3 or 4 times recommended levels may be associated with improved rates of response. As discussed previously the use of Derm Caps with the antihistamines clemastine and chlorpheniramine can have a synergistic effect. In addition, Derm Caps have allowed a reduction of approximately 50% in the dose of alternate day prednisone required to control atopic dogs (Miller, 1989). Side effects from fatty acid supplements have been very limited. The most serious is the possibility of pancreatitis in animals predisposed to it. One investigator (Kwochka, 1992) reported that two schnauzers developed pancreatitis when fatty acids were added to their diets. Diarrhoea is an infrequent problem and may be alleviated by reducing the amount of fat in the diet or reducing the amount of supplement. When large doses are utilised the increase in caloric intake may need to be offset by administering a lower fat content diet or decreasing the total food intake.

Hyposensitisation

Hyposensitisation, (immunotherapy, biological therapy), is a form of therapy that attempts to modify the patient's immune response to allergenic challenge. The mechanism of action is not understood. The classical theory is that it induces the production of IgG "blocking" antibodies to the specific allergen. This IgG antibody will bind (block) allergen making less available for binding with IgE on mast cells. The hyposensitisation solution should be selected by the practitioner or specialist who has developed an interest in intradermal testing and hyposensitisation. If it is the intent of the reader to prescribe hyposensitisation, select antigens and completely manage the patient without help from a specialist then other references should be consulted for more detail (Reedy and Miller, 1989; Halliwell and Gorman, 1989). The use of hyposensitisation is predicated upon intradermal skin testing or in vitro testing which determines the specific allergens to which the patient is sensitive. The results of hyposensitisation are affected by several factors: accuracy and quality of the skin test; method, type and dose of hyposensitisation extract; control of other environmental and intrinsic pruritic factors (fleas, dry skin, food allergy) and secondary pyoderma. No studies have been undertaken to determine whether glucocorticoids affect response to hyposensitisation. During the first two weeks on hyposensitisation the author prefers to avoid using systemic glucocorticoids. Hyposensitisation is reported to be effective in 50% to 80% of atopic dogs. There are differences in grading schemes, antigen sources and treatment protocols in these studies. Only one double blind, placebo controlled study has been reported (Willemse *et al*, 1984). The placebo contained aluminium hydroxide, an immune adjuvant, which may have contributed to the 20.8% favourable response in the placebo treated group. The treatment group had 59.3% response which was significantly better than the placebo group. Hyposensitisation is the most effective alternative to treatment with systemic glucocorticoids in the USA. Approximately 75% of atopic dogs have no need for systemic glucocorticoids when hyposensitisation is combined with other non-steroidal treatments. Hyposensitisation may be more economical than antihistamines and other treatment options, especially in large dogs. It is usually less labour intensive than oral and topical treatments after maintenance therapy is reached. The client must be informed that improvement is gradual with obvious benefit taking as long as 9 months to occur. It is important to stress that this therapy is not completely curative and most dogs need to have booster injections every 2-4 weeks for life. It is best if the client is willing to learn how to give the subcutaneous hyposensitisation injections so that they can be administered at home without the need for frequent clinic visits. It is imperative that recheck visits be kept as many cases require adjustments in their hyposensitisation protocol. In other cases the client may feel the hyposensitisation is not helping when in reality it is, but pyoderma or another complicating factor is present. After patients have been on hyposensitisation therapy for four months they should be evaluated. Within the first 2-4 months clients will often notice a partial response to the hyposensitisation injections. This will be noted as a decrease in overall pruritus or, more commonly, a temporary reduction in pruritus for several days following the injection. In these cases, the frequency of injections is increased. The author will increase from an injection every 20 days to as frequent as every 10 days without changing the dose. If pruritus continues to recur earlier than 10 days following the injection then the frequency is increased further but the strength is also reduced. When pruritus increases following an injection then the dose is decreased or the pet is pre-treated with hydroxyzine 30 minutes prior to the injection. In rare cases that develop pruritus following an injection, the volume of antigen given may have to be lowered and may never reach the normal maintenance dose. In some cases, pretreatment with antihistamines may not be effective and treatment with oral prednisone (0.5mg/kg) one hour prior to the injection may be required.

Even in patients showing no response to hyposensitisation recheck appointments and phone calls are encouraged as clients will need the support. A major cause of treatment failures is clients discontinuing hyposensitisation therapy without having persisted with treatment for long enough to achieve a response. This group of failures may be minimised with good client communication. It is most important that the clinician realise hyposensitisation therapy is an art where treatment is based on each individual patient's response with the majority of patients receiving modifications of the standard treatment protocols. The major drawback of hyposensitisation is that it is more expensive, compared to alternative treatments; evaluation of efficacy can take 6-9 months. The expense of skin testing and initial therapy with only 60%-80% success discourages many clients from pursuing hyposensitisation. When approached carefully the success and long term savings are usually worth the economic risk that it may not be as effective as lifelong systemic glucocorticoids. Serious side effects are uncommon and will usually occur in the first or second month of therapy. Anaphylaxis is the primary life threatening side effect. Usually there will be less severe reactions to the injections preceding the development of anaphylaxis. In the author's experience over 10 years, two of five cases that developed anaphylaxis had hives or anangioedema previously. Other less specific signs to watch for include: weakness, panting, diarrhoea, anxiousness or hyperactivity. Most dermatology specialists have only seen a few anaphylactic reactions in their careers and the vast majority of patients survive. Less serious but more common side effects are an exacerbation or worsening of the dog's clinical signs. This can usually be controlled by changing the hyposensitisation protocol or pretreatment with antihistamines.

Systemic glococorticoids

The effects of glucocorticoids are numerous (Chapter 27). The basis for using glucocorticoids in atopic disease is for the anti-inflammatory effects of the drugs. Though glucocorticoids have numerous effects at the doses used for management of pruritus, inhibition of phospholipase A_2 and arachidonic acid metabolism are likely to be the major desired effect. The use of glucocorticoids is associated with many adverse effects which are beyond the scope of this chapter so this discussion will be limited to their proper use for the management of atopic disease.

Treatment of atopic disease requires long term therapy and therefore short acting oral glucocorticoids (prednisone, prednisolone or methylprednisolone) are preferred. Methylprednisolone (Medrol [USA]; Medrone V [UK]) may be used in cases where polydipsia and polyuria (PD/PU) or incontinence are a problem (Griffin, 1987). It is not routinely used because it is more expensive. The following discussion relates to prednisone but prednisolone or methylprednisolone may be substituted. When substituting methylprednisolone 4mg is equivalent to 5mg of prednisone. Prednisone should be given on alternate days at approximately the same time to minimise adrenal suppression from long term therapy. The disease must first be in remission before initiating alternate day therapy. When initially trying alternate day therapy many clinicians become dissatisfied and frustrated because they do not initially control the disease prior to starting alternate day therapy. Initially, the daily prednisone dose should be halved and given every 12 hours until a favourable response is seen, usually in around two days. The next step is to switch the total daily dose to once every 24 hours. This daily dose should be continued for two to three treatments. The dosage is then converted to every other day. This is done gradually by slowly decreasing every other treatment dose while keeping the alternate every other treatment the same. Generally, after each reduction the new dose is kept the same for two treatment cycles (4 days). As long as the symptoms remain controlled the dosage is decreased until the animal is on the original once daily dose being given only every other day. This dosage is then gradually tapered until the lowest effective dose is reached.

Many clinicians will use long acting injections instead of the tapering regimen of oral therapy and then start alternate day prednisone one to four weeks later. Although this may be effective for some cases the author has seen many referrals where it was not effective. Optimal therapeutic dosages cannot be predetermined and depend on individual responses. The following guidelines may be helpful: antipruritic therapy 0.5 mg/kg/day; anti inflammatory therapy 1.1 mg-1.5 mg/kg/day. The maintenance dose should be the least dose that is effective. Trial therapy with oral triamcinolone acetonide (Vetalog; Ciba-Geigy) is indicated for cases poorly responsive to or requiring greater than 1.0 mg/kg of prednisone every two days. Oral triamcinolone acetonide usually does not cause PD/PU or increased appetite as often as prednisone.

Dogs that do not respond well to one type of glucocorticoid may respond better to another type. Occasionally a patient's signs may be controlled with a lower dose of oral triamcinolone than the equivalent dose of prednisone. Oral triamcinolone is about 2-5 times as potent as oral prednisone therefore a dose of 0.2mg is equivalent to 1mg of prednisone. When oral triamcinolone is effective at 0.2 mg/kg in animals whose signs were not controlled with prednisone at 1 mg/kg there may be a relative steroid sparing effect which may help alleviate some of the side effects and risks. Since oral triamcinolone suppresses the adrenal glands for 24-48 hours the drug should optimally be given at a maintenance dose every three days (Chen, 1990). Some dogs given alternate day oral triamcinolone had improved clinical results with less side effects than the doses of prednisone needed to achieve the same effect.

Animals need to be monitored for the diverse and numerous side effects that may be seen with glucocorticoid therapy. The problems the author sees most commonly include: poor, dry coat; dry skin; thin skin; muscle wasting; gastrointestinal disturbances; bacteriuria and recurrent pyoderma. Other side effects seen less frequently include: secondary bacterial or fungal infections; demodicosis; liver disease; pancreatitis; gastrointestinal ulceration and behavioural changes. The most important aspect of monitoring long term therapy is observation of the patient. Physical examinations should be done every 6-9 months if the client is not noticing any problems. Initially urine cultures should be done at least yearly as the incidence of bacteriuria is 40% (Ihrke et al, 1985). In animals that develop bacteriuria recurrence is common so urine cultures may be required more frequently than yearly. Serum chemistry values should be acquired every 12 to 24 months. Elevated liver enzyme values are usually seen and should be interpreted in conjunction with physical examination findings and previous chemistry results. The patient should be re-evaluated if problems are observed or the signs are recurrent.

REFERENCES

CHEN, C.L. (1990). Pharmacokinetics of one-day and eight-day oral administration of triamcinolone acetonide in the dog. *Veterinary Reports* **3**, 1.

GRIFFIN, C.E. (1987). Proceedings of the 11th Annual Kal Kan Symposium for the Treatment of Small Animal Diseases. Medical Management of Pruritus, Ohio State University. p 41.

GRIFFIN, C.E. (1992). Atopic disease. In: *Current Veterinary Dermatology*, (Eds., Griffin, C.E., Kwochka, K.W. and MacDonald) Mosby.

HALLIWELL, R.E.W. and GORMAN, N.T. (1989). *Veterinary Clinical Immunology*. W. B. Saunders, Philadelphia.

IHRKE, P.J., NORTON, A.L., LING, G.V. and STANNARD, A.A. (1985). Urinary tract infection associated with long-term corticosteroid administration in dogs with chronic skin disease. *Journal of The American Veterinary Medical Association.* **186**, 43.

LLOYD, D.H. (1989). Essential fatty acids and skin disease. *Journal of Small Animal Practice* **30**, 207.

LLOYD, D.H. and THOMSETT, L.R. (1989). Essential fatty acid supplementation in the treatment of canine atopy: a preliminary study. *Veterinary Dermatology*, **1**, 41.

MILLER, W.H., GRIFFIN, C.E., SCOTT, D.W., ANGARANO, D.K. and NORTON, A.L. (1989). Clinical trial of DVM Derm Caps in the treatment of allergic disease in dogs, a nonblinded study. *Journal of the American Animal Hospital Association.* **25**, 163.

MORIELLO, K.A., FEHRER-SAWYER, S.L., MEYER, D.J. and FEDER, B. (1988). Adrenocortical suppression associated with topical otic administration of glucocorticoids in dogs. *Journal of The American Veterinary Medical Association* **193**, 329.

PARADIS, M., SCOTT, D.W. and GIROUX, D. (1991a). Further investigations on the use of nonsteroidal and steroidal anti-inflammatory agents in the management of canine pruritus. *Journal of The American Animal Hospital Association* **27**, 44.

PARADIS, M., LEMAY, S. and SCOTT, D.W. (1991b). The efficacy of clemastine (Tavist), a fatty acid containing product (Derm Caps), and the combination of both products in the management of canine pruritus. *Veterinary Dermatology* **2**, 17.

REEDY, L.M. and MILLER, W.H. (1989). Allergic Sin Diseases of Dogs and Cats. W.B. Saunders, Philadelphia.

SCARFF, D.H. and LLOYD, D.H. (1989). Double-blind, placebo-controlled cross-over study of evening primrose oil in the treatment of canine atopy. *Veterinary Record*, **131**, 97.

SCOTT, D.W. and BUERGER, R.G. (1988). Nonsteroidal anti-inflammatory agents in the management of canine pruritus. *Journal of the American Animal Hospital Association* **24**, 425.

SCOTT, D.W. and MILLER, W.H. (1990). Nonsteroidal management of canine pruritus: chlorpheniramine and a fatty acid supplement (DVM Derm Caps) in combination and a fatty acid supplement at twice the manufacturer recommended dosage. *Cornell Veterinarian* **80**, 381.

SHOULBERG, N. (1990). The efficacy of fluoxetine (Prozac) in the treatment of acral lick and allergic-inhalant dermatitis in canines. Proceedings American Association of Veterinary Dermatologists and American College of Veterinary Dermatologists annual members' meeting. San Francisco, p 31.

WILLEMSE, A., VAN DEN BROM, W.E., RIJNBERK, A. (1984). Effect of hyposensitisation on atopic dermatitis in dogs. *Journal of The American Veterinary Medical Association* **184**, 1277.

MANAGEMENT OF IMMUNE MEDIATED DISORDERS

Wayne S Rosenkrantz

INTRODUCTION

Management of immune mediated skin diseases requires changing, varying or adjusting the immune response by pharmacological therapy. Suppressing the immune response is often easy to do; however, controlling the degree of immunosuppression can occasionally be difficult. Generally it is easier to suppress an abnormal immune response than the normal immune response.

Many immunosuppressive drugs function by affecting specific stages of the cell cycle. The response of cells to the drug will vary and depends on the stage in the cell cycle. The most sensitive cells are those that are rapidly proliferating. Some immunosuppressive drugs may also function by lymphokine regulation.

Prior to utilising an immunosuppressive drug there are important pretreatment considerations:

First, ensure that the diagnosis is correct. One of the most important diagnostic tests to perform when dealing with a suspected immune mediated skin disease is a skin biopsy. Direct immunofluorescence or immunoperoxidase techniques can occasionally be of value. Routine laboratory screens (clinical haematology, plasma biochemistry and urinalysis) and antinuclear antibody testing (ANA) are also important tests to consider. Performing basic skin scrapings, cytology and fungal and bacterial cultures is essential to rule out major differentials. Using an immunosuppressive drug in a case of demodicosis that was misdiagnosed as an immune mediated disease could be devastating.

Secondly, a pretreatment data base should be established, which should include a complete blood count and chemistry screen. This may uncover pre-existing conditions that would make a specific therapy contraindicated.

Third, many cases of immune mediated skin diseases are complicated by secondary pyoderma and it is common to utilise antibiotics prior to or initially with immunosuppressive therapy. Antibiotic selection is usually based on empirical selection of agents effective against coagulase positive staphylococci (Chapter 25).

The most common immune mediated skin diseases are pemphigus foliaceus (Plates 38 and 41), discoid lupus erythematosus (Plate 42) and pemphigus erythematosus. Other forms of pemphigus (vulgaris and vegetans), systemic lupus erythematosus, bullous pemphigoid and immune mediated vasculitis are less commonly recognised. This chapter will deal with drugs that can be utilised for most of these diseases, but will emphasise those useful for pemphigus foliaceus and discoid lupus erythematosus.

INITIAL MANAGEMENT

GLUCOCORTICOIDS

Systemic

Prednisone, prednisolone and Methylprednisolone. Of the various immunosuppressive agents used to treat immune mediated skin diseases, systemic glucocorticoids (in the form of prednisone) are the most common. Induction dosages of 2.2 to 3.3 mg/kg bid (Muller *et al.*, 1989) are generally used, although Griffin (1986) and Rosenkrantz (1988) have both had success at lower dosages, 1.1 mg/kg bid. Methylprednisolone can be used in animals that have polyuria-polydipsia on prednisone. Methylprednisolone has less mineralocorticoid side effects and, particularly in smaller breed dogs, may produce less polyuria-polydipsia. The tablets are available in 4 and 16 mg sizes, equivalent to 5 and 20 mg of prednisone respectively. The induction dosage is 0.8 to 1.5 mg/kg bid. The major disadvantage of methylprednisolone is expense; even the generics are more costly than prednisone. Cases that fail to achieve full remission at these induction dosages within 14 days are candidates for other, more potent oral glucocorticoids or combination immunosuppressive therapy. Long term response to systemic glucocorticoids is generally favourable in 30% to 40% of the pemphigus foliaceus and discoid lupus erythematosus cases (Ihrke *et al.*, 1985). Once remission is obtained, oral prednisone or methylprednisolone is tapered to approximately 0.2 to 0.5 mg/kg on alternate days for long term management.

Tapering to a long term maintenance dosage is best achieved over an 8 to 10 week period. An example for a 40 kg dog, with pemphigus foliaceus, would include an initial induction of 50 mg prednisone bid for 14 days, followed by 7 days of 100 mg once a day. In subsequent weeks the alternate day dosages would be lowered by 20 mg a week - ie. week 1 (Mon) 100 mg/(Tues) 80 mg (Wed) 100 mg (Thurs) 80 mg, etc.; week 2 (Mon) 60 mg (Tues) 100 mg (Weds) 60 mg, etc.; week 3 (Mon) 100 mg (Tues) 40 mg, etc. Once an alternate day regimen is reached, the tapering should continue, again lowering 10 to 20 mg per week - (Mon) 100 mg (Tues) 0 (Wed) 100 mg, etc. for week 5; (Mon) 80 mg (Tues) 0, etc. for week 6; (Mon) 60 mg (Tues) 0, etc. for week 7.

When 1 mg/kg on alternate days is reached, the tapering process can be much slower. Dosage reduction should be at every 2 to 4 weeks, 5 to 10 mg per week. Most cases will require a minimum maintenance of 0.5 mg/kg on alternate days. If cases flare up during tapering, induction needs to be restarted; or an alternative mode of therapy needs to be utilised if the flare-up occured at too high a maintenance dosage. If glucocorticoids are used as the sole therapy, bi-yearly to yearly complete blood counts, plasma biochemistry and urine cultures should be performed to monitor for common side effects. Periodic ACTH stimulation tests can also be utilised to monitor adrenal gland atrophy. Common "Cushingoid" changes may require discontinuation of the glucocorticoid and a change in the immunosuppressive therapy. If significant side effects develop, alternative therapy will need to be considered.

Alternative Oral Glucocorticoids. The use of other, more potent, oral glucocorticoids can also be tried for induction and maintenance regimens. Oral triamcinolone at 0.2 to 0.3 mg/kg bid or dexamethasone at 0.1 to 0.2 mg/kg bid can be used for 14 days for induction, with tapering to 0.1 to 0.2 mg/kg every two or three days (triamcinolone) and 0.05 to 0.1 mg/kg every two or three days (dexamethasone). As with prednisone, monitoring for side effects needs to be performed. These glucocorticoids are more potent and have a longer half-life than prednisone, and side effects can be produced more readily. For this reason it is important to strive for an every third day administration. However, some cases will be readily maintained, with minimal Cushingoid complications, on an alternate day administration schedule.

Parenteral Glucocorticoids. In severely affected cases of pemphigus, lupus or bullous pemphigoid, parenteral glucocorticoids can be tried as an initial means of ameliorating the disease. This is referred to as "pulse parenteral glucocorticoids" (White, 1985). Success has been reported using suprapharmacological dosages of dexamethasone (1 mg/kg) or methylprednisolone succinate (1 mg/kg) given 2 days consecutively followed by a maintenance oral prednisone or methylprednisolone dosage (White, 1985).

Topical. These may be valuable in the treatment of localised pemphigus foliaceus, pemphigus erythematosus and discoid lupus erythematosus lesions. The potency of the topical glucocorticoid can be geared to the severity of the lesion. Usually a minimum of 2.5% hydrocortisone cream is sufficient, but more potent topical steroids may be needed, such as 0.1% betamethasone valerate (Valisone, USA) creams or ointments, fluocinolone acetonide (Synotic, USA), or 0.1% amcinonide (Cyclocort, USA). Care must be taken with topical steroids, since systemic side effects and localised reactions can occur. Using topicals bid the first week, decreasing to sid the second week, and to alternate days by the third week is recommended. Some cases can be maintained on a application schedule of once or twice a week. In some instances cases brought into remission with systemic glucocorticoids can be converted over to topical glucocorticoid maintenance.

COMBINATION THERAPY

Combinations of glucocorticoids and other cytotoxic drugs are an alternative to treatment with glucocorticoids alone. The following combination regimens may be used successfully:

Azathioprine (Imuran) is an antimetabolite that is transformed into the active agent 6-mercaptopurine, which interferes with DNA and RNA synthesis by inhibiting the enzymes needed for purine synthesis. The immunosuppression results from inhibition of T and B lymphocytes; primarily T lymphocytes are affected. Azathioprine has a slow onset of action, frequently taking 4 to 6 weeks to produce clinical effects. It is available as both 25 and 50 mg tablets (Imuran, Burroughs Wellcome). The dosage is 2.2 mg/kg every one or two days in conjunction with standard glucocorticoid induction dosages. Once remission occurs, both the glucocorticoids and the azathioprine should be tapered to the lowest possible effective alternate day dosage. Azathioprine is the author's first choice cytotoxic drug to use in combination with glucocorticoid therapy for pemphigus and lupus erythematosus. Major side effects include bone marrow suppression, evidenced by leukopenia, thrombocytopenia, or anaemia. Pyoderma, generalised or localised demodicosis or dermatophytosis may be a therapeutic complication. Hence, it is important to perform recheck visits whenever a recurrence of the immune mediated disorder is suspected, since the recurrence may not be pemphigus but a secondary complication. When a secondary opportunistic infection occurs, drug dosages may need to be halved and the appropriate therapy instituted. Initially, complete haematology (including a platelet count) should be performed every 2 weeks for the first 10 to 12 weeks. Once the haematological changes have stabilised, the frequency of monitoring can be decreased to every 2 to 3 months. Periodic plasma biochemistry screens should also be performed, since some cases can develop hepatotoxicity associated with just azathioprine. Cases with marked liver enzyme elevations (ALT levels as high as 5000 ug/dl) have been noted. Most cases respond favourably to drug withdrawal. Azathioprine is not generally recommended for use in cats, since the bone marrow suppression may be marked and fatalities can occur. If used in cats, the dosage should be 1 mg/kg every one or two days.

Chlorambucil (Leukeran) is an alkylating agent that results in misreading of the genetic code as well as DNA breakage and cross-linking. It is the slowest acting and least toxic of the alkylating agents and can be added to a glucocorticoid or azathioprine-glucocorticoid regimen. In cases of feline immune mediated disorders such as pemphigus foliaceus, success with chlorambucil may be seen on an alternate day dosage. Chlorambucil is available as a 2 mg unscored tablet (Leukeran, Burroughs Wellcome). The dosage is 0.1 to 0.2 mg/kg alternate days used solely or with another immunosuppressive agent. Monitoring should be similar to that employed with azathioprine. Side effects relate to myelosuppression and mild gastrointestinal side effects (Rosenkrantz, 1988).

Cyclophosphamide (Cytoxan, Endoxana) is another alkylating agent, considered to be very potent, that can be used individually or in conjunction with glucocorticoids and chlorambucil. It is available as 25 or 50 mg tablets. The dosage is 1.5 mg/kg alternate days. However, the author does not typically use this drug for immune mediated skin disease cases due to its potent myelosuppression and potential for hemorrhagic cystitis and because other therapies are generally effective.

Chrysotherapy, the use of oral and parenteral gold salts, has been shown to have anti-immunological and anti-inflammatory effects. Anti-inflammatory effects include inhibited release of lysosomal enzymes, histamine, and prostaglandins. Gold salts will also have inhibitory effects on complement formation, chemotaxis, phagocytosis, respiratory burst-free radical superoxide release, and hormonal and cellular immunity. Two parenteral compounds are available, aurothiomalate (Myochrysine, Merck Sharp Dohme) and aurothioglucose (Solganol, Schering-Plough). An oral form, auranofin (Ridaura, SmithKline Beecham), is also available. Aurothioglucose is the parenteral form that is preferred. It is available in 10 ml vials of 50 mg/ml. The current protocol is 1 mg/kg/wk intramuscularly. It is recommended that a test dose of 1 to 5 mg be used the first week followed by a second test dose of 2 to 10 mg the second week to rule out idiosyncratic reactions. Some specialists do not do test dosing and start initially with 1 mg/kg/wk. Clinical response is not expected for 6 to 12 weeks, and for this reason the drug is often used in conjunction with oral glucocorticoids initially during the lag phase. If there is no response by the sixteenth week, the dosage can be increased to 1.5 mg/kg/wk. Once a response is seen, the injection interval may be reduced to an as needed basis (ie., every 2 weeks to 2 months). Occasionally the injections can be discontinued, and the disease will remain in remission. This has been seen primarily in cats. Approximately 25% of the cats with pemphigus foliaceus treated with gold have remained in remission for longer than 2 years. Although chrysotherapy has been helpful in dogs, the results have been less successful than in cats. Some investigators have had success with the oral form, auranofin, at 0.1 to 0.2 mg/kg/day. Major side effects of chrysotherapy include hepatic necrosis, thrombocytopenia, toxic epidermal necrolysis, stomatitis, and proteinuria. Minor side effects are sterile abscesses at injection sites and eosinophilia. Platelet counts, complete blood counts, and urinalysis should be performed every 2 weeks during the first 16 weeks. Once remission is seen and maintenance begins, the monitoring can be decreased to monthly and eventually quarterly.

Cyclosporine is a cyclic polypeptide immunosuppressive metabolite of the fungus *Tolypocladium inflatumgams* that inhibits interleukin-2 (T-cell growth factor), thus blocking the proliferation of activated T-lymphocytes. It also blocks gene activation and mRNA transcription and may inhibit the interaction of T-cell antigen receptor with antigen. Cyclosporine also affects other lymphokines, including gamma-interferon. It has had limited success against pemphigus and lupus erythematosus in the dogs and cats (Rosenkrantz *et al.*, 1988). Cyclosporine (Sandimmune, Sandoz) is available in an oral form (100 mg/ml in a 50 ml bottle). The intravenous preparation has a solubilising agent (polyoxyethylated castor oil) that has caused anaphylactoid reactions and is not recommended. The initial induction dosage is 20 mg/kg/day. It is often used in conjunction with oral glucocorticoids and tapered to 10 mg/kg alternate days once remission is obtained. The drug is very expensive, which is a major limiting factor in its clinical use. Adverse reactions include gastrointestinal disturbances, pyoderma, bacteriuria, nephrotoxicity, gingival hyperplasia, papillomatous dermatitis with malignant features, and, in one cat, upper respiratory viral infection (Rosenkrantz *et al.*, 1988).

MISCELLANEOUS THERAPY

Sun avoidance has been advocated because ultraviolet light (UV) exposure has been implicated in the pathogenesis of canine lupus erythematosus and pemphigus erythematosus. In humans, one proposed mechanism for the pathogenesis of cutaneous lupus implicates sunlight. It has been proposed that the ultraviolet radiation causes nuclear and cytoplasmic antigen expression on the surface of the keratinocyte cell membrane. Specific antibodies bind to the antigen surface of the basal cell and initiate a cytotoxic process termed antibody dependent cellular cytotoxicity (Norris and Lee, 1985). The most damaging UV light occurs between 10:00h and 15:00h. Clients should make an effort to keep pets indoors during these hours. If the dog is an "outside dog", shade should be made available and a waterproof sunscreen with sun protection factor (SPF) of 15 or greater applied once to twice a day.

Vitamin E (dl-alpha tocopherol acetate) has been advocated as a safe therapy for discoid lupus erythematosus in one report (Scott *et al.*, 1983). Others have found vitamin E to be rarely effective by itself. There are also some anecdotal reports that topical vitamin E may aid in lesion resolution. The mechanism of action of vitamin E may be related to its role as an antioxidant by stabilising cell and lysosomal membranes against damage induced by peroxides and free radicals. Vitamin E also affects arachidonic acid and prostaglandin metabolism and may enhance immunity and phagocytic function of neutrophils and macrophages. Most agree that vitamin E is a benign drug and may reduce the need for other therapy, allowing reduced amounts of topical and systemic glucocorticoids to be used. It may be tried in cases of discoid lupus erythematosus and pemphigus erythematosus. Aqueous vitamin E (Aquasol) is the formulation of choice, the dosage varying from 400 to 800 IU every 12 hours.

Tetracycline and niacinamide in combination has been described as an alternative treatment for pemphigus foliaceus, discoid lupus erythematosus, pemphigus erythematosus and bullous pemphigoid (White *et al.*, 1992). The study evaluated tetracycline and niacinamide in the treatment of pemphigus foliaceus (n = 8), pemphigus erythematosus (n = 2), discoid lupus erythematosus (n = 20) and bullous pemphigoid (n = 1). Dogs that weighed more than 10 kg were given 500 mg of tetracycline and niacinamide every 8 hours, and those weighing less than 10 kg were given 250 mg of each drug every 8 hours. Niacinamide and tetracycline were effective for DLE, with 40% (8/20) dogs showing an excellent response and 30% (6/20) a good response. Of the dogs with pemphigus foliaceus, 12.5% (1/8) had a good response. One of the dogs with pemphigus erythematosus had a good response. The dog with bullous pemphigoid also had a good response. Based on these results this mode of therapy could be considered in discoid lupus erythematosus, pemphigus erythematosus and bullous pemphigoid cases. However, other practitioners' experiences with tetracycline and niacinamide in treatment of DLE have been less impressive. Only 25% of the author's discoid lupus erythematosus cases have shown any response to this therapy. Side effects are uncommon but can include anorexia, vomiting, and diarrhoea. If these symptoms develop, the niacinamide should be discontinued and the tetracycline continued; some cases may respond to tetracycline alone.

Sulphones and sulphonamides such as dapsone (Avlosulphon, USA) and sulphasalazine (Azulfidine, USA) are the most common sulphones and sulphonamides used in veterinary medicine. Their anti-inflammatory activity is via inhibition of the neutrophil cytotoxicity system and a nonspecific anti-inflammatory effect on cell-mediated immunity. The dosage of dapsone is 1 mg/kg bid-tid, and of sulphasalazine 22 to 44 mg/kg tid (Scott, 1986; Rosenkrantz, 1988). A favourable clinical response should occur in 4 to 6 weeks. A limited number of cases have been treated with these drugs. The author has utilised these drugs in cases of pemphigus foliaceus and immune complexing vasculitis, and minimal responses have been seen. Potential side effects include anaemia, neutropenia, thrombocytopenia, hepatotoxicity, gastrointestinal signs, and skin reactions. Sulphasalazine can cause keratoconjunctivitis sicca, which is generally non-reversible. When this drug is being used Schirmer tear strips should be checked regularly. Complete haematology and plasma biochemistry screens should also be checked every 2 weeks for the first 6 weeks of therapy and reduced in frequency after the dosage has been decreased.

CONCLUSIONS

The initial treatment options for localised immune mediated skin disorders such as discoid lupus erythematosus and pemphigus erythematosus would include tetracycline-niacinamide, vitamin E, sun avoidance or topical glucocorticoids. In more generalised disorders such as pemphigus foliaceus, refractory discoid lupus erythematosus or pemphigus erythematosus, or more severe immune mediated disorders such as systemic lupus erythematosus, bullous pemphigoid and immune complex vasculitis systemic glucocorticoids are indicated. Prednisone or methylprednisolone are the glucocorticoids of choice for initial and long term management. If poor responses are seen, or undesirable side effects occur, then alternative glucocorticoids can be tried (triamcinolone or dexamethasone). Cases refractory to initial therapy will sometimes respond to pulse dosages of parenteral methylprednisolone succinate or dexamethasone, followed by maintenance oral glucocorticoids. Antibiotics should be utilised initially when secondary pyoderma exists. In cases that cannot be controlled at safe, alternate day glucocorticoid dosages, azathioprine should be added. Some investigators suggest starting azathioprine as an initial therapy in conjunction with glucocorticoids. However, the expense of the drug and monitoring are often limiting factors. In addition, 30% to 40% of the cases will not require azathioprine.

If a case cannot be controlled with combination azathioprine and glucocorticoid therapy, chlorambucil should be added to the treatment. If the response is still poor, alternative therapies such as gold salts, cyclosporine, cyclophospamide and sulpha drugs may have to be considered. In refractory cases the primary diagnosis should be reconfirmed, and consultation with a specialist may be advisable. In practice, practitioners may prefer to refer such cases for diagnosis and treatment at an earlier stage than this.

REFERENCES

GRIFFIN, G.E. (1986) Diagnosis and management of primary autoimmune skin diseases: a review. *Seminar of Veterinary Midicine and Surgery (Small Animal)* **2**: 173.

IHRKE, P.J., STANNARD, A.A., ARDANS, A.A. and GRIFFIN, C.E. (1985) Pemphigus foliaceus in dogs: a review of 37 cases. *Journal of the American Veterinary Medical Association.* **186**, 59.

ROSENKRANTZ, W.S., GRIFFIN, C.E. and BARR, R.J. (1988) Clinical evaluation of cyclosporine in animal models with cutaneous immune-mediated disease and epitheliotropic lymphoma. *Journal of the American Animal Hospital Association.* **25**, 377.

MULLER, G.H., KIRK, R. W. and SCOTT, D.W. (1989). Small Animal Dermatology, 4th Edn, W.B. Saunders, Philadelphia.

NORRIS D.A. and LEE L.A. (1985) Pathogenesis of cutaneous lupus erythematosus. *Clinical Dermatology* **3**, 30.

ROSENKRANTZ, W.S. (1988) Immunomodulating drugs in dermatology. In: *Current Veterinary Therapy X* (Ed. R.W. Kirk) W.B. Saunders, Philadelphia.

SCOTT, D.W. (1986) Sulfones and Sulfonamides in canine dermatology. In: *Current Veterinary Therapy IX* (Ed. R.W. Kirk) p. 606 W.B. Saunders, Philadelphia.

WHITE, S.D. (1985) Pulse therapy *Proceedings, Annual members meeting AAVD and ACVD.*

WHITE, S.D., ROSYCHUK, R.A.W., REINKE, S.I. and PARADIS, M. (1992). Use of tetracycline and niacinamide for treatment of autoimmune skin disease in 31 dogs. *Journal of the American Veterinary Medical Association.* **200**, 1497.

LIST OF B.S.A.V.A. PUBLICATIONS

THE JOURNAL OF SMALL ANIMAL PRACTICE

An International Journal Published Monthly   Editor W. D. Tavernor, B.V.Sc., Ph.D., F.R.C.V.S.
Fifteen Year Cumulative Index published 1976
Available by post from: B.S.A.V.A. Administration Office, Kingsley House, Church Lane, Shurdington, Cheltenham, Gloucestershire GL51 5TQ

Manual of Parrots, Budgerigars and other Psittacine Birds
Edited by C. J. Price, M.A., Vet. M.B., M.R.C.V.S.
B.S.A.V.A. Publications Committee 1988

Manual of Laboratory Techniques
New Edition
Edited by D. L. Doxey, B.V.M. & S., Ph.D., M.R.C.V.S.
and M. B. F. Nathan, M.A., B.V.Sc., M.R.C.V.S.
B.S.A.V.A. Publications Committee 1989

Manual of Anaesthesia for Small Animal Practice
Third Revised Edition
Edited by A. D. R. Hilbery, B.Vet., Med., M.R.C.V.S.
B.S.A.V.A. Publications Committee 1992

Manual of Radiography and Radiology in Small Animal Practice
Edited by R. Lee, B.V.Sc., D.V.R., Ph.D., M.R.C.V.S.
B.S.A.V.A. Publications Committee 1989

Manual of Small Animal Neurology
Edited by S. J. Wheeler, B.V.Sc. Cert, V.R., Ph.D., M.R.C.V.S.
B.S.A.V.A. Publications Committee 1989

Manual of Small Animal Dentistry
Edited by C. E. Harvey, B.V.Sc., F.R.C.V.S., Dip.A.C.V.S., Dip.A.V.D.C.
and H. S. Orr, B.V.Sc., D.V.R., M.R.C.V.S.,
B.S.A.V.A. Publications Committee 1990

Manual of Small Animal Endocrinology
Edited by M. F. Hutchinson, B.Sc., B.V.M.S., M.R.C.V.S.
B.S.A.V.A. Publications Committee 1990

Manual of Exotic Pets
New Edition
Edited by P. H. Beynon, B.V.Sc., M.R.C.V.S.
and J. E. Cooper, B.V.Sc., D.T.V.M., C.Biol., F.I.Biol., Cert. L.A.S., M.R.C.Path., F.R.C.V.S.
B.S.A.V.A. Publications Committee 1991

Manual of Small Animal Oncology
Edited by R. A. S. White, B.Vet.Med., Ph.D., D.V.R., F.R.C.V.S., Dip.A.C.V.S.
B.S.A.V.A. Publications Committee 1991

Manual of Canine Behaviour
Second Edition
Valerie O'Farrell, Ph.D., Chartered Psychologist
B.S.A.V.A. Publications Committee 1992

Manual of Ornamental Fish
Edited by R. L. Butcher, M.A., Vet.M.B., M.R.C.V.S.
B.S.A.V.A. Publications Committee 1992

Manual of Reptiles
Edited by P. H. Beynon, B.V.Sc., M.R.C.V.S.
J. E. Cooper, B.V.Sc., D.T.V.M., C.Biol., F.I.Biol., Cert. L.A.S., M.R.C.Path., F.R.C.V.S.
and M. P. C. Lawton, B.Vet.Med., Cert.V.Ophthal., Cert.L.A.S., G.I.Biol., F.R.C.V.S.
B.S.A.V.A. Publications Committee 1992

Manual of Small Animal Dermatology
Edited by P. H. Locke, B.V.Sc., M.R.C.V.S.
R. G. Harvey, B.V.Sc., Cert.S.A.D., C.Biol., M.I. Biol., M.R.C.V.S.
and I. S. Mason, B.Vet.Med., Ph.D., M.R.C.V.S.
B.S.A.V.A. Publications Committee 1993

Manual of Small Animal Ophthalmology
Edited by S. M. Petersen-Jones, D.Vet.Med., D.V.Opthal., M.R.C.V.S.
and S. M. Crispin, M.A., Vet.M.B., B.Sc., Ph.D., D.V.Ophthal., M.R.C.V.S.

B.S.A.V.A. VIDEO 1 (VHS and BETA)
Radiography and Radiology of the Canine Chest
Presented by R. Lee, B.V.Sc., D.V.R., Ph.D., M.R.C.V.S.
Edited by M. McDonald, B.V.Sc., M.R.C.V.S.
B.S.A.V.A. Publications Committee 1983

An Introduction to Veterinary Anatomy and Physiology
By A. R. Michell, B.Vet.Med., Ph.D., M.R.C.V.S.
and P. E. Watkins, M.A., Vet.M.B., M.R.C.V.S., D.V.R.
B.S.A.V.A. Publications Committee 1989

Proceedings of the B.S.A.V.A. Symposium "Improved Healthcare in Kennels and Catteries"
Edited by P. H. Beynon, B.V.Sc., M.R.C.V.S.
B.S.A.V.A. Publications Committee 1991

Practical Veterinary Nursing
Second Revised Edition
Edited by C. J. Price, M.A., Vet.M.B., M.R.C.V.S.
B.S.A.V.A. Publications Committee 1991

Practice Resource Manual
Edited by D. A. Thomas, B.Vet.Med., M.R.C.V.S.
B.S.A.V.A. Publications Committee 1992

Members Information Service
Edited by D. A. Thomas, B.Vet.Med., M.R.C.V.S.
B.S.A.V.A. Publications Committee 1993

AVAILABLE FROM BOOKSELLERS

Canine Medicine and Therapeutics
Third Edition
Edited by E. A. Chandler, B.Vet.Med., F.R.C.V.S.,
D. J. Thompson, O.B.E., B.A., M.V.B., M.R.C.V.S.,
J. B. Sutton, M.R.C.V.S.
and C. J. Price, M.A., Vet.M.B., M.R.C.V.S.
Blackwell Scientific Publications 1991

Feline Medicine and Therapeutics
Second Edition
Edited by E. A. Chandler, B.Vet.Med., F.R.C.V.S.,
C. J. Gaskell, B.V.Sc., Ph.D., D.V.R.,. M.R.C.V.S.
and R. M. Gaskell, B.V.Sc., Ph.D., M.R.C.V.S.
Blackwell Scientific Publications 1993

An Atlas of Canine Surgical Techniques
Edited by P. G. C. Bedford, Ph.D., B.Vet.Med. (D.V. Ophthal), F.R.C.V.S.
Blackwell Scientific Publications 1984

Jones's Animal Nursing
Fifth Edition
Edited by D. R. Lane, B.Sc., F.R.C.V.S.
Pergamon Press 1989